Models of Obesity

From Ecology to Complexity in Science and Policy

Taking a comparative approach, this book investigates the ways in which obesity and its susceptibilities are framed in science and policy and how they might work better. Providing a clear, authoritative voice on the debate, the author builds on earlier work to engage further in ecological and complexity thinking in obesity. Many of the models that have emerged since obesity became a population-level issue are examined, including the energy balance model, and models used to examine human body fatness from a range of perspectives including evolutionary, anthropological, environmental and political viewpoints. The book is ideal for those working on, or interested in, obesity science, health policy, health economics, evolutionary medicine, medical sociology, nutrition and public health who want to understand the shifts that have taken place in obesity science and policy in the past 40 years.

Stanley J. Ulijaszek is Professor of Human Ecology at the University of Oxford and Director of the Unit for Biocultural Variation and Obesity there. He was recently appointed Honorary Professor of Health Research in the Humanities at the University of Copenhagen. His work on nutritional ecology and anthropology has involved fieldwork and research in Papua New Guinea, the Cook Islands and South Asia, while his interests in dietary transitions have led him to examine the evolutionary basis and cultural drivers of obesity.

Cambridge Studies in Biological and Evolutionary Anthropology

Consulting editors

C.G. Nicholas Mascie-Taylor, *University of Cambridge*

Robert A. Foley, *University of Cambridge*

Series editors

Agustín Fuentes, *University of Notre Dame*

Nina G. Jablonski, *Pennsylvania State University*

Clark Spencer Larsen, *The Ohio State University*

Michael P. Muehlenbein, *The University of Texas at San Antonio*

Dennis H. O'Rourke, *The University of Utah*

Karen B. Strier, *University of Wisconsin*

David P. Watts, *Yale University*

Also available in the series

53. *Technique and Application in Dental Anthropology* Joel D. Irish and Greg C. Nelson (eds.) 978 0 521 87061 0

54. *Western Diseases: An Evolutionary Perspective* Tessa M. Pollard 978 0 521 61737 6

55. *Spider Monkeys: The Biology, Behavior and Ecology of the Genus Ateles* Christina J. Campbell 978 0 521 86750 4

56. *Between Biology and Culture* Holger Schutkowski (ed.) 978 0 521 85936 3

57. *Primate Parasite Ecology: The Dynamics and Study of Host-Parasite Relationships* Michael A. Huffman and Colin A. Chapman (eds.) 978 0 521 87246 1

58. *The Evolutionary Biology of Human Body Fatness: Thrift and Control* Jonathan C.K. Wells 978 0 521 88420 4

59. *Reproduction and Adaptation: Topics in Human Reproductive Ecology* C.G. Nicholas Mascie-Taylor and Lyliane Rosetta (eds.) 978 0 521 50963 3

60. *Monkeys on the Edge: Ecology and Management of Long-Tailed Macaques and their Interface with Humans* Michael D. Gumert, Agustín Fuentes and Lisa Jones-Engel (eds.) 978 0 521 76433 9

61. *The Monkeys of Stormy Mountain: 60 Years of Primatological Research on the Japanese Macaques of Arashiyama* Jean-Baptiste Leca, Michael A. Huffman and Paul L. Vasey (eds.) 978 0 521 76185 7

62. *African Genesis: Perspectives on Hominin Evolution* Sally C. Reynolds and Andrew Gallagher (eds.) 978 1 107 01995 9

63. *Consanguinity in Context* Alan H. Bittles 978 0 521 78186 2

64. *Evolving Human Nutrition: Implications for Public Health* Stanley Ulijaszek, Neil Mann and Sarah Elton (eds.) 978 0 521 86916 4

65. *Evolutionary Biology and Conservation of Titis, Sakis and Uacaris* Liza M. Veiga, Adrian A. Barnett, Stephen F. Ferrari and Marilyn A. Norconk (eds.) 978 0 521 88158 6

66. *Anthropological Perspectives on Tooth Morphology: Genetics, Evolution, Variation* G. Richard Scott and Joel D. Irish (eds.) 978 1 107 01145 8

67. *Bioarchaeological and Forensic Perspectives on Violence: How Violent Death is Interpreted from Skeletal Remains* Debra L. Martin and Cheryl P. Anderson (eds.) 978 1 107 04544 6

68. *The Foragers of Point Hope: The Biology and Archaeology of Humans on the Edge of the Alaskan Arctic* Charles E. Hilton, Benjamin M. Auerbach and Libby W. Cowgill (eds.) 978 1 107 02250 8

69. *Bioarchaeology: Interpreting Behavior from the Human Skeleton*, 2nd edn. Clark Spencer Larsen 978 0 521 83869 6 & 978 0 521 54748 2

70. *Fossil Primates* Susan Cachel 978 1 107 00530 3

71. *Skeletal Biology of the Ancient Rapanui (Easter Islanders)* Vincent H. Stefan and George W. Gill (eds.) 978 1 107 02366 6

72. *Demography and Evolutionary Ecology of Hadza Hunter-Gatherers* Nicholas Blurton Jones 978 1 107 06982 4

73. *The Dwarf and Mouse Lemurs of Madagascar: Biology, Behavior and Conservation Biogeography of the Cheirogaleidae* Shawn M. Lehman, Ute Radespiel and Elke Zimmermann (eds.) 978 1 107 07559 7

74. *The Missing Lemur Link: An Ancestral Step in Human Evolution* Ivan Norscia and Elisabetta Palagi 978 1 107 01608 8

75. *Studies in Forensic Biohistory: Anthropological Perspectives* Christopher M. Stojanowski and William N. Duncan 978 1 107 07354 8

76. *Ethnoprimatology: A Practical Guide to Research at the Human-Nonhuman Primate Interface* Kerry M. Dore, Erin P. Riley and Agustín Fuentes 978 1 107 10996 4

77. *Building Bones: Bone Formation and Development in Anthropology* Christopher J. Percival and Joan T. Richtsmeier 978 1 107 12278 9

Models of Obesity

From Ecology to Complexity in Science and Policy

STANLEY J. ULIJASZEK

University of Oxford

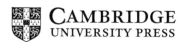

CAMBRIDGE
UNIVERSITY PRESS

CAMBRIDGE
UNIVERSITY PRESS

University Printing House, Cambridge CB2 8BS, United Kingdom

One Liberty Plaza, 20th Floor, New York, NY 10006, USA

477 Williamstown Road, Port Melbourne, VIC 3207, Australia

4843/24, 2nd Floor, Ansari Road, Daryaganj, Delhi – 110002, India

79 Anson Road, #06–04/06, Singapore 079906

Cambridge University Press is part of the University of Cambridge.

It furthers the University's mission by disseminating knowledge in the pursuit of
education, learning, and research at the highest international levels of excellence.

www.cambridge.org
Information on this title: www.cambridge.org/9781107117518
DOI: 10.1017/9781316338650

First published 2017

Printed in the United Kingdom by Clays, St Ives plc

A catalogue record for this publication is available from the British Library.

Library of Congress Cataloging-in-Publication Data
Names: Ulijaszek, Stanley J., author.
Title: Models of obesity : from ecology to complexity in science and policy / Stanley J. Ulijaszek.
Other titles: Cambridge studies in biological and evolutionary anthropology.
Description: Cambridge, United Kingdom ; New York, NY : Cambridge University Press, 2017. |
Series: Cambridge studies in biological and evolutionary anthropology | Includes bibliographical
references and index.
Identifiers: LCCN 2017025805 | ISBN 9781107117518 (Hardback : alk. paper)
Subjects: | MESH: Obesity | Models, Statistical | Energy Metabolism–physiology
Classification: LCC RA645.O23 | NLM WD 210 | DDC 362.1963/980021–dc23
LC record available at https://lccn.loc.gov/2017025805

ISBN 978-1-107-11751-8 Hardback

Contents

Acknowledgements and Influences   *page* viii

1.   **Introduction**   1

2.   **Rationalities and Models of Obesity**   23

3.   **Energy Balance, Genetics and Obesogenic Environments**   35

4.   **Governance through Measurement**   53

5.   **Inequalities**   71

6.   **Food and Eating**   94

7.   **Global Transformations of Diet**   111

8.   **Obesity Science and Policy**   133

9.   **Complexity**   150

10. **Systems and Rationalities**   168

     References   183
     Index   226

Acknowledgements and Influences

In research and academia, huge thanks go to Georg Gottlob for discussions of his early work on expert systems, to Thorkild Sorensen and his critical dissection of energy balance models and to Bruno Latour for conferring a secular blessing upon the Unit for Biocultural Variation and Obesity, which I founded at the University of Oxford in 2007. Great thanks go to many friends and colleagues for their help and willingness to join in discussion about obesity and obesity-related things. In no particular order, they include Caroline Potter, Karin Eli, Megan Warin, Michael Goran, Geof Rayner, Steve Woolgar, Michael Marmot, Avner Offer, Harry Rutter, Michele Belot, Finn Rasmussen, Mike Rayner, Tenna Jensen, John Komlos, Paulina Nowicka, Philip James, Astrid Jespersen, James Stubbs, Line Hillesdal, Boyd Swinburn, Vivienne Moore, Michael Davies, Elizabeth Ewart, Fredrik Karpe, Jimmy Bell, John Cawley, Adam Drewnowski, Amandine Garde, Berit Heitman, Karen Throsby, Jean-Michel Oppert, Steve Simpson, Barry Popkin, Shelley Fox, Anne Katrine Kleberg Hansen, Emma-Jayne Abbotts, Jonathan Wells, Claudio Franceschi, Tanja Schneider, Gabriella Morini, Javier Lezaun, Kaushik Bose and Annamaria Carusi. Particular thanks go to Shira de Bourbon Parme, who made me aware of polyrationality. Thanks go to the more junior scholars with whom I have shared ideas and food across the past decade: Amy McLennan, Nadine Levin, Marisa Macari, Michelle Pentecost, Mel Wenger, Daniel Schwekendiek, Jonas Winther and Tess Bird among them. Apologies to anyone I have left out.

Beyond academia, this volume was influenced by many sources. Pirandello's 'Six Characters in Search of an Author' was a starting point, soon followed by Seurat's 'La Grande Jatte', Georgio Morandi's still lifes of bottles, jars and containers, Luciano Berio's 'Visages', Joseph Beuy's 'Fat Chair', Annie Catrell's 'Pleasure/Pain', and Jake and Dinos Chapman's 'CFC76311561'. The works of Jenny Saville (Plans), Jessica Charlesworth (Food Activism), Andrew Carnie (Irrigate) and Amy Sharrocks (Museum of Water) also became part of what I call my obesity collection, as I prepared and wrote this book. A walk through this collection of different art forms speaks to cacophony, matters of scale, classification, the clatter and uncontrollability of late modernity, the materiality of fat bodies, of classification, boundaries and structure, of the social disconnects created by modernization and globalization, of networks and phylogenies, all of which are attached to obesity as an object of study. With the emergence of obesity as a matter of complexity, other works entered the collection: Caspar David Friedrich's 'Wanderer above the Sea of Fog' and Christoffer Eckersberg's 'View of the Park of Liselund Manor on the Island of Mon', as early modern nineteenth-century rational mappings of the sublime and of the material world. Viewing major exhibitions of the former artist in Hamburg in 2006 and the latter artist in Copenhagen in 2015 inspired me to read about rationality as framed by Immanuel Kant, Max Weber and others, and to consider how their timeless work might be applied to help organize the varied and often seemingly cacophonous endeavours in science and policy in trying to understand and regulate obesity.

1 Introduction

Books on obesity have proliferated in the past three decades, along with the scientific literature, as obesity rates across the world have risen. How is this book different from the others? By looking at how obesity is framed, with different models, world views or rationalities, it is hoped that this book will make some of the issues that structure obesity science and policy more obvious. Since the emergence of obesity as a population-level issue, many models have been developed to explain its causation, emergence and rapid increase (Ulijaszek 2008). These include models that describe thrifty genotypes, obesogenic behaviour, obesogenic environments and nutrition transition, as well as biocultural models that examine interactions of genetics, environment, behaviour and culture (Ulijaszek 2007a). Models for obesity interventions and regulation are also many fold, and include ones that underpin biomedical treatment, epidemiological monitoring, public health approaches (including multilevel models), social marketing and economic regulation, as well as health and nutrition promotion and education. None can hope to be individually correct, given the complexity of the issue (Finegood 2011). Examining the rationalities that underpin different models of obesity (Chapter 2) should help reveal why some interdisciplinary approaches to obesity work better than others.

The view that all models are wrong, but some are useful, attributed to British statistician George E.P. Box (1919–2013), rings true for obesity. All obesity models are conditional, or wrong, in Box's formulation, but are useful for ordering what is currently known about obesity. Models of obesity are not neutral, nor are the facts that emerge from them. Tables 1.1 and 1.2 show two versions of what can be taken as fact about obesity now, based on different world views. The 'ten facts about obesity' given by the World Health Organization (2014) reflect the remit of this particular institution. These facts are largely epidemiological and scientific, and focus largely on prevention. Alternatively, the 'facts about obesity' from the perspective of a writing group that includes very senior obesity researchers almost exclusively in the United States (US) (Casazza et al. 2013) are more treatment-focused, with some emphasis on weight management through individual, familial and pharmaceutical manipulations, as well as on surgical interventions. This reflects the commercial interests and US orientation of much of the authorship of this writing group (Casazza et al. 2013). Such commercial orientation may carry a bias, as is the case with research funded by the pharmaceutical industry more broadly (Lexchin et al. 2003). These two sets of facts about obesity have different framings of what is considered important: predominantly for treatment in the case of Casazza et al. (2013), and

Table 1.1. Ten facts about obesity throughout the world

	Fact	Commentary
1	Overweight and obesity are defined as 'abnormal or excessive fat accumulation that may impair health'	Body mass index (BMI) – weight in kilograms divided by the square of the height in metres (kg/m^2) – is a commonly used index to classify overweight and obesity in adults. The World Health Organization defines overweight as a BMI equal to or more than $25\ kg/m^2$, and obesity as a BMI equal to or more than $30\ kg/m^2$
2	More than 1.4 billion adults were overweight in 2008, and more than half a billion were obese	At least 2.8 million people each year die as a result of being overweight or obese. The prevalence of obesity nearly doubled between 1980 and 2008. Once associated with high-income countries, obesity is now also prevalent in low- and middle-income countries
3	Globally, over 40 million preschool children were overweight in 2008	Childhood obesity is one of the most serious public health challenges of the twenty-first century. Overweight children are likely to become obese adults. They are more likely than non-overweight children to develop diabetes and cardiovascular diseases at a younger age, which in turn are associated with a higher chance of premature death and disability
4	Overweight and obesity are linked to more deaths worldwide than underweight	Sixty-five per cent of the world's population live in countries where overweight and obesity kill more people than underweight. This includes all high-income and middle-income countries. Globally, 44 per cent of diabetes, 23 per cent of ischaemic heart disease, and between 7 and 41 per cent of certain cancers are attributable to overweight and obesity
5	For an individual, obesity is usually the result of an imbalance between calories consumed and calories expended	An increased consumption of highly calorific foods, without an equal increase in physical activity, leads to an unhealthy increase in weight. Decreased levels of physical activity will also result in an energy imbalance and lead to weight gain
6	Supportive environments and communities are fundamental in shaping people's choices and preventing obesity	Individual responsibility can only have its full effect where people have access to a healthy lifestyle, and are supported to make healthy choices. The World Health Organization mobilizes the range of stakeholders who have

Table 1.1. (*cont.*)

	Fact	Commentary
		vital roles to play in shaping healthy environments and making healthier diet options affordable and easily accessible
7	Children's choices, diet and physical activity habits are influenced by their surrounding environment	Social and economic development as well as policies in the areas of agriculture, transport, urban planning, environment, education, food processing, distribution and marketing influence children's dietary habits and preferences as well as their physical activity patterns. Increasingly, these influences are promoting unhealthy weight gain, leading to a steady rise in the prevalence of childhood obesity
8	Eating a healthy diet can help prevent obesity	People can: maintain a healthy weight; limit total fat intake and shift fat consumption away from saturated fats to unsaturated fats; increase consumption of fruit, vegetables, pulses, whole grains and nuts; and limit their intake of sugar and salt
9	Regular physical activity helps maintain a healthy body	People should engage in adequate levels of physical activity throughout their lives. At least 30 minutes of regular, moderate-intensity physical activity on most days reduces the risk of cardiovascular disease, diabetes, colon cancer and breast cancer. Muscle strengthening and balance training can reduce falls and improve mobility among older adults. More activity may be required for weight control
10	Curbing the global obesity epidemic requires a population-based multisectoral, multidisciplinary and culturally relevant approach	The World Health Organization's *Action Plan for the Global Strategy for the Prevention and Control of Noncommunicable Diseases* provides a roadmap to establish and strengthen initiatives for the surveillance, prevention and management of non-communicable diseases, including obesity

From World Health Organization (2014).

predominantly for reporting and prevention in the case of the World Health Organization (2014). They also differ in where responsibility is placed for the rise in obesity rates and for their possible reduction (Chapter 8).

Models of obesity must represent the phenomenon of obesity as accurately as possible. Much obesity science is observational and correlational, as for example in

Table 1.2. Facts about obesity in the US

	Fact	Commentary
1	Although genetic factors play a large role, heritability is not destiny; moderate environmental changes can promote much weight loss	If we can identify key environmental factors and successfully influence them, we can achieve clinically significant reductions in obesity
2	Diets (reduced energy intake) very effectively reduce weight, but trying to go on a diet or recommending that someone go on a diet generally does not work well in the long term	Recognizing this distinction helps our understanding that energy reduction is the ultimate dietary intervention required and that approaches such as eating more vegetables or eating breakfast daily are likely to help only if they are accompanied by an overall reduction in energy intake
3	Regardless of body weight or weight loss, an increased level of exercise increases health	Exercise offers a way to mitigate the health-damaging effects of obesity, even without weight loss
4	Physical activity or exercise in a sufficient dose aids long-term weight maintenance	Physical activity programmes are important, especially for children, but for physical activity to affect weight, there must be a substantial quantity of movement, not mere participation
5	Continuation of conditions that promote weight loss promote maintenance of lower weight	Obesity is best conceptualized as a chronic condition, requiring ongoing management to maintain long-term weight loss
6	For overweight children, programmes that involve the parents and the home setting promote greater weight loss or maintenance	Programmes provided only in schools or other out-of-home structured settings may be convenient or politically expedient, but programmes including interventions that involve parents and are provided at home are likely to yield better outcomes
7	Provision of meals and use of meal replacement products promote greater weight loss	More structure regarding meals is associated with greater weight loss, as compared with seemingly holistic programmes that are based on concepts of balance, variety and moderation
8	Some pharmaceutical agents can help patients achieve clinically meaningful weight loss and maintain the reduction as long as the agents continue to be used	While we learn how to alter the environment and individual behaviours to prevent obesity, we can offer moderately effective treatment for obese people
9	In appropriate patients, bariatric surgery results in long-term weight loss and reductions in the rate of incident diabetes and mortality	For severely obese persons, bariatric surgery can offer life-changing, and in some cases life-saving, treatment

Adapted from Casazza et al. (2013).

the study of the relationships between obesity rates and socioeconomic status (SES) (Sobal and Stunkard 1989; Sobal 1991). Hypothesis testing is integral to some models of obesity, such as those involving macronutrient intake and energy balance (Schutz 1995). Models for obesity regulation are usually predictive and involve hypothesis testing, as for example with the prediction across time of the efficacy of taxation of sugar-sweetened beverages on an obesity-related outcome such as change in sugar consumption. The understanding of the underlying world views, or rationalities, of models of obesity demands two things. The first is an understanding of how obesity is framed as a problem by the makers and/or users of any particular model. This sets the parameters for what is to be understood, and how. The second is an understanding of the values underpinning a model, because any model makes explicit these values in its use. This book contends that it is important to frame, comparatively, the rationalities of different models of obesity if obesity science and policy are to function as interdisciplinary endeavours.

Framing Obesity as a Problem

Extreme body fatness was known in ancient Greece (Bevegni and Adami 2003), and appears as a pathological category in writings ascribed to Hippocrates, between around 440 and 370 BCE (Gilman 2010). As a category of pathology, the cause of extreme body fatness in the ancient world was viewed in holistic ways. This approach persisted until the eighteenth-century Enlightenment, when changing understandings of disease reframed obesity as a problem of the individual body (Gilman 2010). This understanding has continued in medical practice and now informs most policy responses to obesity. While obesity was also common among the English upper classes in the late eighteenth century (Trowell 1975), it only emerged as a population phenomenon among North American men in the nineteenth century (Kahn and Williamson 1994). Obesity increased in successive surveys in both the US and United Kingdom (UK) across the twentieth century (Garrow 1978), its accelerating rates corresponding largely to the rise of global capitalism and neoliberalism from the 1980s onwards (Finucane et al. 2011; Stevens et al. 2012). This period has been characterized as late modernity (Giddens 1990, 1998), additionally involving increased privatization of services in most nations, and the almost universal expansion of computing and information technology to serve most aspects of life. The global nature of obesity was recognized in the 1990s (Popkin and Doak 1998), while obesity was formally classified as a disease by the World Health Organization *Consultation on Obesity* in 1997 (World Health Organization 2000). Since then, a number of agencies in the US have declared or accepted obesity as disease. These include the National Institutes of Health (in 1998), the Internal Revenue Service (in 2002), the Centers for Medicare and Medicaid Services (in 2006), the Food and Drug Administration (in 2012), the American Association of Clinical Endocrinologists (in 2012), the American Medical Association (in 2013), the US Office of Personnel Management (in 2014) and the US Department of Labor (in 2015) (Mechanick et al. 2012; Kahan and Zvenyach 2016). Obesity also became a matter for economic concern in the US in the 1990s (Philipson and Posner 1999, 2008), as rates accelerated (Flegal et al. 1998, 2002), and when the direct health costs (Allison et al. 1999), health consequences (Mokdad et al. 2003) and possible demographic changes (Olshansky et al. 2005) associated with it became apparent. Its expense alone has made it a priority for action by several governments (Colditz 1999; Fry and Finley 2005).

Federal government concern about obesity in the US was only expressed in 2001, with *The Surgeon General's Call to Action to Prevent and Decrease Overweight and Obesity* (US Department of Health and Human Services 2001). This noted the health consequences of obesity to be among the greatest faced by the country, in its associations with premature death, disability, additional health-care costs, lost work productivity and social stigma. The *Surgeon General's Vision for a Healthy and Fit Nation 2010* (US Department of Health and Human Services 2010) noted the continued rise of overweight and obesity, reviewing its causes and health conse-quences, and offering 'opportunities for prevention'. In acknowledging the broad-ranging nature of population obesity, it saw obesity prevention interventions as requiring attention to individual behaviours, biological traits, and aspects of social and physical environments that impact on health outcomes. While also acknowledg-ing the economic burden of rising obesity rates, the idea of prevention through the regulation of corporations whose products and services can contribute to obesity was conspicuously absent.

In the UK, obesity was first noted in 1991 as being a health issue of significant magnitude to warrant policy action (Department of Health 1992; Jebb et al. 2013), and was subsequently singled out for specific policy concern with the National Audit Office (2001) report *Tackling Obesity in England* (Chapter 4). Health policy documents of the previous decade only paid oblique acknowledgement to obesity and its dietary risk factors. These included cross-governmental policies published in 1992 and 1999 – *The Health of the Nation* strategy (Department of Health 1992) and *Saving Lives: Our Healthier Nation*, respectively (Her Majesty's Government 1999). The *National Service Framework for Coronary Heart Disease*, released in 2000, also made reference to obesity as a risk factor for chronic disease (Department of Health 2000). The National Audit Office (2001) report was the first to give authoritative estimates of the costs and consequences of obesity for the UK. It also emphasized the need for greater effort to be placed on establishing an evidence-based approach to obesity for greater consistency of management by the health services, and for more extensive joint work on obesity across government, both nationally and locally. Anti-obesity policy in the UK took on a more urgent note when the House of Commons Health Committee (2004) framed obesity as being ungovernable in both economic and health terms. The following year, the Department of Trade and Industry (2005) viewed the rising costs of obesity with alarm, noting that in 1998 the National Audit Office estimated the cost of obesity to the National Health Service to be £480 million, while in 2002 the Health Select Committee placed this cost at more than double the earlier amount, at between £990 and £1125 million. The 2002 Health Select Com-mittee placed the indirect costs of obesity to the economy at £2 billion a year, rising to £3.6 billion by 2010. The Department of Trade and Industry (2005) report viewed the health and economic costs of obesity to the country as being compelling reasons for addressing obesity seriously. This increasing sense of urgency carried into the UK government Foresight project *Tackling Obesities: Future Choices*, as the annual direct costs of treating obesity and its related morbidities to the National Health Service in England were revised upwards to £4.2 billion per year in 2007 (Butland et al. 2007). Estimates of the indirect costs (arising from the impact of obesity on the wider economy from, for example, loss of productivity) were calculated to be several times higher, rising from £2.6 billion per year in 1998 (National Audit Office 2001) to £15.8 billion per year in 2007 (Butland et al. 2007).

Although obesity has been problematized in many ways, the dominant frameworks are medical, public health and economic, all ultimately based on the energy balance model of obesity. In Chapter 3, the energy balance model and the genetic systems that regulate its physiology are described. Energy balance models, framed in terms of physiological homeostasis, have the deepest history in obesity science. Early energy balance research focused on whole-body physiology, using both human and animal models in studying relationships between macronutrient intake and energy expenditure. While seemingly straightforward, decades of work have revealed the relationships between intake and expenditure to be ever more entangled, with genetic and environmental factors influencing many aspects of the energy balance model. Human genetics may have undergone selection for traits that promote energy intake and storage and that minimize energy expenditure (Rosenbaum and Leibel 1998), thus favouring obesity production in most populations. This view has been contested by alternative framings of obesity genetics (Chapter 3). Regardless of which view of evolutionary genetics of obesity is correct, obesity genotypes and energy balance susceptibilities to obesity can only be expressed in positive energy ecologies, where it is easy for energy intake to exceed energy expenditure. Such ecologies have been vaguely defined as obesogenic environments, and Chapter 3 continues by describing how they are framed in science and policy. Environments and ecologies favouring population obesity have been created, largely unwittingly, with the neoliberal turn in politics since the 1980s, and the concurrent growth of global financialization of markets. From the 1960s onwards, motorized transport has been privileged in many wealthy or high-income countries (HICs), as have the roads and highways that serve it, thus marginalizing physically active transport. Obesogenic environments are served by industrialized and globalized food supplies, both of which shape eating patterns of populations almost everywhere, supplying energy-dense foods at lower prices than more nutrient-dense foods such as fruit and vegetables. Although obesogenic environments have emerged in late modernity, no single modernizing force or outcome can be held responsible for this changing ecology. Rather, it is argued in this book that obesogenic environments are produced by the entanglement of expert systems (Chapter 3), including those of food, transport and urban planning, none of which has sought obesity as an outcome.

From a strictly medical perspective, Bray (2004) has argued that obesity is a chronic relapsing neurological disease, which requires lifelong treatment or management. Similarly, Casazza et al. (2013) argue that it should be conceptualized as a chronic condition requiring ongoing management. Alternatively, a public health framing of obesity views it as a chronic disease risk factor, alongside high blood pressure, tobacco use, high blood glucose and physical inactivity (World Health Organization 2009a). The World Health Organization (2009a) has placed obesity among the leading global risks of mortality, considering it to be responsible for 5 per cent of all deaths globally. Public health approaches to obesity emphasize prevention as being the only feasible way to resolve population obesity (Visscher and Seidell 2001; Lobstein et al. 2004), usually through state policy (Nestle and Jacobsen 2000; Kumanyika et al. 2002). The costs of obesity to the economy are usually the most politically compelling, however (Rashad and Grossman 2004; Mazzocchi et al. 2009; Cawley 2010; Grossman and Mocan 2011). Obesity has clear economic costs, and both economic and public health framings of obesity are related to each other with their roles in state regulation.

Medical and economic framings of obesity reflect the dominant institutions of late modern society. There are other framings of body fatness that make obesity, as a category, problematic (McCullough and Hardin 2013). Critics of the medicalization of body fatness reject the term 'obesity', many favouring the term 'critical fat studies' as a way of distancing themselves from the pathologization of oversized bodies. While some critical fat studies scholars do not deny the materiality of the body (Guthman 2013), there is a clear difference between those who see obesity as a physical reality, and those who see it as being socially constructed (Warin et al. 2015). The American Medical Association's resolution to recognize obesity as a disease in 2013 (Table 1.3) acknowledges both the material reality of obesity and obesity as a disease state with multiple pathophysiological aspects. This has led to recommendations for intervention that largely emphasize treatment. Questioning the notion of obesity as a disease, de Vries (2007) has asserted that if some bodily conditions either confer evolutionary or biological advantage or are common to a species, they should not be regarded diseases; only if bodily conditions are rare and fall out of the range of morphological normality should they be considered diseases. With respect to obesity, bodily fatness is typical of the human species, is usually within the range of normality and cannot be considered to be a disease by these criteria, except at the extremes. However, when societal aspects of obesity are considered, de Vries (2007) argues that it can be framed as disease because it represents bodily deviation from norms and social desirability. Beyond treating obesity as a disease, some of the medical preoccupation with obesity seeks to correct unwanted or immoral behaviour (Crossley 2004; Gard and Wright 2005). Moral judgement has been argued to be implicit in some medical approaches to obesity (Aphramor 2005; Gard and Wright 2005; Monaghan 2005; Evans 2006; Colls 2007; Evans and Colls 2009; Gard 2011a). With respect to childhood obesity, de Vries (2007) sees its medicalization as confronting children and their parents with a societal expectation that they will recover from this stigmatized condition. Failure to 'recover' in this sense is morally judged by society as weakness on the part of the child and potentially as child abuse on the part of their parents, as they deny their obese child a normal life (de Vries 2007).

Table 1.3. American Medical Association resolution to recognize obesity as a disease

AMERICAN MEDICAL ASSOCIATION HOUSE OF DELEGATES Resolution: 420 (A-13)

Introduced by: American Association of Clinical Endocrinologists; American College of Cardiology; The Endocrine Society; American Society for Reproductive Medicine; The Society for Cardiovascular Angiography and Interventions; American Urological Association; American College of Surgeons

Subject: Recognition of Obesity as a Disease

Referred to: Reference Committee D (Douglas W. Martin, MD, Chair)

Whereas, Our American Medical Association's Council 1 on Science and Public Health Report 4, A-05, has identified the following common criteria in defining a disease: 1) an impairment of the normal functioning of some aspect of the body; 2) characteristic signs or symptoms; and 3) harm or morbidity; and

Whereas, Congruent with these criteria there is now an overabundance of clinical evidence to identify obesity as a multi-metabolic and hormonal disease state including impaired functioning of appetite dysregulation, abnormal energy balance, endocrine dysfunction including elevated leptin levels and insulin resistance, infertility, dysregulated adipokine signaling, abnormal endothelial function and blood pressure elevation, nonalcoholic fatty liver disease, dyslipidemia, and systemic and adipose tissue inflammation; and

Whereas, Obesity has characteristic signs and symptoms including the increase in body fat and symptoms pertaining to the accumulation of body fat, such as joint pain, immobility, sleep apnea, and low self-esteem; and

Whereas, The physical increase in fat mass associated with obesity is directly related to comorbidities including type 2 diabetes, cardiovascular disease, some cancers, osteoporosis, polycystic ovary syndrome; and

Whereas, Weight loss from lifestyle, medical therapies, and bariatric surgery can dramatically reduce early mortality, progression of type 2 diabetes, cardiovascular disease risk, stroke risk, incidence of cancer in women, and constitute effective treatment options for type 2 diabetes and hypertension; and

Whereas, Recent studies have shown that even after weight loss in obese patients there are hormonal and metabolic abnormalities not reversible by lifestyle interventions that will likely require multiple different risk stratified interventions for patients; and

Whereas, Obesity rates have doubled among adults in the last twenty years and tripled among children in a single generation and a recent report by the Robert Wood Johnson Foundation states evidence suggests that by 2040 roughly half the adult population may be obese; and

Whereas, The World Health Organization, Food and Drug Administration (FDA), National Institutes of Health (NIH), the American Association of Clinical Endocrinologists, and Internal Revenue Service recognize obesity as a disease; and

Whereas, Obesity is recognized as a complex disease by CIGNA, one of the nation's largest health insurance companies; and

Whereas, Progress in the development of lifestyle modification therapy, pharmacotherapy, and bariatric surgery options has now enabled a more robust medical model for the management of obesity as a chronic disease utilizing data-driven evidenced-based algorithms that optimize the benefit/risk ratio and patient outcomes; and

Whereas, The suggestion that obesity is not a disease but rather a consequence of a chosen lifestyle exemplified by overeating and/or inactivity is equivalent to suggesting that lung cancer is not a disease because it was brought about by individual choice to smoke cigarettes; and

Whereas, The Council on Science and Public Health has prepared a report that provides a thorough examination of the major factors that impact this issue, the Council's report would receive much more

Table 1.3. (*cont.*)

of the recognition and dissemination it deserves by identifying the enormous humanitarian and economic impact of obesity as requiring the medical care, research and education attention of other major global medical diseases; therefore be it

RESOLVED, That our American Medical Association recognize obesity as a disease state with multiple pathophysiological aspects requiring a range of interventions to advance obesity treatment and prevention.

Received: 05/16/13

From American Medical Association (2013).

Medicine is not the only domain in which obesity is morally judged. Such judgement exists as stigma and discrimination in a wide range of other institutional contexts, and is especially strong in employment, in the workplace and in media representations (Chapter 5) (Puhl and Brownell 2003). Stigma also accompanies the weighing and quantification of fat bodies (Chapter 4) that is a precondition to the framing of obesity as a medical, economic and public health problem. The standardized metric of obesity since the year 2000 is the body mass index (BMI). This measure was adopted by the World Health Organization (2000) for use by governments and international agencies primarily because of its positive association with mortality and morbidity, and with the future morbidity of children. The BMI cut-off for classifying obesity among adults has been set at 30 kg/m^2, while that for overweight has been set at between 25 and 30 kg/m^2 (World Health Organization 2000). The internationally accepted classificatory cut-offs for childhood obesity and overweight are age-specific measures of BMI that pass through 25 and 30 kg/m^2, respectively, at the age of 18 years (Cole et al. 2000). Both classifications are used consistently when discussing or describing overweight and obesity of adults and children in this book. Such epidemiologically determined obesity rates are used to make a case for, and monitor, public health and economic interventions against obesity. There are other measures of obesity (Chapter 4), but BMI is the most widely used in epidemiological mapping and econometric modelling of obesity. While the BMI cut-offs for obesity in adults (World Health Organization 2000) have strong relationships with mortality at the population level (Berrington de Gonzalez et al. 2010; Flegal et al. 2007), they cannot be used to predict mortality either among different adult age groups (Winter et al. 2014), or among some regional populations of the world (Wen et al. 2009). Furthermore, epidemiological studies relating body fatness (by the proxy of BMI) and mortality have methodological biases, including reverse causation and confounding by related factors such as smoking (Hu 2008).

Economics and Obesity

Econometric models start with the assumption that individuals practise rationality in choice, action, preference and belief (Chapter 2). Economic rationality is central to contemporary mainstream economics (Foley 1998). It requires consistency of action

(Weirich 2004), which, in relation to the production of healthy bodies, can include appropriate nutrition in pregnancy and infant feeding, good maternal care of children, a good balance between physical activity and food intake, and an anticipation of the future outcomes of all of these actions. Eating and maintenance of a healthy body weight can be seen as economic decisions, with people trading the utility from current food intake against the associated monetary expense and potential disutility of future weight gains (Ruhm 2010). There are models of rational choice for a number of health behaviours, including the consumption of addictive substances (Becker and Murphy 1988), and such models should be well suited to evaluating food choices, since everyone has great experience in eating and most adults know the consequences of overeating (Ruhm 2010). With a rational consumption model, obesity can be viewed as being an outcome of consistent actions if individuals have incomplete or out-of-date information with which to guide their actions. For example, advice about healthy eating has changed across decades, and past choices and actions that have subsequently led to obesity may have been shaped by information that was shaped by the best evidence of the time but in the decades prior to the rapid rise in population obesity. Before the 1980s, obesity rates were generally low, concerns about it were few and health promotion was aimed at other targets. The rational consumption model would predict that when better knowledge of obesity was gained in subsequent decades, such removal of informational constraints would have resulted in reduced obesity rates, primarily because few people want to be obese. This prediction was not fulfilled, however, suggesting a breakdown of this model. According to Offer (2016), the theory of consumption in economics may not work for obesity, which is at least in part an outcome of difficulties in reconciling conflicting objectives, especially if the payoffs occur at different times. The immediate gratifications of eating may be inconsistent with the longer-term gratification of health and achieving normative bodily ideals (which in most HICs is slimness).

Rational consumption may thus be bounded by the context in which it is practised, with constraints of information and time (Simon 1955). Such is the case when people feel stressed or are insecure, have precarious lives and low wages, and must make food choices with limited time and money. Economic decisions made under such circumstances are considered to involve bounded rationality, whereby decisions leading to optimal solutions are less possible than ones that lead to satisfactory ones (Simon 1956). The idea of obesity as a product of convenience (Ulijaszek 2007b) is a model that relies on assumptions of bounded rationality, in that decisions made under conditions of limited time, information or money are unlikely to seek obesity as an outcome. Simon (1956) noted that time-limited decisions are made less time-limited with the possession of greater economic resources. People with more economic resources have more relaxed time limits, and are therefore less bounded and more likely to make better economically rational decisions. In wealthy nations, those of high SES are less economically bounded and are less likely to make decisions that predispose or lead to obesity than among those of low SES (Chapter 5). Although behaviour that leads to obesity may not be economically rational in the formal sense, other forms of rationality might better explain the emergence of population obesity.

Such rationalities include evolutionary (Speakman 2013) and psychological (Manktelow and Over 1993) ones among others, and Chapter 2 turns to alternative framings of rationality in relation to obesity.

Regulating Obesity

Rates of adult obesity have increased in most regions of the world since the 1980s (Stevens et al. 2012; Ng et al. 2014), with the global rise in the average BMI of adults being about 1.1 kg/m² per decade between 1980 and 2008. This is equivalent to an average increase in body weight of around one-third of a kilogram per person per year, globally (Finucane et al. 2011). For many populations, this increased body fatness represents the embodied rise out of poverty, but for some it has meant emergent and increasing population obesity. Among children and adolescents, rates of overweight and obesity appear to have plateaued in some HICs (Rokholm et al. 2010; Olds et al. 2011; Schmidt Morgen et al. 2013; Wabitsch et al. 2014), although this effect has been shown mostly in studies of short duration (Lissner et al. 2013; Visscher et al. 2015). Where rates of childhood and adolescent obesity have been shown to plateau, socio-economic inequalities in obesity rates have persisted or increased (Ulijaszek et al. 2016a), as in the US (Singh et al. 2010; Frederick et al. 2014) and the UK (Stamatakis et al. 2010). Figures 1.1 and 1.2 show this effect for children in England between 2007 and 2014 (Public Health England 2016). Figure 1.3 presents these data as percentage differences in obesity rates between the least and most deprived Local Authority Districts in England, showing fairly consistent increases in childhood

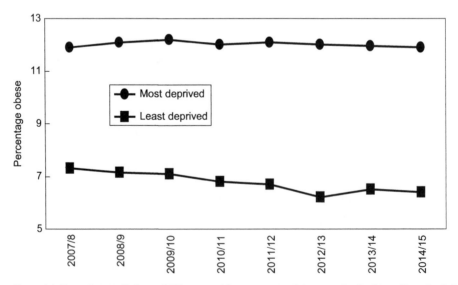

Figure 1.1. Prevalence of obese children aged between 4 and 5 years, in the least (first decile) and most (tenth decile) deprived Index of Multiple Deprivation Local Authority Districts based on school postcode in England, between 2007/8 and 2014/15 (adapted from Public Health England 2016).

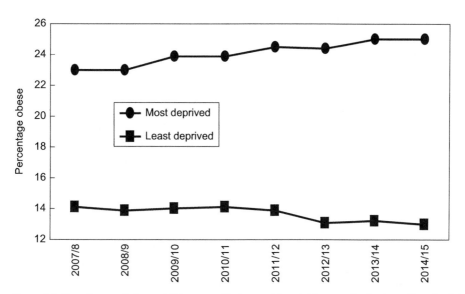

Figure 1.2. Prevalence of obese children aged between 10 and 11 years, in the least (first decile) and most (tenth decile) deprived Index of Multiple Deprivation Local Authority Districts based on school postcode in England, between 2007/8 and 2014/15 (adapted from Public Health England 2016).

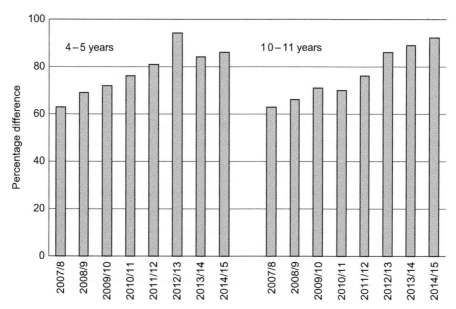

Figure 1.3. Percentage difference in obesity rates between the least (first decile) and most (tenth decile) deprived Index of Multiple Deprivation Local Authority Districts based on school postcode in England, between 2007/8 and 2013/14, for children aged between 4 and 5 years, and between 10 and 11 years (adapted from Public Health England 2016).

obesity inequality between 2007 and 2015. The simple explanation of why obesity rates continue to rise much more than they appear to plateau is one of positive energy balance (Swinburn et al. 2011), but this fact alone does not translate easily into obesity reduction policy. When seen at the macro-level as an unwanted outcome of interactive expert systems (Chapter 10), the potential intractability of obesity as an object for intervention becomes more visible.

An expert system is defined by the complex task it is developed to perform, with the aim of replacing or aiding human expertise. As a contributor to obesity, the global food system (Chapter 6) is considered to be expert because it involves many different processes and materialities, and a wide range of organizations and people with diverse expertise. It involves different forms of food production across the world, using many different technologies. It also involves the primary processing of food, its storage and transportation, and its secondary processing into food products. Furthermore, it involves responsibility for food safety, the prevention of contamination, transportation of food to retail outlets, and its sale, dealing with waste in every part of the system. Expert systems emerged as a field in computation in the 1970s as a way of problem solving that could deal with complexity and self-organization (including human intelligence and behaviour) (Feigenbaum 2003), problems that ecologists and biological systems theorists have been interested in since the 1930s (Bertalanffy 1969). Expert systems software, successful in analysing complexity (Luger and Stubblefield 2004) was put to social and economic purpose. Hayes-Roth et al. (1983) have identified various categories of application for expert systems methodology, including interpretation, prediction, diagnosis, design, planning, monitoring, instruction and control. Expert systems methods underpin the smooth running of everyday life, especially in HICs, including the provision of ever-available water, electricity, food, transport, communication, health, welfare and employment. Expert systems methods have been developed for a large number of practical purposes, many of which are summarized in Table 1.4. Agriculture, construction, retail, transportation, epidemiology, urban planning, engineering, distribution planning, public transport, medical management and medical diagnosis are areas that benefit from expert systems methods, and which have some relationship to obesity. Expert systems are all around us, silent and invisible, and generally helpful. They interact with each other, often to good purpose, but sometimes with negative outcomes, as with rising obesity rates. Such systems operate as ecologies and are difficult to understand, let alone regulate.

The pervasiveness and resistance of obesity to intervention may make it less an object for eradication than for control. Bray's (2004) framing of obesity as a chronic relapsing condition has parallels elsewhere in public health, as for example in the changing discourses surrounding both malaria and HIV infection – for control rather than eradication in the first case (Lancet Editorial 2011), and as a chronic disease in the second (Deeks et al. 2013). An acceptance of this view would make obesity a matter for long-term regulation. This is implicit in governmental and international monitoring of obesity rates. Chapter 4 describes obesity measures – especially BMI – that underpin the health and economics approaches that are at the core of such regulatory processes. Quantification precedes almost any intervention at the nation state level, and both epidemiology and economics employ standardized and institutionalized methods for

Table 1.4. The development of methods for expert systems: some examples

System	Reference
Agriculture	McKinion and Lemmon (1985)
Construction	McGartland and Hendrickson (1985)
Retail	Jones and Ledger (1986)
Transportation	Lukka and Lukka (1988)
Epidemiology	Cristea and Zaharia (1988)
Urban planning	Kim et al. (1990)
Engineering	Gottlob and Nejdl (1990)
Factory management	Meyer (1990)
Distribution planning	Chen et al. (1993)
Weather forecasting	Kumar et al. (1994)
Waste management	Basri and Stentiford (1995)
Recycling	Tandler et al. (1995)
Public transport	Mackett and Edwards (1996)
Predicting year-on-year climate variation	Rodionov and Martin (1999)
Medical management	Pandza and Masic (1999)
Work productivity analysis	Rao and Miller (2004)
Traffic management	Wen (2010)
Non-destructive testing of welds in shipping and aircraft	Valavanis and Kosmopoulos (2010)
Medical diagnosis	Keles et al. (2011)
Fashion colour trends	Yu et al. (2012)
Food safety	Filter et al. (2016)

understanding problems, and for identifying ways in which they might be regulated. The standardization of obesity measurement using BMI has allowed sense to be made of population obesity more easily through the practice of epidemiology. BMI measurement involves anthropometry, and this has an historical basis. This is described in this chapter, as are critiques of BMI as used in obesity work. Obesity rates across nations have also been modelled according to welfare provision, and this chapter also describes this work.

Chapter 5 considers inequalities in obesity rates within – and across – nations. When considering obesity rates in relation to the wealth of nations, this book uses the World Bank classification according to income: HICs, upper middle-income countries (UMICs), lower middle-income countries (LMICs) and low-income countries (LICs). It deviates only when reporting on country data that are classified otherwise. There are other classifications. The United Nations classification is based on the World Bank classification, but omits a number of small countries. The Organization for Economic Cooperation and Development (OECD) classification divides nations into two groups: category I (high income by the threshold used by the World Bank) and category II (low and middle income combined). The OECD and World Bank schemes show disagreement with respect to the classification of a number of geographically smaller countries, such as those in the Middle East, the Caribbean and the Pacific. For the sake of comparison, Table 1.5 shows the World Bank classification of nations by

Table 1.5. Nations according to status, according to income (World Bank) and Human Development Index (United Nations Development Programme), 2015

		Human Development Index				
		Very high	High	Medium	Low	Not classified
World Bank: income	High	Belgium, Brunei Darussalam, Canada, Chile, Croatia, Cyprus, Czech Republic, Denmark, Estonia, Finland, France, Germany, Greece, Hong Kong, Hungary, Iceland, Ireland, Israel, Italy, Japan, Kuwait, Latvia, Lichtenstein, Lithuania, Luxembourg, Malta, Mauritius, Netherlands, New Zealand, Norway, Poland, Portugal, Qatar, Republic of Korea, Saudi Arabia, Singapore, Slovak Republic, Slovenia, Spain, Sweden, Switzerland, Taiwan, UK, United Arab Emirates, US	Oman, Russia, Seychelles, St Kitts and Nevis, Trinidad and Tobago, Uruguay, Venezuela	Equatorial Guinea		Bermuda, Cayman Islands, Channel Islands, Curacao, Faeroe Islands, French Polynesia, Greenland, Guam, Isle of Man, Macao, Monaco, New Caledonia, Northern Mariana Islands, Puerto Rico, San Marino, Sint Maarten (Dutch), St Martin (French), Turks and Caicos Islands, Virgin Islands (US)
World Bank: income	Upper middle	Cuba	Belarus, Belize, Bosnia and Herzegovina, Botswana, Brazil, Bulgaria, China, Colombia, Costa Rica, Domenica, Dominican Republic, Ecuador, Fiji, Grenada, Iran, Jamaica, Jordan, Kazakhstan, Lebanon, Libya, Macedonia, Mexico,	Gabon, Iraq, Maldives, Mongolia, Namibia, Paraguay, South Africa, Turkenistan		Marshall Islands, Tuvalu

World Bank: income						
Lower middle	Montenegro, Palau, Panama, Peru, Romania, Serbia, St Lucia, St Vincent and the Grenadines, Suriname, Thailand, Tunisia, Turkey, Sri Lanka, Ukraine	Equatorial Guinea, Georgia	Kosovo	Bhutan, Bolivia, Botswana, Cabo Verde, Congo, Republic, Egypt, El Salvador, Ghana, Guatemala, Guyana, Honduras, India, Indonesia, Kiribati, Kyrgyz Republic, Lao, Micronesia, Moldova, Morocco, Nicaragua, Philippines, Samoa, Sao Tome and Principe, Syria, Tajikistan, Timor-Leste, Uzbekistan, Vanuatu, Vietnam, West Bank and Gaza, Zambia	Cameroon, Cote d'Ivoire, Djibouti, Kenya, Lesotho, Mauritania, Myanmar, Nigeria, Pakistan, Papua New Guinea, Senegal, Solomon Islands, Sudan, Swaziland, Yemen	
Low				Cambodia	Benin, Burkina Faso, Burundi, Central African Republic, Chad, Comoros, Democratic Republic of the Congo, Eritrea, Ethiopia, The Gambia, Guinea, Guinea Bissau, Haiti, Liberia, Madagascar, Malawi, Mali, Mozambique, Nepal, Niger, Rwanda, Sierra Leone, Tanzania, Togo, Uganda, Zimbabwe	Democratic Republic of Korea, Somalia, South Sudan

Adapted from Fantom and Serajuddin (2016).

income alongside the United Nations Development Programme's Human Development Index, which is used by McLaren (2007) to describe national patterns of obesity according to SES.

SES refers to the position occupied in a social hierarchy by an individual, family or group, and is broadly synonymous with socioeconomic position. Both SES and socioeconomic position are the outcomes of interactions between the stratification of a social order by powerful social institutions and the active involvement of people in maintaining social hierarchies through cultural and social practices (Graham 2007). The position of people in any social hierarchy is not neutral, cost free or value free, especially in relation to obesity. In HICs, obesity is more common among those of low SES, having been more common among those of higher SES prior to the 1960s. In middle-income countries, obesity is more common in groups of high SES. Differences in body fatness according to SES are often manifest in early childhood (Howe et al. 2010), as is the stigma associated with excess body fatness. The stigma surrounding obesity in most HICs often creates social disadvantages in employment, education, health care and interpersonal relationships (Puhl and Brownell 2001; Brownell et al. 2005), and this chapter goes on to consider these issues. It describes variation in forms of capital that contribute to inequalities in obesity rates (Ulijaszek 2012), and examines the relationships between inequality and insecurity in the production of obesity. It ends by considering the different rationalities that guide the political and economic systems that have contributed to the production of inequalities in obesity rates.

The food system, while under direct corporate control in most countries displaying high rates of obesity, represents an important arena for governmental regulation. It is argued in Chapter 6 that the marketing and provision of cheap, highly palatable energy-dense foods to people who have little resistance to consuming them (contributing to population obesity) represents a failure of regulation. Neoliberal systems and ideology form the discursive basis for many public health interventions (Ayo 2012), which assume that individuals will make rationally 'good' choices, once educated about the health implications of their behaviour – with respect to consuming obesogenic diets, for example. Such assumptions, with respect to food choice and the models of healthy bodies and eating on which they are premised, have been robustly critiqued, however (Guthman, 2011). One branch of obesity science uses physiological models of appetite to link the positive energy balance associated with obesity production with failure to control appetite, despite appetite control being difficult to practise in everyday life. There are good evolutionary reasons why appetite control is difficult. Uncertain and unstable environments in evolutionary time would have made food security precarious, and being able to eat plentiful amounts of energy-dense foods very quickly when available would have favoured survivorship, and by extension, reproduction. Overweight and obese women in the US have been shown to reproduce at higher rates than women of normal weight or below, at least prior to 1980 (Ellis and Haman 2004). Keith et al. (2006) have suggested that the relationship between obesity and fecundity is a two-way one: both from obesity predisposition to fecundity, and from fecundity to obesity. The latter relationship is suggestive of energy investment in reproduction post-conception. Gorging and overeating, and the positive energy balance that can come of them, is in this example evolutionarily rational (Chapter 3). Calls from public health for individual self-control in eating do not consider such rationality, giving prime importance to the Weberian formal rationality that underpins governmental regulation more broadly (Chapter 2), including that of obesity.

Market systems of food processing and delivery, which make palatable energy-dense foods cheap and extensively available, are fundamental to the creation and maintenance of obesogenic environments. A dominant explanatory framework for the emergence of obesogenic environments is that of nutrition transition, which in one of its later stages (Pattern Four) relates globalization, urbanization and Westernization to changing food environments among the populations of the world (Table 1.6). An example of Pattern Four nutrition transition can be found in the Cook Islands, where dramatic changes in diet, declining physical activity, increasing body size and rising obesity rates after World War II were experienced, varying by SES (Ulijaszek 2001a, b, c, 2003). Pattern Four nutrition transition models of obesity predominantly focus on economically emerging nations, but there is an acknowledgement that the Western industrialized nations also underwent Pattern Four nutrition transition at an earlier time (Popkin 2004). Pattern Four nutrition transition also affects maternal and child nutrition, and susceptibilities to obesity that are fashioned in early life. Through these early-life processes,

Table 1.6. Patterns of nutrition transition

Pattern	Age	Time	Economy	Diet
One	Food collecting	Pre-12 000 years ago	Hunter-gatherer	High in complex carbohydrates and fibre; low in fat
Two	Famine	Around 12 000 years ago	Origins of agriculture and animal husbandry	Less qualitatively varied; larger variation in seasonal and periodic availability; periods of acute scarcity
Three	Receding famine	Eighteenth and nineteenth centuries	Introduction of agricultural technology; industrial revolution	Increasingly processed; broadly sourced
Four	Degenerative diseases	Twentieth century	Urbanization and economic improvement	Major shift to lower nutrient density, higher energy density; excessively high in fat and sugar
Five	Behavioural change	Twenty-first century	Late modern	According to guidelines, to reduce degenerative diseases and prolong health

Modified from Popkin (2002).

transgenerational effects also influence obesity causation; the profound social changes that have taken place across the twentieth century are likely to have contributed to current obesity rates. Chapter 7 examines Pattern Four nutrition transition in various contexts, as well as in relation to fetal origins, epigenetic, life-course and predictive adaptive response models of obesity. The different rationalities that underpin Pattern Four nutrition transition and the emergence of obesity in this context are also examined here.

Governmental action to regulate obesity requires the best analyses of past circumstances as they relate to obesity production, and the best evidence with which to respond to current obesity-related problems. The translation of science, both biological and social, into good obesity policy is often frustrated by ethical and practical issues as well as by differences in the rationalities that underpin their respective practices. Chapter 8 examines the relationships between obesity science and obesity policy in HICs in recent years, and of the ethics of obesity intervention, before going on to consider how evidence is harnessed towards obesity policy and regulation. While most obesity policy in most places has focused on individual responsibility for its control, one obesity policy initiative dared to be different. The UK government Foresight project *Tackling Obesity: Future Choices* (henceforth Foresight Obesities) (Foresight 2007a, b) led the turn towards complexity in obesity science and policy from 2007. Chapter 9 describes how and why this happened, and shows how this led to an increased interdisciplinary emphasis in obesity science and regulation, mirroring a concurrent call to holistic approaches to society in anthropology (Parkin and Ulijaszek 2007). The resulting *Foresight Obesity Systems Map* describes obesity in the UK as an outcome of several interrelated systems, some expert, some not, operating at different levels of the individual or society, and with different types and degrees of complexity (Table 1.7). These are: a system of genes and their interactions with each other and with the environment; a homeostatic energy balance system; an appetite control system; the food system; the physical transportation system; social systems; and a political system that is either permissive of, or aims to control, obesity. Chapter 9 also examines the policy implications of this and other complexity

Table 1.7. Characterization of systems given in the *Foresight Obesity Systems Map*

System	Complex	Expert	Level
Energy balance	No	No	Individual
Genes	Yes	No	Individual
Appetite	Yes	No	Individual
Social	Yes	No	Society
Food	Yes	Yes	Society
Transportation	Yes	Yes	Society
Political	Yes	Yes	Society

From Foresight (2007a).

models of obesity for understanding the cross-talk between expert systems and the regulation of those systems.

In Chapter 10, it is argued that that the interactions of expert systems, such as food, transport, communications and medicine, have, across several decades, inadvertently contributed to population obesity. Obesity may be complex, but it is argued that understanding complexity alone will not fix obesity. Understanding the rationalities that underpin the various systems that inadvertently produce obesity may help bring potential fixes, however, through polyrational approaches. Polyrationality is a framework that was developed for improving the ways in which urban planning and land and river management are conducted (Davy 1997, 2008, 2013; Hartmann 2012). The structure and function of towns and cities and the relationships between them have been conceived as the products of polyrationality, in which land use involves a variety of practices, values and actors. In this context, land use relations and spatial policy must mediate a multiplicity of demands made by users and owners in very diverse settings. As a case study, Hartmann (2010) describes different types of floodplain management in Germany. Each type of management involves different stakeholders whose interests are underpinned by different rationalities, and who may modify their pattern of use and management in relation to other types of rationality and interest groups. He proposes that each type of interest and rationality, and the dominant cultural bias of each, should be considered in a polyrational land use policy. He calls this a viable clumsy solution composed of a combination of singly rational policies towards a particular problem.

The starting point for a polyrational approach to anything is with 'what is, not with what ought to be'. While it is easy to say that people should not build on floodplains, there may be historical precedent for doing so. For example, the Botley Road area of Oxford, UK, is very prone to flooding, and good flood plain management is essential at certain times of the year. Botley Road was initially developed in the nineteenth century with predominantly working-class housing. A hundred years or so later, this housing is undergoing steady gentrification, but continues to be at risk of flooding. A polyrational approach would not demand that the entire area be demolished, but rather that a systems approach be taken to regulate the water flowing through the rivers, streams and canal of this district under existing circumstances. In this particular case, increasingly accurate weather forecasting and pro-active river management by water containment upstream has mitigated most potential flooding in recent years. Even as a flood relief channel is currently planned for Oxford, polyrational approaches have been used to arrive at the best possible model for avoiding flooding in the future, as climate change is likely to make flooding more frequent. Similarly, with respect to obesogenic environments (Chapter 3), a polyrational approach would not call for a return to a past when obesity was a privilege of a small number of wealthy people. It would build upon and call to change and regulate what already exists. Whether or not 'insurances' might be devised for obesity regulation is an open question, however. This is for the future, as the evidence with which to evaluate such a possibility is absent. This book has much more modest aims than to stake a claim for polyrational approaches to obesity. Rather, in describing various models of obesity, it examines the rationalities of obesity science and policy, with the belief that such understanding can only lead to improved action.

2 Rationalities and Models of Obesity

Why consider models of obesity in relation to their rationalities? The idea of rationality is quite easily understood in terms of everyday practice, for example when considering whether someone is behaving rationally or not. In such a case, rational behaviour might be seen as being internally cohesive to the individual or to the group, and making decisions based on the best possible outcomes using information without emotion. While this serves well for understanding much of human decision making, it cannot explain 'irrationalities' in human behaviour or why people make decisions on the basis of sentiment, attachment or emotion. Nor is it especially useful in relation to higher-order practices involving complex decision making and bureaucracy as in most science and policy. Economics is in the fortunate position of being able to frame its rationality both individually and at higher levels (Chapter 1). This helps higher-level econometric models to be quite easily translatable into policy and to be understood in everyday life. Obesity can result from the breakdown of formal economic rationality (Chapter 1), but most models of obesity do not operate using this, but engage other types of rationality, as better frameworks for understanding the emergence and persistence of population obesity, as well as the predispositions to its development at individual and population levels. The purpose of this chapter is to outline the nature of different types of rationality and how they might be related to models of obesity. It goes on to consider why rationalities are important for understanding how and why obesity is framed differently by different actors.

Rationalities

Rationalities underpin all forms of institutional and organizational behaviour and practice, and models of obesity are implicitly grounded in them. They reflect different orientations to reality that weigh up means and ends of actions in pragmatic ways. When applied to models of obesity, they reflect the different world views that scientists, policy makers, advocacy groups and other people use in framing it as a problem. Different forms of rationality carry different meanings according to discipline, be it economics, psychology, sociology, evolutionary biology or political science.

Rationality is grounded in thinking that emerged in Europe with the rise of modernity from the sixteenth century onwards (Giddens 1998), in a world that was seen as being more open to transformation by human (rather than godly) intervention than ever before. Global transformation from this time onwards increasingly involved the activities of economic and political institutions, of industrial production and of market economies (Giddens 1998). Rationality, as applied in this book to the understanding of obesity, originated with the discourses of Locke (1632–1704), Hume (1711–1776) and Kant (1724–1804) with respect to the moral principles of human decision making and action (Mele and Rawling 2004). By constructing a non-moral rational world characterized by the existence of self-governing reason for all people (and not just for the rich and powerful), Kant (1997) outlined the philosophical basis for social equality as well as for self-directed actions, and individualism. The philosophical principles underpinning present-day individualism are framed by Kant's (1785) instrumental principle towards self-directed actions. This principle is also embedded in normative institutional frameworks and principles to the present day (Korsgaard 1997). Science and technology have been harnessed politically to frame norms and serve regulatory practices from the industrial revolution onwards. With respect to obesity, its framing as a problem for regulation, the identification of its causes by the application of technical criteria, and the call for individualism in its control all involve the application of Kant's instrumental principle. The validity of this principle is in part challenged when the call for individual responsibility for obesity control is challenged (Brownell et al. 2009b) (Chapter 8).

While Locke, Hume and Kant (and others) established rationality as a moral principle in Western societies, Weber (1864–1920) extended the principle to include all forms of practice and thought in the modern world. Weber argued that the principle of rationality should be able to accommodate the global spread of Western thought and practice and the institutions that carry them, including capitalism and bureaucracy (Weber 1978). If Kant's work could be used to explain the rise of individualism and its institutionalization, Weber's work could be used to explain its globalization beyond the West. With respect to population obesity, a Kantian explanation might be sufficient for its understanding in most Western societies, but a Weberian approach might better explain the rise of obesity across the non-Western world (Chapter 7). Kantian rationality has embedded in its logic nineteenth-century social evolutionism, which embraced individualism, capitalism and unilinear progress through the practices of politics and institutions. Weber challenged the completeness of this framing and built upon it, first by proposing two forms of rationality – instrumental and value rationalities – in his *Economy and Society* (Weber 1978), and then subdividing these two into four types – practical, theoretical, substantive and formal – in his *Collected Essays in the Sociology of Religion* (Kalberg 1980; Waters and Waters 2015) (Table 2.1). Instrumental rationality is concerned with the moral principles by which temporary or conditional ends are chosen. Value rationality is concerned with the moral basis of choice of permanent ends that are valuable in themselves. Practical rationality overlaps substantially with his earlier framing of instrumental rationality, while substantive rationality overlaps with his earlier-framed value rationality. Practical rationality prioritizes expediency and pragmatic action in everyday life, weighing up means and ends, while substantive rationality orders action into patterns according to sets of values that vary in comprehensiveness, internal consistency and content. This last type of rationality

Table 2.1. Weber's forms of rationality

Rationality	Description	Example
Practical	A practical rational way of life accepts given realities and calculates the most expedient means of dealing with the difficulties they present. Pragmatic action in terms of everyday interests is dominant, and practical ends are attained by careful weighing and calculation of the most adequate means to attain them	Everyday life
Theoretical	This involves a conscious mastery of reality through the construction of increasingly precise abstract concepts rather than through action. Since a cognitive confrontation with experience prevails in this form of rationality, such thought processes as logical deduction and induction, the attribution of causality and the formation of symbolic meanings are typical. More generally, all abstract cognitive processes denote theoretical rationality	Science
Substantive	Substantive rationality directly orders action into patterns in relation to a past, present or future value postulate. A value postulate implies entire clusters of values that vary in comprehensiveness, internal consistency and content. Thus, this type of rationality is a manifestation of the capacity for value-rational action. A substantive rationality may be circumscribed, organizing only a delimited area of life and leaving all others untouched. Friendship, for example, whenever it involves adherence to such values as loyalty, compassion and mutual assistance, constitutes a substantive rationality. Communism, feudalism, hedonism, egalitarianism, Calvinism, socialism, Buddhism, Hinduism and the Renaissance view of life, as well as all aesthetic notions of 'the beautiful', are also examples of substantive rationalities, however far they may diverge in their capacity to organize action as well as in their value content. In all cases, substantive rationality is considered to be a valid canon or unique standard against which reality's flow of unending empirical events may be selected, measured and judged. Values are not demonstrable by the methods of science. Even the most precise technically correct rationalization within, for example, economics, cannot be said to be legitimate and valid as progress, at the level of values	Culture
Formal	This generally relates to spheres of life and structures of domination that acquired specific and delineated boundaries only with industrialization, most significantly in economic, legal and scientific spheres, and with the growth of bureaucracies. Whereas practical rationality always indicates a tendency to calculate and to solve routine problems by means–end rational patterns of action in reference to pragmatic self-interests, formal rationality legitimates a similar means–end rational calculation by reference to universally applied rules, laws or regulations. To the degree that calculation in terms of abstract rules dominates, decisions are arrived at without regard to persons	Bureaucracy

Adapted from Kalberg (1980).

prioritizes action in relation to sets of values that can include attributes such as loyalty, trust and mutual assistance, which cannot, according to Weber (1946), be demonstrated by scientific methods. Theoretical rationality involves conscious mastery of reality through the construction of precise abstract concepts rather than through action (a particular property of science). It privileges logical deduction and induction, attribution of causality and the attachment of symbolic meanings to abstract concepts. Formal rationality includes systems of economic, legal and scientific practice, and the bureaucratic forms that link them. This form of rationality emerged, according to Weber (1946), only with industrialization, and differs from practical rationality in its legitimation of means–end rational calculations in relation to universally applied rules, laws or regulations. Decisions made using such calculations are arrived at without regard to persons (Kalberg 1980), a key feature of the modern bureaucracies that emerged in the nineteenth century and which have proliferated since.

All models of obesity are underpinned by some form or forms of rationality, and one purpose of this book is to make them explicit. Kantian rationalities are deeply embedded in scientific method (Friedman 2002), principles of individualism (Johnston 2005) and institutional practice (Kant 1891). Kantian rationality also informs Weber's practical and formal rationalities (Kalberg 1980). Although his framing of rationality is not used explicitly in relation to models of obesity in this book, Kant's ghost walks through every chapter. Table 2.2 shows relationships among the different forms of rationality considered in this volume, and how they might translate into everyday obesity-related constructs. In obesity science, the formulation of hypotheses belongs to the domain of Weberian theoretical rationality, while experimental scientific procedures involve Weberian formal rationality. Obesity intervention and regulation engage both bureaucratic forms of domination and economics, and are practically and substantively rational in the Weberian sense. Economic rationality emerged from Jevons' (1866, 1871) work on rational choice theory, and takes individual behaviour as the starting point for economic analysis (Green and Shapiro 1994); in Weberian terms, it embraces both Weberian practical and formal rationalities. Economics is practically rational when people and organizations take the most appropriate courses of action to meet their economic aims, and is formally rational in its use of institutions and bureaucracies in meeting practical aims. In circumstances of bounded rationality (Simon 1955), limitations of time and information make it impossible to make decisions that conform to rational choice theory (Chapter 1). The idea of bounded rationality emerged in reaction to modern (unbounded) versions of economic rationality (Gigerenzer 2010). In psychology, rationality is a normative concept that is used to examine reasoning and decision making (Samuels and Stitch 2004), which informs both bounded rationality and behavioural economics (Kahneman 2003).

Psychological rationality involves coherence to individual norms and to normative theories of individualized behaviour involving logical reasoning, probabilistic thinking and decision making (Shafir and LeBoeuf 2002), and is underpinned by Weberian practical rationality. It has been invoked in evolutionary explanations of human behaviour.

Table 2.2. Some forms of rationality as they might apply to obesity

| | | Form of rationality | | | | | | |
| | | Weberian practical | Economic | Weberian formal | Psychological | Weberian theoretical | Evolutionary | Weberian substantive |
Overlap with other forms of rationality		Economic	Weberian substantive and psychological	Economic	Weberian practical		Weberian practical and substantive	
Everyday construct	Government	X	X	X	X			
	Corporations	X	X	X	X			
	Public health	X	X	X				
	Medicine	X	X	X				X
	Science	X	X			X		
	Individualism	X	X		X		X	
	Groups of people	X	X		X		X	X
	Interest groups	X	X					X
	Religion[a]							X

[a] Included because it can shape or pattern human behaviour.

In his social brain hypothesis, Dunbar (1998) attempted to reconcile two extremes of sociality (unequal and equal) in a human evolutionary framework. Where long-term reciprocity can help ensure evolutionary success, cooperation, reciprocation, honouring commitments and keeping promises can be considered substantively rational in the Weberian sense. Such behaviour can also be explained as an outcome of self-interested choices, even among the most selfishly incentivized persons (Bicchieri 2004), and is therefore also economically rational. While psychological rationality can encompass Weberian substantive rationality as well as economic rationality at the level of the individual, it may also require coherence of behaviour in relation to individual and group norms. Such coherence of behaviour varies with context, however. According to Shafir and LeBoeuf (2002), many studies have documented the various ways in which decision making does not cohere, nor follow basic principles of logic. Rather, people regularly use intuitive strategies that are effective for much of the time, but which also produce biases.

Such biases exist in perception of risk. For example, a study of emotion and risk in the United States (US) after the 11 September attacks in 2001 showed fear to increase estimates of everyday risk and anger to reduce them (Lerner et al. 2003). Furthermore, the perceived everyday risks of handguns, cars and nuclear power in the US are more closely related to the general dread they arouse than to risk statistics (Fischhoff et al. 1978). As with dread and risk of accident by nuclear power, motor cars and handguns, so with food and eating (Chapter 6). Ecological decisions involving the obtaining of food and eating involve perceptions of risks and benefits. While eating behaviours may be evolutionarily rational, risks attached to changing consumption patterns in relation to changed ecological circumstances are not easily intuited by people. Without feeding there is no survival, and neocortical feed-forward mechanisms have evolved to create and maintain associative pleasures in food. Humans express such mechanisms to a degree that no other species can, in support of the ecologically based drive to eat. The pleasure of eating and overeating often foregrounds any perceptions of risk of obesity in the future. In addition to risk, human food consumption is considered economically rational, and more or less bounded according to circumstance (Chapter 1).

The model of bounded rationality has been adapted for regulatory processes that involve structuring human behaviour. By linking ideas from cognitive psychology and psychological rationality to those of bounded rationality (Chapter 1), Kahneman and Tversky (1972) put in place the framework for behavioural economics (Thaler 2015), of which nudge theory is an off-shoot (Thaler and Sunstein 2008). The nudge approach, which uses modified choice architecture as a mechanism by which to govern human behaviour, has been favoured by the United Kingdom and other governments for obesity prevention and control. Nudge is used in policy by either harnessing unconscious biases or encouraging individuals to be more reflective in their choices (Lodge and Wegrich 2016). There are advocates both for (Oliver 2011) and against (Rayner and Lang 2011) its use in the regulation of obesity. Nudge is acknowledged by its authors as being a libertarian paternalistic approach to present-day problems (Thaler and Sunstein 2008), but the nudge approach does not apply bounded rationality to itself. The manipulation of the bounded rationality of individuals towards behaviours deemed by governments to promote well-being and obesity reduction is often in contradiction to governmental permissiveness of the market forces that have promoted obesity in the first place (Chapter 8).

Bounded rationality cannot adequately explain all aspects of seemingly irrational behaviour in relation to models of obesity. The decisions that individuals make about eating and personal body weight, for example, fail to account for biology, where cognitive decision making is accompanied by biologically based emotional and impulsive responses (Ruhm 2010). Emotion is strongly implicated in overeating (Macht 2008) and obesity production (Zeeck et al. 2011), as well as in decision making in many other aspects of life (Finucane et al. 2000). People rely on affective reactions, positive or negative, to speed up judgements and decision making (Finucane et al. 2000), and these can sometimes predispose to obesity. Food consumption patterns that involve overeating can be considered rational in evolutionary terms, but they can also predispose to obesity. Biology is unconcerned about health and well-being beyond its contribution to reproductive fitness and reduced mortality, however, and the procurement, processing and consumption of food are all evolutionarily rational practices that influence reproductive success and survival. Lambert (2009) has argued that physiological fitness (homeostasis) must be considered quite separately from reproductive (Darwinian) fitness, acknowledging that these two models often recruit different types of rationality (in most cases, of either the Weberian theoretical or evolutionary type).

Models and Obesity

All models are simplifications of reality and are therefore wrong (Chapter 1). They are, however, among the most fundamental instruments of science, and are useful in constructing formal systems that will not produce theoretical consequences that do not contradict empirical reality (Hacking 1983). Models of obesity do mostly representational work, for the understanding and prediction of almost any cause and effect relationship, and vary widely in range and complexity. Predictions or other statements drawn from models mirror or map the real world only as far as they are demonstrated to hold true (Ritchey 2012). To understand obesity models, it is important to consider some general principles that govern the development and use of models more generally. However, until very recently, there were no general theories of models. After investigating the epistemological, methodological and operational aspects of scientific modelling, Ritchey (2012) offers criteria for what a general theory of modelling should contain (Table 2.3). This includes having operational definitions and employing generality, from which properties can be abstracted that can show how models do their work. These criteria also include the provision of a framework for the successful application of different modelling methods for hypothesis production and of common modelling language and terminology. Furthermore, models should be operational, not merely representational. Models of energy balance, for example, should be able to describe the dynamics of

Table 2.3. If there were a general theory of modelling, what would it involve?

It would provide an operational definition of the concept of a model that informs about how models are developed and how they operate. This is in contrast to a nominal definition of a model such as 'a model is an abstract representation of the thing being modelled'

The definitional framework of a model should be as general as possible, to include the main types and forms of modelling methods employed in science

The operational definition should either include, or make it possible to abstract, a set of properties or parameters that indicate how models do their work, and by which different modelling methods can be classified, exemplified, compared and otherwise scrutinized

It would provide a framework for identifying the requirements for the successful application of different modelling methods for different tasks and objects of scientific enquiry

It should offer a basis for treating models and modelling both as a means of representation and as epistemic tools for hypothesis and theory generation

It should provide a common modelling language and terminology

Adapted from Ritchey (2012).

energy balance, and not be merely static representations (Chapter 3). They should also be instruments for hypothesis and theory generation. The operational definition of a model should include a set of properties or parameters that show how it does its work. In obesity science, this might involve mapping cause and effect relationships in appetite regulation, for example. It should also be possible to test the applicability of a modelling method by relating its methodological limits to the properties of the object being modelled. This could be done, for example, when comparing econometric models of different food taxation regimes on energy intake (Chapter 4). Obesity models should strive for common modelling language and terminology, as, for example, in the use of epidemiological data in econometric modelling of obesity (Chapter 4).

Different approaches to obesity employ a wide range of models – animal, human physiological, genetic, epidemiological, economic, psychological, geographical, biocultural, social and complex. They vary, as all models do, according to their specification, directionality, quantifiability, relationality and types of connectivity (Ritchey 2012). Variables in any model may be internally specified, containing a well-defined range of ordered or non-ordered values or states, or unspecified and treated as black boxes. Furthermore, connections between variables may be directed or non-directed, and the relationships between them may be expressed in either quantified or non-quantified ways. Relationships between variables can be mathematical, probabilistic (statistical), quasi-causal (implying influence only) or non-causal (implying logical or normative relations). Furthermore, models can be cyclic or acyclic.

Quantified models of obesity are usually made operational by overlaying statistical or mathematical models on them. Such overlays form the basis for analysis and inference. The assumptions made when, for example, an experimental model of obesity is built must be as robust as the assumptions that must be met in statistical analysis.

With respect to statistical models alone, the standard method for evaluating outcomes in clinical interventions, the randomized controlled trial (Schultz et al. 2010), has known limitations (Grossman and McKenzie 2005), including statistical ones. Assmann et al. (2000) found that half of 50 such studies examined for their rigor of use of statistical methods incorrectly used significance tests for baseline comparison. Furthermore, they found that methods of randomization and/or data stratification were often poorly described, and that there was little consistency in the use of covariate adjustment. Speaking to statistical practice in scientific research more broadly, Ioannidis (2005) has viewed most published research to be false on the basis of statistical procedure alone. This is because the probability of a research claim being true depends on (among other things) study power and bias, the number of other studies on the same question, and the proportion of true to not true relationships among the relationships examined in a scientific field. Ioannidis (2005) goes on to say that research findings are less likely to be true when, among other circumstances, the number of studies carried out in a field is low, when effect sizes are small, where there is great flexibility in study design, analysis and outcomes, when there is great financial interest and prejudice, and when there are many teams in a scientific field chasing statistical significance.

Models of obesity that employ statistics may often be questioned for the reasons given by Assmann et al. (2000) and Ioannidis (2005). Scales of analysis and multiple abstractions may also obscure meaning that might be taken from quantitative obesity models. For example, the genetics of human population obesity is commonly inferred from variations in the make-up of the genome within a sample of people. Such a sample of people usually varies to some unknown extent in its representativeness of a population. Inferring obesity-related meaning from such genetic variation involves characterization of this sample of individuals according to obesity phenotypes such as the body mass index (BMI) or waist circumference. Such phenotypes vary in the extent to which they represent risk – of disease, mortality and/or poor economic output, for example. To relate variations in these phenotypes and genotypes, other models, statistical or mathematical, are overlaid, adding abstraction to uncertainty. Statistical and mathematical analysis might present a convincing narrative of the genetics of obesity, but the meaning of this narrative remains open to interpretation, if only from a methodological perspective.

Another abstraction in some types of obesity model involves the use of animals in experimentation. Before the 1980s, there were many categories of animal model used to examine biological and environmental factors that might contribute to obesity (Sclafani 1984) (Table 2.4). The exploratory nature of obesity research at that time is reflected in the aetiological classification of animal models of obesity then: neural, endocrine, pharmacological, nutritional, environmental, seasonal and genetic. Most of the animal models presented in Table 2.4 are of obesity causation, while two of them, endocrine and pharmacological, are models for treatment. The uses of animal models in obesity research have changed as dominant ideas about obesity have changed; by the 2000s, they overwhelmingly reflected genetic, physiological and developmental foci.

Table 2.4. Aetiological classification of animal models of obesity in the 1980s

Type	Characterization
Neural	Hypothalamic
	Midbrain
	Chronic lateral hypothalamic stimulation
	Olfactory bulbectomy
	Amygdala–temporal lobe lesions
	Unilateral abdominal sympathectomy
Endocrine	Ovariectomy
	Chronic insulin treatment
	Chronic glucocorticoid treatment
Pharmacological	Cyproheptadine treatment
	Clonidine treatment
	Chlordiazepoxide treatment
Nutritional	Force feeding
	Meal feeding
	Diet-induced (high-fat diet, high-sugar diet, cafeteria or supermarket diet)
	Post-natal overnutrition
	Pre-natal undernutrition
Environmental	Physical restriction
	Tail pinch
Seasonal	Pre-hibernation
	Pre-migration
Genetic	Single gene, dominant (yellow mouse, adipose mouse)
	Single gene, recessive (obese mouse (*ob*), diabetes mouse (*db*), fat mouse, fatty rat)

Adapted from Sclafani (1984).

The abstract nature of many models of obesity, created using structural realist approaches (Worrall 1989) common to most obesity science, usually incorporating statistical models, is difficult to translate into everyday practice. This is because such translation involves the deployment of different rationalities – which overlap imperfectly, if at all – from Weberian theoretical approaches in obesity science, to Weberian practical and formal approaches in obesity intervention and policy. The more abstract a model of obesity, the less open it is to common sense and everyday scrutiny, and the greater the need for translation into common understanding for policy makers, practitioners and everyday people to gain value from it. Abstraction in obesity science has increased as complexity approaches to obesity became possible in the 2000s (Chapter 9). Obesity science only recently began to engage in complexity through multilevel modelling (Lopez 2007; Rundle et al. 2007), complex systems modelling (Hammond 2009; Finegood et al. 2010) and simulation modelling (Levy et al. 2011), but not yet agent-based modelling (although such methods are in place for modelling interactions between nutrients (Simpson et al. 2010)). The study of society is not usually amenable to structural realist approaches, however, and this is one reason why the different framings of obesity in the biological and social sciences do not easily overlap or integrate.

Models of obesity offer no moral guide to the use of the facts emerging from their use (Nagel 1997), nor do they necessarily relate to the social realities of obesity production in different populations (Chapter 5). Obesity policy, however, relies on the social realities of politics, institutions, human behaviour and practice to enact the moral principles that underlie decisions about obesity intervention (Chapter 8), as well as the enactment of such intervention itself. For example, an econometrics model of obesity reduction via taxation might give insight into consumption patterns and human behaviours that might offer possible interventions. Whether or not such intervention through taxation (Chapter 4) should be enacted rests on assumptions about the moral correctness of such an intervention (Chapter 8), in addition to its likely impacts. Is it morally acceptable for such taxation, if it only indirectly targets obesity but more directly increases economic inequality in a population? Alternatively, is it morally acceptable to measure heights and weights of all children in primary school, to be used in epidemiological and econometric modelling (Chapter 4), with the knowledge that this may promote weight stigma (Chapter 5)?

Rationalities in Models of Obesity

The rationalities that underpin different models of obesity are multiple and sometimes contradictory. Models of obesity can differ enormously in their theoretical underpinnings and objectives, and there are multiple and often conflicting rationalities even on a single branch of obesity science. This is one reason why turning obesity science into policy and practice has been difficult (Chapter 8). For example, the rationalities of consumer choice and behaviour in relation to food (Chapter 6) are not only economic, but also Weberian substantive, evolutionary and psychological. Meanings of obesity are also highly contested (Warin et al. 2015) across the biological and social sciences, and this often reflects the engagement of different rationalities in the different sciences. Gard (2011a) has identified two broad camps competing for legitimacy in obesity studies – alarmists and sceptics. Alarmists include those epidemiologists, public health and medical specialists who claim that a health crisis is upon us, and that the health and mortality risks associated with a looming global obesity epidemic are fast growing. They are overwhelmingly driven by Weberian practical rationality, although their practices involve Weberian theoretical and formal rationalities. Alternatively, sceptics (usually embracing critical fat studies) repudiate the idea of obesity as a 'risk factor' or disease. In this field, obesity research includes feminist scholarship, fat activism, critical dietetics, cultural studies, sexual diversity studies, anthropology, sociology and social geography, and world views are overwhelmingly based in Weberian substantive rationality. It is rare to find critical fat scholars engaging with emerging scientific insights into obesity. According to Gard (2011b), most social science that has critiqued mainstream obesity research has paid little attention to what has actually been published by such obesity science. It has been simply added to the list of sexist, racist and classist scientific discourses that is the usual focus of academic critiques of science. There is no definitive standpoint among either alarmists or sceptics. With different rationalities underpinning what obesity and body fatness are for either broad camp, it is not surprising that alarmists and sceptics rarely see eye to eye.

Beyond the alarmist–sceptic divide, various scientific models of obesity – genetic, epigenetic, developmental, obesogenic behavioural, obesogenic environmental, nutrition transition, biocultural and complexity – engage with different rationalities, especially when they also engage in policy, where multiple, often competing rationalities are in play. This idea is developed across this book. Late modernity (Chapter 1) has penetrated most of the world, and expert systems operate nearly everywhere. Exceptions lie where tradition prevails, and the production of obesity may involve rationalities invoked in mutual assistance and loyalty, for example, according to conditions of modernity or tradition. In many low-income and lower middle-income countries, the production of body fatness may be guided more by aesthetics and reproductive success. The former involves Weberian substantive rationality, while the latter involves evolutionary rationality. This is the case with respect to the ritual fattening of Massa and Mussey men in rural Cameroon (de Garine and Koppert 1991). Obesity among urban males in Cameroon, however, at 6.3 per cent in 2003 (Kamadjeu et al. 2006), is an outcome of modernity, and is largely a product of the formal rationality that largely underpins modernity. The rationalities that underpin different expert systems (Chapters 1 and 10) may be congruent, but may also differ in some respects. Corporations, governments, medicine and public health generally share economic, Weberian practical and Weberian formal rationalities (Table 2.2). Interest and advocacy groups may to some extent share many of the rationalities that underpin governments and corporations, but their activities may also be underpinned by Weberian substantive rationality.

The dominant icon of obesity modelling is that of energy balance, which provides the underpinning logic to many other scientific models of obesity, including genetic, epigenetic, developmental, behavioural, environmental, biocultural and complexity models. It is also the basic logic that many obesity interventions draw on, whether it be weight management, dietary restriction, pharmaceutical intervention or obesity surgery. The energy balance model is underpinned by, and engaged with, many forms of rationality in its scientific and policy use, and the next chapter turns to this, as well as to the genetic and environmental models that directly relate to it.

3 Energy Balance, Genetics and Obesogenic Environments

Energy balance is the central concept in the physiological study of obesity – at its simplest, a long-term outcome of excess dietary energy consumed relative to physical and metabolic energy expended. While easy to comprehend, this model of obesity invokes a wide range of rationalities in its scientific and policy operationalizations. When framed as a scientific model of individualized obesity causation, energy balance is underpinned by Weberian practical and theoretical rationalities (Chapter 2). When used to frame obesity policy and regulation (Chapter 8), it is formally rational in the Weberian sense. Genetic predispositions and ecology both influence energy balance (Neel et al. 1998; Bouchard 2008), while developmental programming and epigenetics (Chapter 7) have been more recently co-opted as modifiers of energy balance. The population genetics of obesity are shaped by evolutionary ecological forces that act through differential selection for metabolic efficiency and fat storage (Barsh and Schwartz 2002), appetite (Yeo and Heisler 2012), taste sensitivity (Drayna 2005) and cold adaptation (Sellayah et al. 2014), making the energy balance model also evolutionarily rational. The environments in which obesity emerges and persists have been characterized as being obesogenic (Swinburn et al. 1999a) in very particular structured and geographical ways, usually involving aspects of urbanism. Despite the widespread use of the term, obesogenic environments are difficult to define (Jones et al. 2007), because all urban environments reflect their design and use assemblages, past and present, and do not automatically predispose to obesity. The sociodemographic structures of urban environments modulate the extent to which they predispose to obesity, as does the availability of affordable energy-dense foods and the extent to which such environments are structured to encourage physical inactivity and convenience. These prerequisites of obesogenicity in urban environments are often produced inadvertently by expert systems (Chapters 1 and 10) that more generally deliver objects and services (including water, sanitation, food, shelter, electricity, transport, communication and leisure) that on balance contribute to either health and well-being, or alternatively illness and chronic disease, in human populations. A geographical location may become labelled obesogenic when the expert systems that ensure the smooth running of everyday life there also contribute to the production of obesity. This chapter examines how models of obesity based on energy balance and the genetics that underpin it have become naturalized forms in obesity science and policy. It goes on to consider the obesogenic environments construct using the case study of Geelong, a small industrial city in Australia, in the 1990s and 2000s.

Energy Balance

The word 'energy' (in Greek, *enérgeia*) was coined by Aristotle (384–322 BC) as representing something 'being at work'. Energy, to the ancient Greeks, was an observed but unmeasurable force and a link between human function and pleasure. Energy became a phenomenon of scientific enquiry only in the nineteenth century, once it became measureable (Smith 1998), and once Kelvin (1824–1907) demonstrated the interchangeability of its different forms, which were subsequently formalized in laws of thermodynamics. Kelvin's conceptualization of energy was significant in defining the concept of physical force in nature, but it removed bodily experience (such as pleasure and pain) from the consideration of energetics as a physiological process. The field of energetics has since been used instrumentally in human physiological study of pregnancy, lactation, growth and development, undernutrition (Ulijaszek and Strickland 1993; Ulijaszek 1995), obesity (Ulijaszek and Lofink 2006), and in exploring human ecological relationships in evolutionary frameworks (Ulijaszek 1992, 1995; Leonard and Ulijaszek 2002).

The homeostatic principle that underpins the idea of energy balance predates Socratic philosophy, with the doctrine of balance of opposite qualities being its direct ancestor. Humoral theory, based on the equilibrium of dissimilar elements and opposite qualities, followed from Hippocrates' (460–370 BC) work, and formed the basis of Western medicine into the eighteenth century. While humanistic Western medical practice increasingly relied on understandings of pathology and deviation from norms by which to define illness, the notion of the balance of opposites has never disappeared from Western medicine. It can be found, for example, in the blood sugar balance discourse of Type 2 diabetes management (Clarke and Foster 2012), and in energy balance discourses surrounding the personal control of body weight for the prevention or management of obesity (Yates-Doerr 2013). The ideas of physiological homeostasis and energy balance are usually taken to be synonymous, as both are concerned with energy flow through living systems by the process of metabolism, or energy transformation within biological systems. But while homeostasis is fundamental to physiological explanations of nutritional health, biological energy systems are not ultimately homeostatic. According to Wallace (2010), competition for limited energy resources is the basis of natural selection – within any species, those that are more effective at acquiring and/or expending available energy will sustain their energy flux and thus survive and reproduce. Life is largely conducted under non-equilibrium conditions, and organisms, groups of organisms or species that may seem to be in energy balance across the course of a day may not be across years, centuries or millennia. There are many examples in biology of attempts to use equilibrium constructs under non-equilibrium conditions (Morowitz 1991). While short-term physiological homeostasis can be demonstrated in humans under laboratory conditions, free-living humans, like other species, show only a semblance of longer-term energy homeostasis and then only if the non-homeostatic processes of reproduction and physical growth and development are ignored. Positive energy balance is associated with pregnancy, lactation and bodily growth, while energy

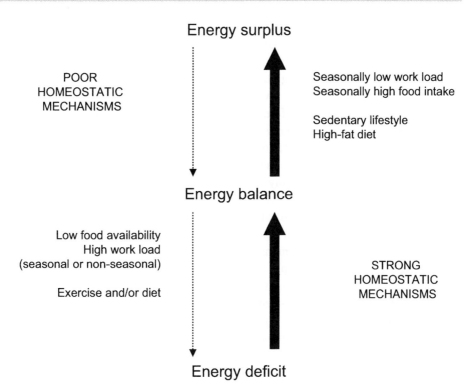

Energy surplus

POOR
HOMEOSTATIC
MECHANISMS

Seasonally low work load
Seasonally high food intake

Sedentary lifestyle
High-fat diet

Energy balance

Low food availability
High work load
(seasonal or non-seasonal)

Exercise and/or diet

STRONG
HOMEOSTATIC
MECHANISMS

Energy deficit

Figure 3.1. Changing bodies: weight regulation in ecological context (adapted from Ulijaszek 2002a).

imbalance, both positive and negative according to ecological circumstances, contributes to the selective forces that have driven human evolution.

While seemingly straightforward, decades of study have shown the relationships between energy intake and expenditure to be complex and intertwined. Eating and physical activity are both strongly implicated in the regulation of body weight, with homeostatic physiological mechanisms defending the body against changes in energy balance (Figure 3.1). Energy brought into the body by food consumption must balance energy expended in bodily maintenance, reproduction and physical activity (and in children, physical growth and development), if either undernutrition or obesity is to be avoided. Human physiology is much better able to strike such a balance in ecologies of low food availability than in ones with plenty. Where food availability is low, physiological energy deficits can lead to weight loss initially, but energy balance recalibrates at lower levels of intake and expenditure as a consequence of physiological and behavioural adaptations (Ulijaszek 1996a), which defend body size and composition. When food is plentiful, only very weak homeostatic mechanisms exist to restore individual energy balance in the face of ecological energy surplus (Webber 2003). In the absence of increased reproduction, increasing body size and fatness may result. Obesity at the population level has emerged in societies where low or declining reproductive rates have coincided with good or improving food security in the past 60 years or so (Chapter 7). Energy balance models of obesity may therefore have a misplaced focus on the individual or nation state as the unit of study, rather than the family or other reproductive grouping.

Various types of energy balance model have been developed, including set-point, energy density, protein leverage and brown fat models. All of them relate the ecological structuring of energy intake and expenditure to the individual physiological regulation of energy input and output at the whole-body level (Mayer 1955; Rothwell and Stock 1981; Prentice and Jebb 2003; Simpson and Raubenheimer 2005; Nedergaard et al. 2007). The set-point model is based on epidemiological observations that show that many people have more or less constant body weight across adult life (Muller et al. 2010). This model views body weight and body fatness as being maintained homeostatically by internal endocrine regulatory factors, involving either glucostatic or lipostatic mechanisms (Mayer 1955). Tests of this model show the set point in humans to have upper and lower limits, rather than being under tight control. For example, the fluctuation in body weight that results from either under- or overfeeding requires a considerable change to the hypothetical set point, at least after starvation, re-feeding and overeating (Muller et al. 2010). In a review of studies of body weight regulation through energy balance, Muller et al. (2010) conclude that there is strong biological control of body weight and weight stability when experimental subjects eat boring but healthy chow diets. Most studies supporting the set-point hypothesis have been carried out under such conditions. The strong biological control that preserves weight stability (Muller et al. 2010) is lost when subjects eat more palatable energy-dense diets, and thus the set-point model of energy balance has little explanatory value in the context of high availability of palatable energy-dense foods to free-living people, as in most high-income countries (HICs) now, and increasingly across the rest of the world.

Scientifically demonstrating clear set points in different people has proved difficult, and the set-point model has been modified to take account of some of the inconsistencies associated with it. One modification has involved amending the set-point idea to one of a range of 'settling points' at any of several body weight steady states, without feedback control of energy intake (Hall and Heymsfield 2009). Another modification has involved incorporation of the idea of a threshold control system that only responds to negative energy balance (Leibel 2008). Two further modifications of the set-point model involve energy balance in relation to consumption of specific macronutrients. These are the energy density (Prentice and Jebb 2003) and protein leverage (Simpson and Raubenheimer 2005) models of obesity, respectively. The macronutrient composition of diet and its effects on satiation (physiological cues to terminate eating) and satiety (the feeling of fullness after eating) can vary enormously. High-fat foods have weak effects on satiation and satiety compared with refined carbohydrates, while protein has the strongest effects on both (Lawton et al. 1993; Stubbs et al. 2000; Stubbs and Whybrow 2004). Furthermore, energy-dense, fat-rich foods have been shown to have lower satiation and satiety effects than bulky, hydrated foods that are high in protein, fibre or water content (Drewnowski 1998). In general, diets that are more energy dense have lower effects on satiation and satiety, making it easier to overeat passively and gain weight (Gerstein et al. 2004). Across the world, the contribution of different macronutrients to total daily dietary energy intake is highly variable, with population means ranging between 19 and 35 per cent for protein, 22 and 40 per cent for carbohydrate and 28 and 58 per cent for fat (Cordain et al. 2002). The effects of such differences in macronutrient composition of diets on satiation and satiety thus also vary considerably and, it has been argued, so do the set points for energy balance (Prentice and Jebb 2003).

Simpson and Raubenheimer's (2005) protein leverage model of obesity posits that when humans trade off their protein intake against carbohydrate and fat on nutritionally unbalanced diets, physiological regulatory mechanisms prioritize protein when regulating food intake, maintaining appetite for further consumption of food until protein needs are met. In relation to possible dietary causes of obesity, these authors note that changing patterns of fat and carbohydrate consumption may drive population obesity precisely because humans seek to obtain a constant level of intake of protein, even when its density in the diet is low. They have formalized their model mathematically, relating changes in protein availability across nations between 1970 and 2000 to obesity rates in the early 1990s in 13 HICs – Australia, Canada, Denmark, Finland, France, Germany, Italy, the Netherlands, New Zealand, Spain, Sweden, the United Kingdom (UK) and the United States (US). They showed that obesity rates are highest where protein intakes have declined most (the US) and lowest where they have increased the most (Denmark). The protein leverage model has also been tested experimentally. A randomized controlled laboratory-based study shows that dietary dilution of protein with carbohydrate and fat in meals promotes the overconsumption of dietary energy more generally (Gosby et al. 2011). Furthermore, in a free-living population followed longitudinally in the Philippines, Martínez-Cordero et al. (2012) found that intakes of calories from protein remained more constant over time, while intakes of calories from carbohydrates or fat varied, even when corrected for the low proportional contribution of protein to dietary energy. The protein leverage model of obesity causation is difficult to demonstrate with diets that are low in protein, however, and it is unclear whether low protein intake would cause overeating, or would be an outcome of overeating on carbohydrate and/or fat (Martens et al. 2013).

Another energy balance model of obesity, associated with the function of brown adipose tissue (BAT), was proposed in the 1970s. BAT has great capacity to generate heat and is an important site of diet-induced thermogenesis (energy expenditure due to the digestion of food) (Dulloo 2013). Differences in BAT activity were initially considered to be a partial explanation of why some people can eat plentifully and not put on weight while others cannot (Nicholls and Locke 1984). The extent to which BAT is involved in the regulation of energy balance has been well studied in rodents, with overfeeding activating heat production through the stimulation of the sympathetic nervous system (Seale et al. 2007). Processes attributed to active BAT in experimental animals (mainly rodents), including non-shivering thermogenesis (cold-induced energy expenditure that does not involve shivering) and diet-induced thermogenesis, both of which reduce the possibility of weight gain, were previously considered either absent or attributable to unknown alternative mechanisms in humans (Nedergaard et al. 2007). Saito et al. (2009) challenged this view when they demonstrated, in Japanese subjects, greater activation of BAT in winter compared with summer, and an inverse relationship between BAT activity and body mass index (BMI), as well as total and visceral fat, in their subjects. Cold-induced activation of oxidative metabolism in BAT (associated with increased energy expenditure) has since been confirmed in humans (Ouellet et al. 2012; van der Lans et al. 2013), the quantitative contribution of brown fat metabolism to human energy expenditure being uncertain but impressive (Dulloo 2013).

Energy balance models of obesity mostly conform to the criteria that should underpin obesity models more broadly (Chapter 2). They all offer means of representation, with clear operational definitions, common modelling language and terminology, but vary in the degree of generality they employ. Some of these models have also been used for hypothesis generation. The original set-point model does not employ a high degree of generality, however, nor does the brown fat model of energy balance. The settling-point modification of the set-point model has a higher degree of generality, gained at the cost of possible hypothesis generation. The protein leverage hypothesis is the best framed of all energy balance models, because it offers high generality and a good framework for hypothesis generation. No energy balance model has been successful in demonstrating causality in obesity production, however, and Sorensen et al. (2012) have questioned the implicit causality of energy balance models often assumed by their proponents. They argue that the translation of energy balance theory to testable scenarios about development of obesity has largely failed, because energy balance theory has not translated successfully into an explanation of obesity at the population level.

The failure of translation of energy balance theory into the biological phenomenon of obesity perhaps also lies with a misunderstanding of the thermodynamics of non-equilibrium systems, especially in relation to reproduction and evolution. Many physiological processes are homeostatic, but their homeostasis cannot be used to explain evolutionary processes, since evolution is not homeostatic (Wallace 2010). It is precisely what is not homeostatic in nature that drives the development of more complex structures with increased energy flow, of greater diversity both within organisms and in ecosystems, and with more hierarchical levels at all levels of biological organization (Toussaint and Schneider 1998). Long-term energy imbalance is a fundamental property of biology, ecology and evolution. In this framing, obesity is an emergent property of evolved human biological systems, under the very particular circumstances of assured food security and declining fertility rates in the late twentieth century.

There are mundane issues of measurement that also make energy balance models problematic. While the relationship between energy expenditure and energy intake can be measured accurately enough to detect energy imbalance over periods of days or weeks under tightly controlled laboratory conditions (Dulloo 2006), this is much more difficult to do in free-living people. This is largely because of systematic bias in everyday self-reported food intake (Schoeller 1990), and only moderate precision in the measurement of energy expenditure in free-living conditions. The most precise measure of energy expenditure, the doubly labelled water method, has a precision of around 5 per cent (Schoeller 1990). This translates into a measurement error of energy expenditure in excess of 100 kilocalories per day for most individuals. Combined with bias in energy intake measures, the combined error of assessing energy imbalance can easily be 1000 kilocalories per day, which is around 36 per cent of the recommended daily allowance (RDA) for energy for a very inactive but average-sized adult male (of BMI 27.4 kg/m^2) in England in 2013, and around 24 per cent of the RDA for energy for an extremely active one (World Health Organization/Food and Agriculture Organization/United Nations University 2001; Craig and Mindell 2014). If this English adult male had a BMI of 21 kg/m^2, then the combined error of assessing energy imbalance would be around 42 per cent of RDA if he were very inactive and 28 per cent if he were extremely active. This level of inaccuracy prevents any evaluation of impacts of any potential energy balance-based interventions designed to give small incremental weight loss over time (Hall et al. 2012). An alternative way of observing positive energy imbalance is to measure change in weight or body fatness across a period of time. The amount of body fat gained on a daily basis is so small, however, that it cannot be measured daily among free-living subjects by any available technique (Sorensen et al. 2012). But if it were possible to measure the components of energy balance exactly, it would only confirm that the energy balance theory is valid, but without knowledge of what causes energy imbalance (Sorensen et al. 2012).

Availability of dietary energy to satisfy increased dietary needs is, of course, a prerequisite for obesity development – obesity does not develop during famine – and in this way it may be considered a necessary, but not sufficient, cause of obesity. Both set-point and settling-point energy balance models frame body weight as being in homeostasis at varied levels according to energy ecology or the plane of energy nutrition. In societies of abundance, a prudent lifestyle (involving high cognitive control of food intake) is seen as being a precondition for efficient biological control, stable body weight and maintenance of a set point (Muller et al. 2010). Decades of individualized and population-based applications of health-promotion models for obesity control have had limited success in applying this principle, however.

A further failure of energy balance models, according to Sorensen et al. (2012), concerns the impossibility of separating out cause and effect. As obesity may take years to emerge in any individual, behavioural and metabolic feedback mechanisms between components of energy balance become increasingly entangled. Physiologically, regulation of energy balance involves afferent signals from the body's periphery about the state of energy stores, and efferent signals that influence energy intake through appetite, energy expenditure and physiological mechanisms such as diet-induced thermogenesis (Hill et al. 2012). With increasing body fatness in an individual, there is an expansion of adipose tissue and a build-up of metabolically active, energy-demanding lean tissue (visceral organs, skeletal muscles and bones) and a consequent increase in energy expenditure. This by itself leads to increased demand for energy intake to remain in energy balance (Sorensen et al. 2012). Physical activity becomes more difficult as body fatness increases and moves into the clinical zone of obesity, most commonly for mechanical reasons associated with carrying more body weight. Physical activity generally declines with increasing obesity, reducing the dietary energy needed to maintain neutral balance per unit of body size. The components of energy balance can also be influenced physiologically by changes in each other, as a consequence of either positive or negative energy balance. These physiological shifts act to defend body energy stores, maintain energy balance and prevent shifts in body mass. If energy balance were not controlled by such a system, and were responsive only to behavioural mechanisms controlling food intake and volitional energy expenditure, most people would routinely experience wide swings in body weight over short periods of time, which they do not (Hill et al. 2012). The observation that obese people eat more and move less than non-obese people, and that energy balance is under physiological control (Hill et al. 2012) cannot therefore be used to make any inference about obesity causation (Sorensen et al. 2012).

Employing an energy balance rationale in obesity management results in only modest weight loss with exercise (Thomas et al. 2012) and dietary restriction (Wu et al. 2009) interventions, respectively, but only slightly greater weight losses when exercise is combined with dietary restriction (Wu et al. 2009). This has opened to question the usefulness of energy balance models as the basis for weight-loss interventions, because interventions that reduce body fat stores without dealing with physiological compensatory responses that promote the recovery of lost fat are more likely to fail than those that do (Guyenet and Schwartz 2012). Long-term success of obesity interventions based on energy balance models is possible, if such interventions are performed rigorously and include strong cognitive restraint against overeating. Meta-analyses of randomized controlled trials show that all types of intervention can produce weight loss in their first 6 months of operation, of between 2.4 and 8.7 per cent of initial body weight (Figure 3.2) (Franz et al. 2007). This is within the range of usual seasonal weight change experienced by people living in traditional subsistence economies (of between 0.2 and 9.3 per cent) (Ulijaszek and Strickland 1993) and lies within the range of acceptable 6-monthly weight loss for humans. Interventions involving diet only, or diet plus exercise, or pharmaceuticals plus diet, have been shown to produce weight loss that is sustainable beyond a year (Franz et al. 2007), but this requires strong reinforcement not to overeat.

There is a possibility that energy balance models of obesity, when applied to obesity interventions, might actually contribute to increasing obesity in some people. Most people who are able to lose weight and maintain that weight loss for 2 years are generally able to remain at their lower body weight across subsequent years (Wing and Phelan 2005). However, about a third of dieters fail to adapt to lower levels of energy intake, instead gaining weight after dieting as a consequence of a mix of reduced energy expenditure, increased consumption of calories from fat, decreased dietary restraint, and increased hunger, dietary disinhibition and binge eating (McGuire et al. 1999). From an evolutionary perspective, increased post-dieting appetite, raised food consumption and weight gain are adaptations that defend body size and reproductive ability (Ulijaszek and Bryant 2016) (Chapter 6). Younger adults have greater reproductive potential than older ones, and are several

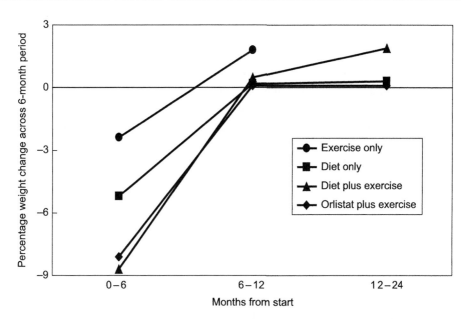

Figure 3.2. Weight-loss outcomes from a systematic review and meta-analysis of weight-loss clinical trials with a minimum 1 year follow-up. Results are shown as percentage change across each period (calculated from data by Franz et al. 2007).

times more likely to binge eat (Hudson et al. 2007). Defence of body weight through increased appetite and binge eating while attempting to lose weight (McGuire et al. 1999) may therefore contribute to continuing increases in obesity (Ogden and Carroll 2010) for evolutionarily rational reasons (Chapter 6).

The past 40 years or so of energy balance research has been driven, in large part, by the promise of novel pharmacological solutions to obesity. Coupled with dietary control, pharmaceuticals have the same potential to induce weight loss as the control of dietary intake while increasing physical activity (Franz et al. 2007). In 2010, there were three drugs approved by the US Food and Drug Administration (FDA) specifically for weight loss, all of which have either significant side effects or poor longer-term efficacy (Tseng et al. 2010). One of these, silbutramine, has since been withdrawn from use in the US and the European Union, while a second, phentermine, has been withdrawn in the UK. The pursuit of new anti-obesity drugs in the US has had the blessing of the FDA since 2012 (Chapter 1). Medical approaches to obesity treatment link the Weberian theoretical rationality of science to the economic and Weberian formal rationalities (Chapter 2) of the pharmaceutical industry.

Genetic and Evolutionary Influences on Obesity

At the aggregate level, energy metabolism varies within and across populations, and genetic predispositions to positive energy balance also vary. Such predispositions have evolved, and this section turns to evolution and the genetics of obesity. Larger body mass and a greater ability to accumulate fat in seasonal ecologies (when the circumstances allow) relative to other non-human primates are two key adaptive features in human ecology (Aiello and Wells 2002). In nature, body fatness is a good thing. Energy stored in adipose tissue buffers against risk of mortality soon after birth and at weaning, when nutrition is often disrupted (Kuzawa 1998). Fatness in human females is linked to fertility (Brown and Konner 1987; Norgan 1994), ovarian function being particularly sensitive to ecological energy balance and energy flux (Ellison 2001). At any BMI, females have a greater proportion of body weight as fat and a greater proportion of fat in the lower body than males. Fat in the lower body is much less readily available for everyday energetic needs than either upper body or abdominal fat, but is mobilized more readily during pregnancy and lactation (Garaulet et al. 2000; Ulijaszek and Lofink 2006), buffering against variation in ecological energetic resource availability (Ellison 2001).

Since energy stores are vital to survivorship and reproduction, the ability to conserve energy as adipose tissue would have conferred selective advantage in the limited ecological energetic circumstances that early *Homo sapiens* would have been periodically exposed to. Seasonality of food availability is likely to have been a major environmental pressure in hominin evolution (Foley 1993), and this continues to be common in the subsistence ecologies of primates (Hladik 1988) and humans (de Garine and Harrison 1988). The tendency to overeat in response to food portion size, palatability and energy density is a general mammalian evolutionary trait that is favoured in seasonal environments and in the ecological energetics of scarcity. The fact that most mammals are able to overeat to high levels of body fatness (Kanarek and Hirsch 1977) suggests that some of the genetic basis for human obesity lies in evolutionary time that is deeper than that of the hominin–chimpanzee divergence of over 7 million years ago (White et al. 2009). Furthermore, the biological drives of feeding, hunger and the dietary regulation of macronutrient intake have shared physiological and behavioural bases with other animals, beyond primates (Ulijaszek 2002a; Berthoud 2004), as does the social facilitation of food intake, where social interaction increases the amounts of food eaten, when it is plentiful (Harlow and Yudin 1933; Tolman 1964; de Castro 1994).

The idea that obesity may have a genetic basis is almost as old as Mendelian genetics itself, although this was initially poorly elaborated. In 1907, Carl von Noorden delineated two types of obesity: exogenous and endogenous (Jou 2014). In this formulation, the exogenous form of obesity, which was seen as being the most common at that time, was the consequence of external factors such as excessive food consumption. Endogenous obesity was seen as being usually caused by physiological disorders such as hypometabolism or other thyroid disorders (Jou 2014), and was taken to be innate or, in present-day terms, genetic. Energy balance models of obesity dominated medical research in obesity for the first half of the twentieth century (Pennington 1953) and into the 1980s (Jou 2014). Modern genetics, post-Watson and Crick (1953), had little influence on obesity research initially, perhaps because obesity was not viewed as a pressing medical problem in the 1950s and 1960s. The shift to modern genetics thinking in obesity science was initiated by the work of James Neel (1915–2000), who put forward the thrifty genotype hypothesis for understanding the emergence of Type 2 diabetes in modernizing populations (Neel 1962). Neel (1962) viewed the (then undiscovered) genes that could predispose to Type 2 diabetes as having been advantageous to individuals and populations prior to modernization, but becoming detrimental thereafter. By the end of the 1970s, significant rates of Type 2 diabetes and obesity had been observed together in populations outside of the Euro-American mainstream, on Samoa and the Cook Islands (McGarvey and Baker 1979; Prior and Tasman-Jones 1981), among non-white South Africans (Walker 1981) and in remote-dwelling Indigenous Australians (Edwards et al. 1976), lending observational support to Neel's (1962) hypothesis.

Genetic research into obesity from the 1980s onwards primarily involved the development of an understanding of the genetics of energy balance, initially using monogenic rodent models of obesity. Linkages between the genetic and physiological study of obesity became possible with the identification of the *ob* gene product, leptin (Zhang et al. 1994), the leptin receptor (Tartaglia et al. 1995) and the agouti gene and agouti-related protein (Zemel et al. 1995; Mizuno et al. 2003). Subsequent modification of the thrifty genotype hypothesis (Neel et al. 1998) formally considered conditions associated with diabetes – including body fatness – to have been adaptive in the remote past but to have become disadvantageous to health in recently changed environments. Type 2 diabetes, obesity and hypertension then came to be described as 'syndromes of impaired genetic homeostasis', 'civilization syndromes' and 'altered lifestyle syndromes' (Neel et al. 1998). Maladaptive traits associated with the modified thrifty genotype hypothesis included the tendency to overeat as well as obesity; the environments in which these maladaptive traits presented were subsequently described as being obesogenic (Swinburn et al. 1999a). Neel et al. (1998) argued that thrifty genotypes were multiple, having undergone selection in different ways in different populations and in response to different kinds of environmental pressure. An alternative to the thrifty genotype idea was developed in the 2000s, the 'drifty genotype', which posited that most mutations in obesity susceptibility genes are neutral, having drifted over evolutionary time (Speakman 2006, 2008, 2013), and had not undergone natural selection, as proposed by Neel (1962) and Neel et al. (1998).

The drifty genotype model of obesity does not contradict the thrifty genotype hypothesis with respect to homeostasis and ecological energy balance, but suggests that there could be many pathways to the genetic regulation of energy balance, and speaks to the large number of genotypes now known to be linked to energy imbalance and obesity (Albuquerque et al. 2015). Since all aspects of metabolism are under genetic control, and the expression of obesity phenotypes is much more limited than the expression of peptides that regulate metabolism, it has been argued that natural selection for the capacity to save and store energy is likely to have taken place for different genes with the same phenotypic result (Lev-Ran 2001). Speakman (2013) also considers the possibility that obesity may never have existed in human evolutionary history except in individuals with unusual genetic modifications, such as those found now in people with monogenic forms of obesity.

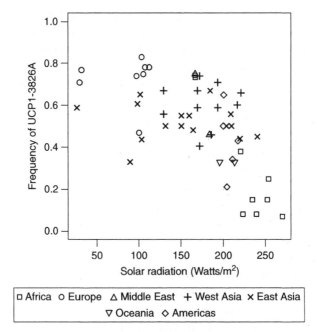

Figure 3.3. Variation in human population frequencies of uncoupling protein 1 (UCP1-3826A) in different geographical regions according to ecology and climate (solar radiation). From Hancock et al. (2011) by permission of Oxford University Press.

Another perspective, which has followed in response to Speakman (2013), is another modification of the thrifty genotype hypothesis in which genes that predispose to obesity are seen as being maladaptive by-products of positive selection on another advantageous trait (Albuquerque et al. 2015). An example of such selection might be for differences in bodily BAT content and composition due to differential exposure to cold, hot and temperature-seasonal environments of ancestral modern humans between 70 000 and 20 000 years ago (Sellayah et al. 2014). According to these authors, genes essential to survival, especially in new-born or young children, such as those that control thermoregulation, would have been of greater importance than thrifty genes because they would have allowed survival to reproductive age. One such gene, essential for body temperature maintenance in cold climates, is *UCP1*, encoding uncoupling protein 1, which is highly expressed in BAT (Sellayah et al. 2014).

Sellayah et al. (2014) also view different susceptibilities to obesity between geographical populations as being due to differential exposures to climatic selection events that began when modern humans migrated out of Africa around 70 000 years ago. This position is supported by an analysis of population genetic variation in the *UCP1* gene (Hancock et al. 2011). Figure 3.3 shows a plot of population frequencies of a single nucleotide polymorphism of UCP1 associated with thermogenesis, UCP1-3826A, against a measure of climate (solar radiation) in populations from different global regions (Hancock et al. 2011). The symbol for each point represents the major geographical region with which each population is associated – Africa, Europe, the Middle East, West Asia, East Asia, Oceania and the Americas. The frequency of UCP1-3826A is highest in European populations, clustering at the latitudes with the least solar radiation, showing them to be most cold adapted. Migration to northern latitudes would have necessitated the selection of genes for cold adaptation, such as those that enhance thermogenesis. Due to their secondary effects on metabolism, adiposity and energy expenditure, they would have become key to the low genetic predisposition to obesity in Western populations now (Sellayah et al. 2014). East Asian populations cluster at similar latitudes to Europeans, but have lower frequencies of UCP1-3826A, suggesting that they are less cold adapted by this mechanism, and perhaps more predisposed to obesity. By the same measure, African populations are the least cold adapted and perhaps the most susceptible to obesity (Sellayah et al. 2014).

Famines are unlikely to have been selective pressures prior to the origins of agriculture (Prentice et al. 2008), although Speakman (2007) views this selective pressure to have been as equally absent after the origins of agriculture as before it. He has suggested that genes predisposing to fat gain would have arisen through random mutations and drift following the removal of predation pressure from around 2 million years ago, with increased ecological control that would have come with the development of more complex social behaviour, weapons and fire. Prentice et al. (2008) argue that natural selection for efficient metabolism took place, but was overwhelmingly due to differential fertility, in contrast to Sellayah et al.'s (2014) view that survivorship and differential mortality would have been more important. Prentice et al. (2008) see differential fertility to have been the dominant selective pressure after the origins of agriculture, drawing from observations of present-day Gambia and Bangladesh, where conceptions during the annual hungry season are greatly reduced. These authors draw on Fisher (1930), who viewed the intensity of selection by differences in fertility to be enormous relative to selective intensities due to mortality, in producing large evolutionary changes in relatively short time frames. Fisher's view came from observations in zoology more broadly, rather than of human populations, where natural selection due to differential fertility does not seem to exceed that of differential mortality.

Various evolutionary demographic studies of traditional societies show both differential fertility and mortality to be important selective pressures, however. Using Crow's index (I_t) of the opportunity for natural selection due to mortality (I_m) prior to reproductive age, and to differences in fertility (I_f) among women who have reached reproductive age (Crow 1958), Kapoor et al. (2003) found fertility selection to be higher than mortality selection in 24 Himalayan rural agricultural populations. Furthermore, in a comparison of 22 caste and seven tribal populations in India, Prakash and Sudhakar (2011) found average fertility selection to be higher than mortality selection for caste populations (I_f = 0.352; I_m = 0.295) and tribal populations (I_f = 0.571; I_m = 0.384). In a comparison of 95 rural populations across India, Kapoor and Kaur (2012) found no overall difference between average fertility selection (I_f = 0.314) and mortality selection (I_m = 0.316). In combination, these studies show that both differential fertility and mortality can exert similar selective pressures on human societies. If this applies to past populations after the origins of agriculture, it weakens Prentice et al.'s (2008) proposed modification of the thrifty genotype hypothesis (that survival advantages were less important than fertility advantages in promoting the spread of thrifty genes), but has no influence on Speakman's (2007) position. But however they are attained, some genotypes are clearly more susceptible to obesity than others, there being high heritabilities for weight and BMI (Carmichael and McGue 1995) as well as for appetite (de Castro 1999) and eating behaviour (Llewellyn et al. 2008).

The Hereditary Basis for Obesity

Predispositions to obesity are both genetic and evolved, epigenetic and developmental (Chapter 7). Gene-based investigations have shown that the vast majority of obesity is related to more than one gene locus, each accounting for only a part of the phenotypic variance (Comuzzie 2002; Albuquerque et al. 2015), although there is one common gene variant that is more closely associated with population obesity than any other. People who are homozygous for a particular allele of the *FTO* gene are 1.67 times more likely to be obese than those not carrying this allele (Frayling et al. 2007); of nearly 39000 study participants, 16 per cent carried this obesity risk allele. There are interactions between different obesity susceptibility genes, as well as gene dosage effects, such that people who are heterozygotes for such genes are likely to be less obese than people who are homozygotes (Farooqi et al. 2001; Chung and Leibel 2005). The search for obesity-related genes using genome-wide association studies (GWAS) has led to the identification of more than 20 obesity-related loci, as determined by their statistical association with the anthropometric body size phenotypes of BMI, body weight, waist circumference and/or waist:hip ratio (Lindgren et al. 2009). More recently, GWAS have identified 39 loci associated with BMI alone (Albuquerque et al. 2015). The functions of obesity-related genes remain poorly understood, however, there being no current consensus concerning the genetic basis of obesity (Walley et al. 2009).

The 20 loci identified by 2009 together explain less than 2 per cent of inter-individual variation in BMI (Lindgren et al. 2009), while in 2015 the proportion of variance in BMI that could be explained by known obesity polymorphisms was between 1 and 4 per cent (Albuquerque et al. 2015). It has been suggested that some of the 'missing' genetic contribution to obesity phenotype variation might be due to the existence of large numbers of low-penetrance common polymorphisms that are associated with BMI; the best effort in finding such 'missing' genetic contributions comes from Yang et al. (2011). These authors included, in analysis, the additive effects of over 500000 autosomal single nucleotide polymorphisms genotyped on 11586 unrelated individuals, which collectively explained 17 per cent of population variance in BMI. This falls far short of the expected variation – the heritability of one obesity phenotype, the BMI, lies between 47 and 90 per cent (Allison et al. 1996; Elks et al. 2012), and a genetic model of obesity should be able to explain such levels of variance. In acknowledgement of this significant gap, obesity geneticists have called for an intensification of the search for genes. For example, Walley et al. (2009) have made a case for developing new models of obesity genetics, saying that the GWAS study design is inadequate for elucidating the genetic architecture of common obesity. They do not suggest what such new models of obesity genetics might look like, however.

Epigenetic regulation of gene expression may modulate obesity risk, and this may explain some of the gap between obesity phenotype heritability and the proportion of obesity phenotype variation currently explicable by molecular genetics. While there are very many genes, of varying penetrance, associated with population obesity, there are also many epigenetic processes mediating their function (Kim et al. 2009). In addition, failures in genomic imprinting that may predispose to obesity by altering expression of growth and cellular differentiation factors can arise from numerous independent genetic events – translocation, inversion, duplication and paternal disomy (Herrera et al. 2011). Childhood developmental processes are responsive to nutrition early in life, as well as to maternal and grandmaternal nutrition, all of which may have consequences for epigenetic regulation (Murgatroyd and Spengler 2011) and predispositions to obesity.

Genetic susceptibilities and epigenetic predispositions have lain dormant in human populations until the emergence of ecologies that predispose to obesity in the past 30 years or so. In HICs, such ecologies make cheap energy-dense food easily available, and frustrate bodily movement with the widespread material presence of the convenience devices of modern society – chairs, cars, computers and mobile phones among them. Genetics and energy balance models of obesity are therefore incomplete without locating them in the context of environmental triggers, past and present, for the onset and continued production of obesity. Ecology and environment are essential for the expression of obesity susceptibility genes, and an understanding of obesogenic environments is a central part of understanding relationships between evolution and genetics in the production of present-day obesity.

Obesogenic Environments

The idea of environmental backgrounds that predispose to obesity (although extremely variant across populations) is encapsulated in the obesogenic environments model of obesity. The model is easily intuited; it includes all aspects of environments, physical and social, that promote gaining weight, and which are not conducive to weight loss (Swinburn et al. 1999a). Obesogenic environments are easily identified by a great preponderance of motorized transport and of sedentary occupations, and the cheap and easy availability of high-fat, high-refined-carbohydrate foods (Booth et al. 2001). They are present in the urban landscapes of most HICs, and it may be that major institutional and structural forces involved in urban planning and regulation in HICs are also involved in obesity production. In general, what makes life convenient and energy efficient at the individual level also promotes obesity (Ulijaszek 2007b). However, establishing causal relationships between environmental factors and obesity is immensely challenging, largely because it is difficult to measure proximate factors that may contribute to obesity, such as population diet and physical activity in everyday life. Neighbourhood factors and local food environments have been related to obesity rates, however (Cummins and Macintyre 2006). It is also difficult to measure social norms as they relate to diet and physical activity (Elinder and Jansson 2009). Furthermore, while many people in HICs live in environments that can be characterized as being obesogenic, not everyone living in such contexts becomes obese. This may be in part due to variation in genetic predisposition and epigenetic susceptibility, but it is also due to variation in environmental exposure and human behaviour.

Obesogenic environments have not always been with us. They have been created, largely unwittingly, in late modern society (Chapter 1). They have come with the marginalization of physically active transportation and with the privileging of the motor car, which has resulted, in many places, in road and highway infrastructure that disadvantages active transport. In Perth, Australia, for example, the older city was restructured using a modernist metropolitan plan based on low-density subur-ban housing, car transport and a freeway system (Stephenson and Hepburn 1955). The city was thus structured around separated land use, with work in one place, and shopping, recreation and sleeping in other locations (Matan and Newman 2016). Signs throughout the city centre at that time stated boldly that 'your car's as welcome as you are' (Matan and Newman 2016). The creation of obesogenic environments has also been helped by the displacement of small local shops that can be walked to, and the simultaneous construction of large supermarkets that require a car for access and which encourage food shopping in bulk. Obesogenic environments have developed with ever-increasing commuting times, and the speeding up of everyday life such that cooking (and eating together) become difficult, even for those heavily committed to the idea. Obesogenic environments can be found across the urban landscape of most HICs, but it is in Australia where the idea was given intellectual form. The concept of the obesogenic environment, and the analytical framework with which it was described, was developed by public health researchers there in the late 1990s in response to an identified need for methods that would allow the environment – which was increasingly being acknowledged as a contributor to population-level obesity – to be rigorously and systematically studied (Ulijaszek et al. 2016b). The Analysis Grid for Environments Linked to Obesity (ANGELO) framework was proposed by Swinburn et al. (1999a) as a tool for systematically describing and analysing obesogenic envir-onments. As a model of obesity, it moved thinking about the environmental contri-bution to obesity in vague terms to the identification of individual factors and features of the environment that could be studied, measured and potentially modified. The obesogenic environments model offers a means of representation through the ANGELO framework, and a high degree of generality, although its use for hypothesis generation is limited (Chapter 2). Early application of the ANGELO framework high-lighted the complexity of factors in the environment that contribute to obesity and health more broadly, as well as the powerlessness of individuals to address many of these factors (Ulijaszek et al. 2016b).

Within Australia, the archetypal obesogenic environment was in the city of Geelong, Victoria, between the 1990s and 2000s; the proposers of this construct (Swinburn et al. 1999a) worked at Deakin University, which has its main campus in Geelong.

In Geelong, as elsewhere in urban HIC settings, obesogenic environments include physical structures, processes and ways of living that developed with the growth of the city. Motor car manufacture underpinned the Geelong economy from the 1920s, and servicemen returning after World War II soon naturalized driving. They had training in, and experience of, motor vehicle use, and rapid expansion of the motor industry after 1945 met the growing demand for cars. With the car came petrol stations and supermarkets, and by the 1960s the sense was that to be modern, convenience should be sought at every opportunity. By the 1980s, shopping malls and strip-land fast-food outlets expanded and extended in Geelong, displacing small shops in the city centre, and changing patterns of food provisioning. Convenience became a marketable commodity in its own right: convenience stores, convenience foods, convenient transport. More generally, the cost of convenience has been the rise of obesity (Ulijaszek 2007b), and Geelong grew to have among the highest rates of obesity in Australia (Pasco et al. 2012). To its credit, the Greater Geelong City Council has since strived to make its city less obesogenic, and the Victorian Population Health Survey of 2014 shows a small decline in adult obesity rates there recently (Healthy Together Geelong 2016), after increases between 2008 and 2011/ 12 (Healthy Together Geelong 2014). And to Perth's credit, in 1993 it was the first city outside Scandinavia to conduct a major 'Public Spaces Public Life' survey by which to improve the walkability of the city (Matan and Newman 2016), a study that was repeated in 2009 (Government of Western Australia Department for Planning and Infrastructure 2009).

It is easy to outline, superficially, the causes of population obesity in Geelong between the 1990s and 2000s, and in towns and cities like it: economic change, economic insecurity, suburbanization, declining traditional industries, the comfort eating that assuages individual insecurity (Chapter 5), the ready availability of cheap, convenient, high-energy-density foods (Chapter 6) and the motorized transport with which to get it. This has happened against a backdrop of almost universal sedentary leisure across Australia, and rising economic inequality (Commonwealth of Australia 2013) that has helped structure the urban environment, such that the lowest in status in Geelong have become the most obese (Brennan et al. 2010) and the most exposed to obesogenic environments, as across the rest of Australia (King et al. 2006) and most other HICs (Chapter 5). Public health responses to widespread obesity in Australia have included a wide range of initiatives promoting good nutrition, activity and maintenance of healthy weight during early childhood and in early childhood settings (Nichols et al. 2011), focusing largely on individual, familial and community resilience against obesogenic environments. However, they usually do not consider structural reasons for obesity, including the creation of obesogenic environments in the first place.

This case study is not exceptional to many others like it in most HICs, and emphasizes the need to study local histories in more global contexts, to understand how the conditions for obesity production come into place. The idea of obesogenic environments as 'triggers for genetic susceptibilities to obesity through energy imbalance' is easy to grasp, and this may be a reason why it is popular among researchers, policy makers, practitioners and other people. Policy approaches to control or regulate aspects of such environments are plentiful (Rabin et al. 2007; Sacks et al. 2008; Story et al. 2008; Dietz et al. 2009; Swinburn et al. 2011; Allender et al. 2012), but they are difficult to coordinate (Mohebati et al. 2007; Shill et al. 2012). Many expert systems (Chapter 1) are involved in building and maintaining urban environments, and the possible obesogenicity of such environments is unplanned for. Expert systems, operating together interactively, create the technological complexity of modern life. This is to a large extent black-boxed, however, and not easily available for governmental regulation, if their operations predispose to obesity. The rationalities that underpin expert systems (Chapter 1) are not immediately apparent, but inevitably involve the intersection and coexistence of sometimes widely differing interests within the same domain. Obesity is one outcome of the interaction of such systems: unwanted, unplanned and unregulated.

Multiple rationalities (Chapter 2) are represented in the production and enactment of obesogenic environments: Weberian formal rationality in bureaucratic management by governments, economic rationality of corporations, and Weberian practical and substantive rationalities of the people that live in them. In policy terms, ameliorating obesogenic environments is difficult, because any major structural change is expensive, can involve many stakeholders and risks affecting people's livelihoods in negative ways. As ecologies, interactive expert systems will always adapt and stabilize in response to regulatory forces, but outcomes of adaptations to new regulation are difficult to envision by anybody. Before effecting change to such systems, there needs to be clear evidence that this will clearly reduce obesity rates. Such evidence is usually either lacking or is conditioned by a range of other factors. With respect to one expert system, the food system (Chapter 6), structural change usually focuses on reformulation of foods and their distribution, and providing information to inform individual choice. Change rarely goes any further, however. People need to eat, and the existing food system is very efficient in delivering food (albeit often of high-energy density and low nutrient content) to those who can afford it. Furthermore, the food industry carries significant economic power and employs great numbers of people; these factors alone make it fairly immune to governmental intervention. The food system is one of several expert systems (Chapter 1) that structure the everyday lives of people. Such systems are minimally touched by regulators, for fear that any tweaking will disturb the networks of relationships between them, potentially making life worse for everyone.

People live in environments that are constructed through social, political and economic processes, both historically and into the present day. What has become obesogenic is often a matter of chance: no individual, agency, corporation or institution planned for obesity. But governments show the seriousness with which they take obesity through population measurement, classification and reporting. This ensures that concerns about obesity (as a measureable outcome) are incorporated into the regulation of systems that are considered to produce it. The next chapter turns to the nation state-based metrics of obesity regulation: anthropometrics and econometrics.

4 Governance through Measurement

The measurement and classification of obesity is fundamental to its regulation, and the disciplines of economics and epidemiology broadly map the obesity landscape to be regulated. Epidemiological data collection and reporting, and the use of obesity epidemiology in econometric modelling of the impacts of obesity, are usually starting points for state-led obesity interventions (Malik et al. 2013). The spur to policy action by most nation states continues to be overwhelmingly economic (Chapter 8), although this has been overlayered by considerations of complexity in some places (Chapter 9). The most persuasive political arguments usually involve framing obesity as a significant burden to the economy and health service, usually through costs to employers, of its medical management and of the chronic diseases associated with it (Wang et al. 2011). Relationships between obesity (and factors presumed to cause it) and economics have been variously demonstrated. Economists have modelled the costs to nations of rising rates of obesity (Wang et al. 2011) and the likely outcomes of economic interventions on these rates (Grossman and Mocan 2011), including the taxation of particular foods and food types (Thow et al. 2010; Novak and Brownell 2011; Jou and Techakehakij 2012; Basu et al. 2014) (Chapter 6). Econometric modelling has also shown technological changes that have lowered the cost of food calories and made work more sedentary to be associated with higher obesity rates (Lakdawalla and Philipson 2002). Furthermore, changes in the price of food have been shown to have small but important effects on body weight and obesity rates (Gelbach et al. 2009; Goldman et al. 2011) (Chapter 5). While the price of food has declined overall since the 1960s (Chapter 6), that of less healthy, more energy-dense food has been shown to have fallen more sharply than that of healthier food, at least in the United States (US) and the United Kingdom (UK) (Mazzocchi et al. 2009). Rising incomes have been shown to have increased the demand for food in economically emerging nations, also leading to higher obesity rates (Popkin 2001). Economists have also shown that in high-income countries (HICs), time has become increasingly scarce (Jabs and Devine 2006), with more people eating highly energy-dense ready-prepared foods, and meals outside the home, both of which are known to lead to increased energy intake (Cutler et al. 2003) and to predispose to obesity. Obesity rates across nations have also been modelled in relation to welfare provision and regime, with Nordic welfare states having lower obesity rates than market-liberal, predominantly English-speaking nations (Lakdawalla et al. 2005; Offer et al. 2010) (Chapter 5).

Both epidemiology and economics employ standardized and institutionalized methods for quantifying matters of importance for governmental regulation. Such

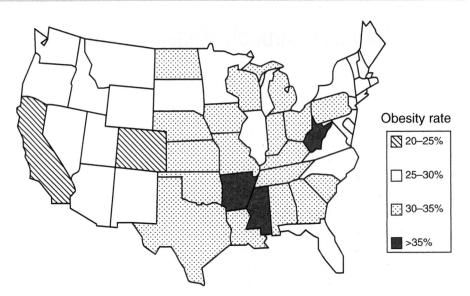

Figure 4.1. Prevalence of self-reported obesity among adults in the US by state, 2014 (adapted from Centers for Disease Control 2016).

measures include population size and distribution, income, birth and death rates, and life expectancy at birth, as well as disease rates and risk factors for chronic disease. In most countries, obesity is reported in terms of the proportion of adults with a body mass index (BMI) greater than 30 kg/m^2 (World Health Organization 2000) (Chapter 1). This cut-off has been repeatedly validated against specific causes of death and total mortality rates (Prospective Studies Collaboration 2009; Flegal et al. 2013). The measurement of obesity rates and its reporting provides evidence for the existence of population obesity and its changing patterns across time, and for identifying possible governmental interventions against it. Speaking to the importance of data collection for childhood obesity policy in Australia, Nathan et al. (2005) have asserted that policy can be made in the absence of strong research evidence, but where powerful and competing groups contest possible policy options, the evidence required needs to be substantial. The most basic form of evidence for obesity policy is nationally representative data on obesity rates across administrative units and across time. Illustrations of this include obesity prevalence maps for the US (Figure 4.1) and England (Figure 4.2), where obesity rates are shown according to within-nation state and local authority, respectively. Year-on-year measurement can be used to construct maps of changing rates of obesity, as has been done by the Centers for Disease Control and Prevention (2016) in the US, for example.

The economic cost of obesity within and across nations varies according to a number of factors including the balance of obesity rates, demographic structure, patterns of employment (including female participation in the workforce), the health burden related to obesity, the extent of privatized medicine, and the market for, and desirability of, non-medical treatments. The political importance of obesity regulation by nation states varies according to the proportion and distribution of the

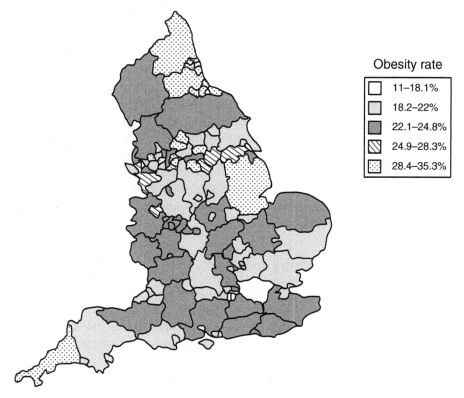

Figure 4.2. Obesity rates in adults, England, 2012 (adapted from Public Health England 2016).

population that is obese, its cost to the economy and ideology. Obesity, in a neoliberal framework, offers significant economic opportunities as well as costs. Medical service provision and the administration of pharmaceutical interventions and surgical procedures are all business opportunities, as are the provision of weight management services and products. In the US, direct obesity costs were US$147 billion in 2008 (Finkelstein et al. 2009), around 1 per cent of gross domestic product (GDP) in that year. In comparison, obesity treatment in the UK in 2007 formed 0.3 per cent of GDP. In the US, 29 per cent of the direct cost of obesity in 2008 was borne by private health care (Finkelstein et al. 2009), making the direct cost of obesity to the state around 0.7 per cent of GDP. This was offset by the US$33 billion per year that citizens of the US spend on weight-loss products (Rashad and Grossman 2004), in addition to the US$43 billion of spending on obesity treatment through private health care. Removing these two off-sets from the direct costs of obesity to the state would make the balance to the US economy a positive one, to the extent of 0.5 per cent of GDP, if there were no indirect costs to the economy such as time taken off work. Such costs move profit into overall marginal loss to the US economy. In the UK, increasing health-care privatization would reduce some of the direct medical costs of obesity to the state (£4.2 billion in 2007; Butland et al. 2007), but the economic opportunity associated with obesity is much lower than in the US. Far less is spent on commercial weight-loss products and services than in the US, although this has increased (Lowe et al. 2001).

All types of economic analysis rely on the best possible representative data on obesity rates at the level of analysis needed (international, national, regional or local), with the possibility of disaggregating those rates into groups (such as gender, age and inequality) that are meaningful for economic understanding and/ or for political action. This chapter examines how and why such numbers are used in support of obesity governance and political regulation. The method of population obesity assessment, anthropometry, is age-old, and this chapter starts by placing the anthropometric measurement and reporting of obesity rates into historical context. It continues with a description of how anthropometric measures of obesity are used in econometric modelling of population obesity.

Political Anthropometry and Obesity

Anthropometry, or the physical measurement of people, has been long used to describe variation in human populations (Tanner 1981), its relative cheapness and simplicity of application being the main motivators for its use relative to other methods. Anthropometric methods have changed little since the nineteenth century, but the meaning and interpretation of anthropometric variation has changed, with new understandings of how human bodily variation is produced and maintained. Between the seventeenth and nineteenth centuries, measures of stature were used as a proxy for health, physical strength and/or economic value of slaves to be taken to the plantations of the US (Engerman 1976) and the Caribbean (Friedman 1982), and of recruits to the armies of Europe and North America (Tanner 1981). Anthropometry was also used in a more limited way to investigate human welfare of both adults and children from the nineteenth century onwards (Tanner 1981), such use accelerating in the second half of the twentieth century, when it became embedded in epidemiological practice, most usually as a proxy for health and nutritional status (Jelliffe 1966).

Anthropometric practice became increasingly an instrument of social welfare when it became known that many environmental factors that influence poor child growth and small body size are conditioned by poverty and low socioeconomic status (SES) (Ulijaszek 2006, 2010), making physique a sensitive marker of the biological quality of life (Tanner 1987). In most countries, there are similar associations between stature and SES, height correlating positively with wealth (Komlos and Lauderdale 2007). While per capita gross national product became accepted as the most widely used measure of the standard of living and of social welfare in the 1930s, global concerns about economic development in relation to human capital from the 1950s onwards encouraged the use of more direct measures of social welfare in econometric modelling. This acknowledged the fact that a wide range of economic outcomes are affected by health (Culyer and Newhouse 2000) and body size (Sunder and Woitek 2005). By the 1970s, anthropometric and nutritional variables were used in econometric modelling of social welfare, alongside existing forms of social accounting, such as national product, population size and distribution, and market prices (Steckel 1998). In 1980, the World Bank initiated the Living Standards Measurement Study, which used the collection of individual, household and community data, including anthropometry, for the assessment of living standards in developing countries (United Nations Statistical Office 1980).

With respect to obesity, body size metrics could only be used in econometric analyses once there was a globally accepted measure of obesity, and a standardized way of reporting it (Chapter 1). This is much as with other variables and indices used in econometric analyses, such as duration and rate of unemployment, the consumer price index, consumer credit, personal income, industrial production, manufacturing and trade sale. For economists, obesity rates, as measured using BMI, are analytically tractable in similar ways to indices expressed in terms of US dollars. The share of countries linking their currency to the dollar in some manner has been stable since 1995, and this group (which includes the US) represents about half of the world's GDP. At around the same time, 1997, just over half of the world's nations agreed to report their obesity rates using BMI to the World Health Organization's (WHO) Global Database on Body Mass Index (World Health Organization 2015a). Various analyses of relations between obesity and economics soon followed (Wolf and Colditz 1998; Allison et al. 1999; Wang and Dietz 2002; Vandegrift and Yoked 2004), with epidemiological data and reporting being used to frame obesity as a global public health and economic problem. While this privileged the use of BMI in obesity reporting, this measure is far from perfect.

Measuring Obesity

BMI has been adopted for epidemiological and public health use because it reflects body energy stores (Norgan 1994) in ecological context, and at the upper end of population distribution shows strong associations with morbidity and mortality from a number of chronic diseases and disorders. Other anthropometric measures such as waist circumference, waist:hip ratio and waist:height ratio compete well with it, however (Visscher et al. 2001; Janssen et al. 2004; Bosy-Westphal et al. 2006; Koziel et al. 2007; Vazquez et al. 2007; Browning et al. 2010; Huxley et al. 2010; Schneider et al. 2010; Liu et al. 2011; World Health Organization 2011). BMI persists as the standard measure of obesity for both pragmatic and historical reasons. It has been used for far longer than any other anthropometric measure, and was the first to be appropriated for the assessment of obesity rates in populations, after measures of stature and weight had been formalized for predicting mortality. There is no alternative measure of obesity that is collected nearly as systematically as BMI, and to change the standard measure of global obesity surveillance would throw the international governance of obesity into disarray at a time when adult obesity rates continue to rise (Stevens et al. 2012).

Classification of childhood obesity using BMI is more problematic than for adults, because of the variability in the growth rates of children both within and between populations. In childhood and adolescence, the non-obese range of BMI changes with changing body proportions with age, making fixed obesity cut-offs inappropriate. Age-specific cut-offs for childhood overweight and obesity that pass through adult classification cut-offs for overweight and obesity were put forward for international use, to allow enumeration of overweight and obesity in childhood and adolescence using normative distributions that vary by age and sex (Cole et al. 2000). While in adults it is possible to establish directly the increased health risks associated with increased BMI, most health effects of childhood obesity (with the exception of risk markers for Type 2 diabetes) only become manifest in adult life and not in childhood (McCarthy et al. 2003).

While relationships between body size and physical condition were adequately known for them to be used in military conscription from the seventeenth century (Tanner 1981) and in the slave trade from the nineteenth century (Steckel 1995), they were only incorporated into life insurance estimation of mortality prediction in the early twentieth century (Tanner 1981). The publication of 'standard height:weight' tables by the life insurance industry began with the *Medico-Actuarial Mortality Investigations of 1912* (Association of Life Insurance Medical Directors 1912; Keys et al. 1972). These tables provided 'ideal' weight for ranges of height for use among insured adults in the US and Canada, according to sex and three categories of body frame. The first version of these standard weight:height tables, based on actuarial data relating to blood pressure, as a proxy for chronic disease risk, was brought into general use for assessing ideal body weight in 1942/43 by the Metropolitan Life Insurance Company in the US (Weigly 1984) (Table 4.1).

Table 4.1. Metropolitan Life Insurance Company table of ideal weight by height for women aged 25 years and over (Weigly 1984), and calculated body mass index (BMI) equivalents of body frame size boundaries

Height (feet and inches)	Weight (lb) by frame size			BMI equivalent (kg/m^2) by frame size		
	Small	Medium	Large	Small	Medium	Large
5'0"	105–113	112–120	119–129	20.57–22.14	21.94–23.51	23.32–25.27
5'1"	107–115	114–122	121–131	20.26–21.78	21.59–23.10	22.91–24.81
5'2"	110–118	117–125	124–135	20.16–21.62	21.44–22.91	22.72–24.74
5'3"	113–121	120–128	127–138	20.07–21.49	21.31–22.73	22.55–24.51
5'4"	116–125	124–132	131–142	20.13–21.70	21.52–22.91	22.74–24.65
5'5"	119–128	127–135	133–145	19.81–21.3	21.14–22.48	22.14–24.14
5'6"	123–132	130–140	138–150	19.97–21.43	21.10–22.73	22.40–24.35
5'7"	126–136	134–144	142–152	19.75–21.32	21.00–22.57	22.26–23.82
5'8"	129–139	137–147	145–158	19.68–21.20	21.90–22.42	23.49–24.10
5'9"	133–143	141–151	149–162	19.69–21.17	20.88–22.36	22.06–23.99
5'10"	136–147	145–155	152–166	19.56–21.14	20.86–22.30	21.86–23.88
5'11"	139–150	148–158	155–168	19.44–20.98	20.70–22.10	21.68–23.50
6'0"	141–153	151–163	160–179	19.13–20.76	20.49–22.12	21.71–24.29

The call for a more universal measure of ideal body size than the Metropolitan Life Insurance Company tables, for use in epidemiological and medical study, came in the 1950s with the first epidemiological description of blood pressure relative to body fatness as determined by different weight:height ratios in a Norwegian population (Boe et al. 1957). Body weight is to some extent related to stature: taller people are generally heavier. This relationship is non-linear, and even direct correction for height does not remove this relationality completely. The height dependency of weight- and stature-based measures of obesity was of concern for Boe et al. (1957), because, if significant, it made it difficult to create a simple universal measure of nutritional status. After examining the height dependency of a number of weight: height indices and ratios, these authors concluded that weight over height squared (W/H^2) gave the best height-independent measure of relative weight. Subsequent studies in British (Billewicz et al. 1962; Khosla and Lowe 1967), Cook Islander (Grimley Evans and Prior 1969) and US (Florey 1970) populations confirmed this view. In an analysis of the relative height independence of body fat prediction using different weight:height ratios (Figures 4.3 and 4.4), Keys et al. (1972) found generally much lower correlations of height with W/H^2 than with either weight over height (W/H) or weight over height cubed (W/H^3). Body fatness, as represented by the sum of triceps and subscapular skinfold thicknesses, was in general equally correlated with W/H and with W/H^2 but much less so with W/H^3. Keys et al. (1972) concluded that, in

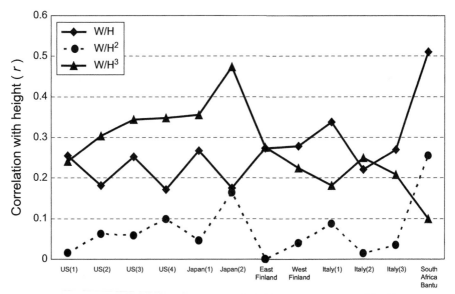

US(1): Minnesota, students; US(2): Minnesota, executives; US(3): sedentary railroad employees; US(4): railroad employees, switchmen; Japan(1): farmers; Japan(2): fishermen; Italy(1): Crevalcore; Italy(2): Montegiorgio; Italy(3): Rome State Railway

Figure 4.3. The observations that led to the proposal that weight over height squared be the standard measure of relative weight across populations (Keys et al. 1972). Correlation coefficients of height among men with weight over height, weight over height squared and weight over height cubed (data from Keys et al. 1972).

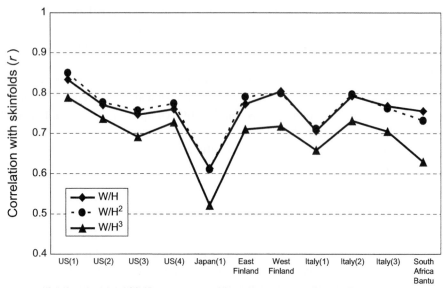

US(1): Minnesota, students; US(2): Minnesota, executives; US(3): sedentary railroad employees; US(4): railroad employees, switchmen; Japan(1): farmers; Italy(1): Crevalcore; Italy(2): Montegiorgio; Italy(3): Rome State Railway

Figure 4.4. The observations that led to the proposal that weight over height squared be the standard measure of relative weight across populations (Keys et al. 1972). Correlation coefficients, in men, of the sum of two skinfold thicknesses at the triceps and subscapular regions of the body, with weight over height, weight over height squared and weight over height cubed (data from Keys et al. 1972).

confirmation of other studies, the ratio W/H^2 was clearly better than other measures of relative weight, and that this ratio should be named the body mass index or BMI.

The cut-offs for ideal weight used in the Metropolitan Life Insurance Company tables are similar to those that were subsequently recommended for the assessment of obesity using BMI by the Royal College of Physicians (1983) in the UK. Figure 4.5 illustrates this for adult women, from calculated BMI equivalents of the upper and lower boundaries of ideal weight for height. The adoption of the closest whole-number BMI equivalent value to the very lowest and very highest boundaries for healthy weight in the Metropolitan Life Insurance Company tables by the Royal College of Physicians (1983) permitted ideal healthy weight to be determined without having to consider or measure frame size (an undefined construct), simplifying the process of obesity assessment (Garrow 1985; James 2004). However, BMI is far from being completely independent of stature. The range of ideal weight according to the Metropolitan Life Insurance Company tables maps better onto the normal range of BMI (20–25 kg/m^2) for shorter individuals than for taller ones (Table 4.1 and Figure 4.5). The standard BMI cut-off for overweight is therefore likely to give underestimates in taller individuals and populations relative to shorter ones, and the same is likely to be true for obesity. Despite this caveat, the BMI cut-offs of 18.5, 17.0 and 16.0 kg/m^2 were accepted for the assessment of chronic energy deficiency in

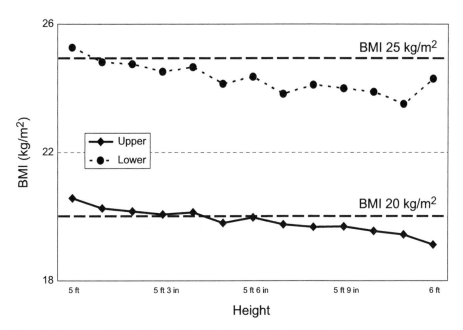

Figure 4.5. Upper and lower limits of ideal body mass index (BMI) for adult women according to height, from calculated BMI equivalents of boundaries of Metropolitan Life Insurance Company table values of ideal weight by height for women aged 25 years and over (calculated from data given by Weigly 1984).

1992 (Shetty and James 1994), while BMI cut-offs of 25 and 30 kg/m^2 were accepted for classifying overweight and obesity, respectively, by the WHO in 1997 (Chapter 1).

Following the acceptance of BMI as the least imperfect measure of relative weight came the standardization of risk of mortality (Calle et al. 1999; McGee 2005; Flegal et al. 2007) and morbidity (Campbell and Ulijaszek 1994; Kennedy and Garcia 1994; Strickland and Ulijaszek 1994; Visscher and Seidell 2001; Canoy et al. 2007) at the lower and higher extremes of BMI. Studies linking BMI to economic productivity (Wolf and Colditz 1998) were also initiated, once BMI was formally accepted by the WHO as the standard measure of both adult undernutrition and obesity (James 2004). In the formalization of BMI for international use for the measurement of obesity (World Health Organization 2000), the overarching aim was to provide simplicity for assessment and monitoring of obesity worldwide. The extent of under-reporting of obesity rates among taller populations was considered of less importance than the possibility of using a standard measure of obesity across the world. Standardized classification of obesity was accepted by the World Health Organization (2000) because it claimed that it allowed meaningful comparisons within and between populations, the identification of individuals and groups at increased risk of morbidity and mortality, the identification of priorities for intervention at individual and community levels, and a firm basis for evaluating interventions. All of these claims can be challenged to some extent.

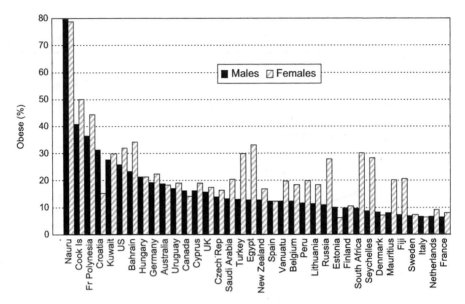

Figure 4.6. Obesity rates by nation in the 1990s and early 2000s (body mass index greater than 30 kg/m^2) for males and females (adapted from Ulijaszek and Lofink 2006).

Initially, the international reporting of obesity using BMI cut-offs of 30 kg/m^2 led to some unexpected observations. For example, Figure 4.6 shows obesity rates of adults across nation states in the 1990s and early 2000s (Ulijaszek and Lofink 2006). Obesity rates in the US were shown to be higher than in European nations, as expected. The extraordinarily high obesity rates shown for some Pacific Island nations (Nauru and the Cook Islands) were also well known. But what also became apparent was that nations such as Kuwait and Saudi Arabia had rates of obesity comparable to those of the US, as did South Africa, Turkey and Uruguay. Such international comparisons allowed obesity to be thought about in more comparable ways, creating the possibility of cross-national approaches to obesity regulation. It also allowed discussions that invoked national particularism in relation to obesity – why should obesity rates be high in the US and low in France (Laurier et al. 1992), for example? National particularism was used to set up obesity in the US as a matter of class, politics, culture, economics (Critser 2003) and morality (Saguy 2006). In contrast, obesity in France was framed as involving both aesthetic and medical issues (Saguy 2006). Another particularism was invoked in the construction of Pacific Islander obesity as an outcome of thrifty genotypes (Joffe and Zimmet 1998). Yet another was the characterization of the people of Nauru as being 'lazy', in partial explanation of the high Type 2 diabetes rates there (Diamond 2003), a quality not evident to anthropologists having worked there (Pollock 1995; McLennan and Ulijaszek 2015). Such particularisms risk making chronic disease epidemiology complicit in stigmatizing the very people they are trying to support (McLennan and Ulijaszek 2015).

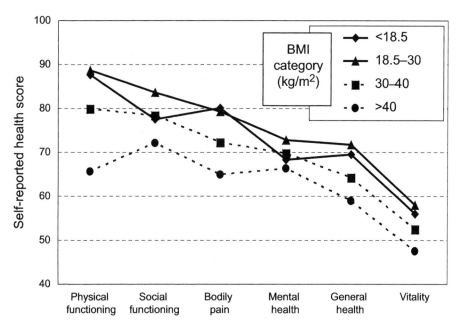

Figure 4.7. Distribution of self-reported health scores by body mass index (BMI) category, after adjusting for age, gender and frequency of health service utilization, in the UK (calculated from Doll et al. 2000).

While BMI cut-offs for obesity classification are viewed as being meaningful according to epidemiological analyses (World Health Organization Expert Consultation 2004), they can differ from individual perceptions of health and well-being. For example, self-reported health status of adults in the UK is lower among obese people than among people categorized as being of normal weight (Figure 4.7), with respect to physical function, bodily pain, general health and vitality, but much less so with respect to social functioning and mental health (Doll et al. 2000). When perceived health and well-being in this sample of UK adults is disaggregated according to chronic disease status, a different pattern emerges (Figure 4.8). All aspects of health and well-being are similar for healthy obese and non-obese subjects, but experience of chronic disease reduces all measures of perceived health and well-being, including social functioning and mental health, to a greater extent among obese subjects than among non-obese ones. Thus, obesity may not be perceived as a problem among those carrying excess body fatness prior to experiencing any of the chronic diseases associated with it (this may be a factor in the obesity scepticism expressed by some healthy obese people).

While the BMI has been universally adopted for obesity assessment, it does not have the best fit for all the purposes to which it has been assigned: individual classification, screening and monitoring for medical purposes, population monitoring for public health purposes, and econometric modelling. As the relationships

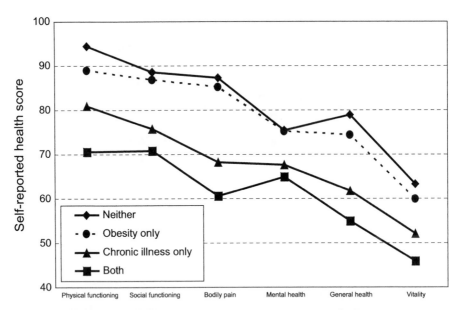

Figure 4.8. Distribution of self-reported health scores (the higher the healthier) according to obesity (defined by body mass index) and chronic illness, after adjusting for age, gender and frequency of health service utilization, in the UK (calculated from Doll et al. 2000).

between BMI, fatness and morbidity vary across populations (World Health Organization Expert Consultation 2004), there remain problems of how best to classify obesity using BMI. Relationships with morbidity and mortality vary according to the measure of obesity used, the population under investigation (e.g. European, Asian or African ancestry, whether it is young or old, male or female), and among the various classificatory boundaries that are used in obesity research and practice (World Health Organization 2000; Zhou 2002; Reis et al. 2009). In some Chinese (Li et al. 2002) and Asian (World Health Organization Expert Consultation 2004) populations, there is increased chronic disease risk at lower levels of BMI than among European populations (Li et al. 2002), and this has prompted the recommendation for lower cut-offs for overweight and obesity for people of Asian origin (World Health Organization Expert Consultation 2004). At the other extreme, Pacific Islander populations generally have lower body fatness relative to lean body mass at any level of BMI, prompting the suggestion that higher BMI cut-offs should be used to assess overweight and obesity in these populations (Swinburn et al. 1999b).

Epidemiological critiques of BMI include its inconsistent relationship with body fatness (Gallagher et al. 1996; Freedman and Sherry 2009), that it does not distinguish between potentially harmful fat in the liver and viscera (Carroll et al. 2008), and that it does not reflect health risk very well, except at the extremes (Lee et al. 2008). Furthermore, anthropometric measurement of obesity has been critiqued by social scientists for its medical distancing of the individual experience of living with

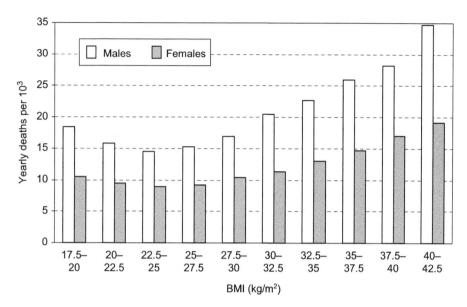

Figure 4.9. All-cause mortality relative to body mass index (BMI) for 894 576 adults in 57 prospective mortality studies in industrialized countries (adapted from Prospective Studies Collaboration 2009).

a fat body (McCullough and Hardin 2013; Yates-Doerr 2013; Forth and Leitch 2014). Bodily measurement in public health practice has also been viewed by social scientists as a way of universalizing the human body by governmental institutions through epidemiological reporting, by relating individuals to norms and health to measurement. Brewis et al. (2011) note the stigma that accompanies the measurement and medicalization of fat bodies (Chapter 5).

Public health and epidemiology argue from the positions of Weberian practical and formal rationalities (Chapter 2) that bodily fatness has a physical reality with economic, social and medical consequences (Chapter 10). The dominant case for obesity as an issue of health and economic consequence comes from epidemiological studies that relate obesity to mortality. There are many of these, to the point that meta-analyses of such work are common. Figure 4.9 shows all-cause mortality according to BMI from the largest of these, the Prospective Studies Collaboration (2009), which included nearly a million adults from 57 prospective studies. This meta-analysis shows that death rates associated with obesity are higher in males than females, relative to BMI norms of 20–25 kg/m^2 (Figure 4.10). Evidence from systematic reviews of adult chronic disease subsequent to childhood obesity shows that there is significantly increased risk of premature mortality with child and adolescent overweight or obesity, as well as significantly increased risk of cardiometabolic morbidity (diabetes, hypertension, ischaemic heart disease and stroke) in adult life (Reilly and Kelly 2011). Cardiovascular disease risk is, however, dependent on the tracking of BMI from childhood to adulthood, with the risk of raised blood pressure in adult life being highest among those at the lower end of the BMI scale in

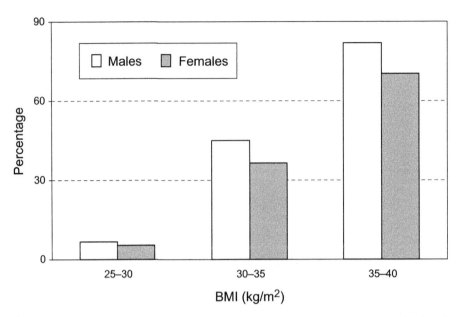

Figure 4.10. All-cause mortality due to obesity, as a percentage above all-cause mortality for adults with body mass index (BMI) between 20 and 25 kg/m^2 (calculated from Prospective Studies Collaboration 2009).

childhood, but overweight in adulthood (Lloyd et al. 2010). This suggests that the period of developmental programming for increased chronic disease risk in adult life (Barker 2004) (Chapter 7) extends beyond fetal and infant development into childhood and adolescence. In another systematic review, Lloyd et al. (2012) observed that the majority of epidemiological studies looking at relationships between BMI and chronic disease across life fail to adjust for adult BMI, and that associations found in various studies may reflect the tracking of BMI across the lifespan rather than direct relationships between childhood obesity and adult chronic disease risk. In studies where adult BMI has been adjusted for, weak negative associations between childhood BMI and metabolic variables have been found, with those at the lower end of the BMI range in childhood but obese during adulthood showing higher risk (Lloyd et al. 2012).

While waist circumference and waist:hip ratio show equally good, if not better, associations with mortality and morbidity risk (World Health Organization 2011), their possible adoption for international comparison would risk delegitimizing programmes and policies for obesity control that have used population monitoring of BMI as the measure of success or failure. This is an important issue, as researchers struggle to determine the effectiveness of obesity policies. When it is not clear how effective anti-obesity policies are, the easiest thing to do is to keep taking measurements. BMI measurement and population monitoring of obesity are practised globally, this approach sitting on the lowest rung of intervention according to the Nuffield public health intervention ladder (Nuffield Council on Bioethics 2007) (Chapter 8).

While there is enormous investment in maintaining programmes that use consistent measures of obesity, this is no different to measures used in a wide range of other globally overseen public health programmes, such as those for the control of HIV (UNAIDS 2013) and of malaria (World Health Organization 2016a), where risk is related to HIV positivity and parasite positivity, respectively. Allowing more categories of risk measurement, such as waist circumference, waist:hip ratio and/or waist:height ratio, would make the understanding of obesity more complex (Chapter 9) and its control more difficult. Good epidemiological science aims to give the best descriptions of the ecological relationships between body fatness and disease, and good obesity policy aims to use such descriptions for best practice in obesity regulation. The next section examines how obesity epidemiology, which generates models of obesity in relation to chronic disease risk, informs obesity policy through econometric modelling.

Obesity and Economics

As the ecology of obesity has become more analytically tractable for economists, a number of issues have emerged to make it much more than a public health issue. Obesity has been shown to be associated with income (Vandegrift and Yoked 2004), especially in women (Lundborg et al. 2006), to carry illness costs (Allison et al. 1999), to be associated with the likelihood of being unemployed (Lundborg et al. 2006) and to carry significant medical costs from childhood and adolescence (Wang and Dietz 2002). In a large study involving data from Sweden, the US and the UK, Lundborg et al. (2014) found a large male labour market penalty in adult life for being overweight or obese as a teenager, reflecting lower skill acquisition among adolescents who are overweight or obese. Obese people are stigmatized against (Puhl and Brownell 2003), carry high chronic disease burdens (Must et al. 1999) and are seen to inhibit economic growth through taking more time off work and performing work less efficiently than non-obese people; they may also be less popular and less motivated to learn and work from childhood onwards (Lundborg et al. 2014).

The possible health-care costs of obesity have been modelled for the US. These show a J-shaped relationship between BMI and projected medical costs, which is higher in men than in women, at both ends of the population distribution of BMI (Figure 4.11). Obesity in the US raises medical expenditures by roughly 75 per cent for males and by roughly 180 per cent for females (Cawley and Meyerhoefer 2012), but BMI-related all-cause mortality is roughly 70 per cent greater for males than females, across most HICs (Figure 4.12) (Prospective Studies Collaboration 2009). The gender difference in medical expenditure in the US is largely due to greater uptake of medical care among women than men at most levels of BMI (Cawley and Meyerhoefer 2012). The gender difference in the overall economic costs of obesity in the US may reflect differences in Type 2 diabetes risk according to BMI, which is more than twofold greater in women than in men from a BMI of 23 kg/m^2 upwards, increasing exponentially for both sexes

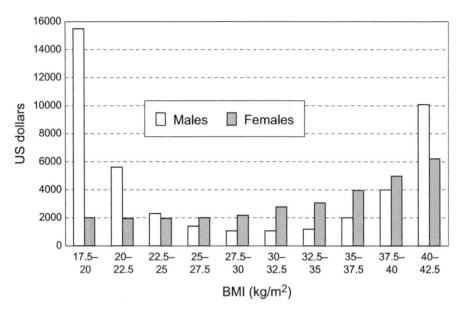

Figure 4.11. Predicted relationship between body mass index (BMI) and annual medical expenditures for all adults with biological children, in the US, shown as expenditures in 2005 in US dollars (data from Cawley and Meyerhoefer 2012).

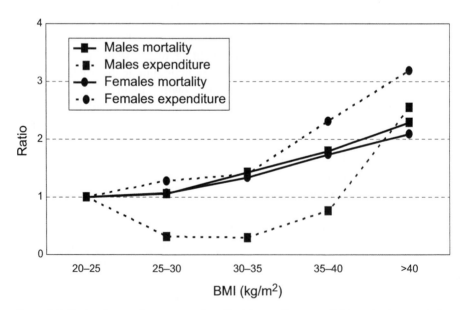

Figure 4.12. Ratio of mortality to annual medical expenditures at different body mass index (BMI) categories, in the US, relative to a BMI of 20–25 kg/m² (calculated from data given in Prospective Studies Collaboration 2009 and Cawley and Meyerhoefer 2012).

(Chan et al. 1994; Colditz et al. 1995). Type 2 diabetes is the fourth greatest cause of death in HICs (Mathers and Loncar 2006), and its treatment and management is expensive. In 2007, the cost of diabetes to the US economy was US$174 billion, one-third of which was indirect and related to disability, work loss and premature death, and two-thirds of which was attributable to its treatment and management (Centers for Disease Control and Prevention 2011a). Differences in bodily aesthetics and health may also influence gender differences in the economic costs of obesity. In the US, women place higher value on bodily aesthetics as a measure of health than men (Saltonstall 1993), while a much higher proportion of women than men actively engage in weight management, most of it involving the use of commercial products and services (Serdula et al. 1999; Bish et al. 2005), thus off-setting some of the medical expense to the state.

While economists accept the epidemiological value of BMI as a measure of obesity (Grossman and Mocan 2011), mortality rates associated with obesity (as measured by BMI) do not map directly to its economic costs. In the US, additional medical expenditure among overweight and obese women relative to women of BMI between 20 and 25 kg/m^2 exceeds their additional mortality rates across the same BMI categories (Figure 4.12), indicating that the illness costs of very high BMI exceed the excess mortality burden associated with it. For males, the illness costs of overweight and moderate obesity are lower than the excess mortality burden in those BMI categories. In the US, death rates due to cardiovascular disease and cancer are consistently higher for men than for women at all levels of BMI (Calle et al. 1999; Prospective Studies Collaboration 2009). Men are less likely to utilize health-care visits to doctors' offices, emergency departments and physician home visits than women; they are also less likely to undertake preventive care, and have fewer hospital discharges and shorter hospital stays than women (Pinkhasov et al. 2010). Thus, women in the US have higher medical care service utilization rates and higher associated charges than men (Bertakis et al. 2000; Pinkhasov et al. 2010), because of gender-based differences in health-seeking behaviours that mediate the relationships between BMI, health risk and medical expenditure.

Epidemiology and economics are linked in their approaches to obesity, and evidence-based policy reflects this entanglement (Chapter 8). The systems of evidence production in obesity epidemiology and economics rely on BMI, which gives an anthropometric approximation of body fatness. This chapter has spoken of many of its limitations, all of which are known by epidemiology, public health and economics. The measure persists in epidemiology and public health practice because it is pragmatically useful in descriptive and predictive modelling of obesity rates. At the national level, obesity rates are also mediated geographically and economically through inequality (Marmot 2004) (Chapter 5). The obesogenic environment model (Chapter 3) privileges structural factors that shape individual predispositions to obesity, and economic improvement should be able to help de-structure obesogenic environments. However, improvements in environmental quality are often linked to changing sociodemographic structures of urban places. According to Guthman

(2011), if the environment changes, it is not appropriate behaviours that will follow, as proponents of the approach suggest, but appropriate people: new inhabitants with a different, perhaps more privileged set of values surrounding health. Without tackling economic inequalities, it is unlikely that inequalities in obesity rates will disappear; they will likely continue to be reproduced, perhaps differently. Obesity and inequality form the basis of the next chapter.

5 Inequalities

Obesity has an impact on national economies (Chapter 4), but the political ecology of obesity is importantly linked to disadvantage in high-income countries (HICs) (Pickett et al. 2005), including lower wages (Sargent and Blanchflower 1994), which reinforce long-term economic inequalities. There are also significant gender differences in the ecological distribution of obesity, both across nations and according to socioeconomic status (SES) (Wells et al. 2012). In most populations across the world, obesity rates are generally higher in women than in men, due to sex differences in body fat distribution (Lovejoy et al. 2009). In lower middle-income countries (LMICs), obesity is more common in groups of higher SES, although this is changing, as modernization and urbanization are changing diets and levels of physical activity across the world (Ulijaszek 1999), and globalization facilitates increased foreign investment in the production and distribution of food products, supermarketization, and the expansion of fast-food chains, especially in countries with largely unregulated markets (Hawkes 2006) (Chapter 6).

Among children, the relationships between SES and obesity only partially map onto those of adults, and differ across the course of childhood. The inverse association between SES and body fatness in HICs is found in both children and adults (Shrewsbury and Wardle 2008), but low SES in early life is usually more closely associated with higher body fatness in adulthood than in childhood (Parsons et al. 1999), following the typical life-course progression of obesity. The co-production of excess body fatness by parents and children also varies by SES (Ulijaszek et al. 2016a). Children of obese parents are more likely to become obese themselves (Lake et al. 1997; Li et al. 2009), and where obesity is highest among those of low SES, this pattern is reproduced across a generation.

Different models of obesity make different inferences about such relationships. The energy balance model (Chapter 3) might infer the mechanism of familial obesity production to be one of similar household environments creating similar patterns of food intake and physical activity among young and old people therein, while a genetics model might infer genetic predispositions to be causally important. The former model would place primacy on SES structuring local ecologies and the household environment, while the latter might assume SES differences in the genetics of obesity susceptibility. A meeting of the two might place reliance on gene–environment interactions (Faith et al. 2004), where, in the absence of evidence for SES-related genotypes, different SES-related environments might lead to different expression of obesity susceptibility genes. Alternatively, a developmental origins model of obesity causation within families would focus on ecologies in transition (Chapter 7). Within families, low grandparental social support combined with low parental SES is closely associated with obesity in preschool-aged children (Lindberg et al. 2015), and an insecurity model of obesity would place emotional and psychological distress central to the link between socioeconomic disadvantage and childhood weight gain, at least in HICs (Hemmingsson 2014).

Socioeconomic influences on body weight are mediated by a wide range of personal and cultural factors, including social attitudes, perceptions of the body and food preferences (Chapter 6), as well as environmental factors including the directly obesogenic ones (Chapter 3), and less obesogenic factors such as the pleasantness and aesthetics of poorer neighbourhoods, and police presence and incidence of violent crime therein (Harrington and Elliot 2009; Kirk et al. 2009). They are also mediated by social capital, social cohesion and collective efficacy – higher levels of which are positively associated with the regulation of weight status, even in poor neighbourhoods (Harrington and Elliot 2009). Within any neighbourhood, access to resources that promote or degrade health is determined by price, proximity, the right to use and informal reciprocity (Bernard et al. 2007). It takes society, not individuals, to create social and economic inequality, and inequalities in obesity rates. As a social and political issue, obesity inequality should also be a matter for policy (Chapters 8 and 10). This chapter describes the political ecology of obesity inequalities according to SES and other forms of capital. It then examines gender inequality in obesity rates and weight bias, and inequality and insecurity in the production of adult and childhood obesity. Inequality has no rationality, but the processes that produce it are driven by various forms of it (Chapter 2).

Inequalities in Obesity Rates

How inequalities are measured and modelled can influence the inferences that can be drawn about their relationships with obesity. In studies of health inequalities, for example, measures such as education, income or occupational class often relate (at least partly) to different causal processes (Geyer et al. 2006). Most research into obesity inequality reduces the range of possible socioeconomic variables to exactly these three measures, however (Drewnowski 2012). The relationships among SES and obesity are powerful and synergistic (Sobal 1991; Marmot et al. 2010), although the components of SES measure different things (Braveman et al. 2005). The economic dimension is represented by financial wealth, while a social dimension can incorporate education, occupational prestige, authority and community standing. Economic status is quite easy to measure (assuming that income is accurately revealed in a survey), but prestige and authority are more difficult to estimate (Haug 1977). While the SES construct is numerically tractable, there is no consensus definition of it, nor is there a commonly accepted way of measuring it (Oakes and Rossi 2003). Education and income (alongside ethnicity) are more usually considered in research into obesity inequality in the United States (US), occupation being considered to offer misleading information about socioeconomic position, or being simply uninformative in this

Table 5.1. Ten-year change in body mass index (BMI) inequality between highest and lowest educational tertiles against 10-year change in adult obesity rates for 26 populations sampled in the World Health Organization MONICA Project

Ten-year change in BMI inequality (number of populations)		Ten-year change in obesity rate (number of populations)	
		Increase	Decrease
Males	Increase	16	1
	Decrease	5	4
Females	Increase	17	6
	Decrease	0	3

Fisher's exact probability test for both males and females: $p = 0.03$.
Data from Molarius et al. (2000).

regard (Drewnowski 2012). Composites of these two (sometimes three) variables are then used to construct social class groupings in epidemiological and public health research (Krieger et al. 1997). In the United Kingdom (UK), SES by occupation is a commonly used measure of inequality (Marshall et al. 1988), alongside SES by level of education and geographical distribution according to urban deprivation. More generally, in the US, there is a tendency to overlook social class as an explanatory factor for variation in obesity rates (Drewnowski 2012), while in the UK, social class differences are more commonly discussed and reported on (Marmot 2004; Public Health England 2015a). Thus, comparisons of within-nation inequalities in obesity rates can only be made cross-nationally with caution, because of differences in underlying assumptions and ways of measurement in different countries.

As obesity rates within and between nations change (Chapter 1), so do social and economic gradients in those rates. One international comparison of 39 centres in 26 nations has shown that as obesity rates have increased over a 10-year period, so too have social gradients (Molarius et al. 2000) (Table 5.1). Across time, the factors that influence inequalities in obesity rates change. For example, growth in global wealth since 2000 (Credit Suisse 2014), increasing income inequality within nations (Milanovic 2016) and the continued secular trend towards increased height and weight in many places (Ulijaszek 1993, 2001d, e) have led to changing SES differentials in a range of life-course factors known to be associated with obesity, including birth weight, nutritional state in utero, and the developmental programming and epigenetic regulation that go with them (Chapter 7), as well as differences in post-natal patterns of physical growth and development.

The relationships between inequality and obesity vary according to economic prosperity and educational status in different ways in different countries. A cross-nation comparison of obesity inequality has been carried out by McLaren (2007), who reviewed 333 published studies on this topic in countries of high, medium and low Human Development Index (HDI), as determined in 2003 (the category of 'very high' was introduced in 2010). The HDI is a composite statistic of life expectancy, education and income measures developed by the United Nations

Development Programme (UNDP) in the 1990s, and offers a measure of national development based on people and their capabilities, in addition to economic growth (United Nations Development Programme 2006). Figure 5.1 shows obesity in high HDI nations to be negatively associated with education for both males and females, and also negatively associated with employment type for females but not for males. Obesity is also negatively associated with income among females but positively associated with income in males in nations with high HDI. In countries of medium and low HDI, obesity and income are positively associated in both women and men (Figure 5.2). Obesity is also positively associated with higher levels of education among men, but not women, in medium and low HDI countries. The observations of McLaren (2007) confirm the views of Geyer et al. (2006) concerning the non-interchangeability of education, income or occupational class as measures of SES with respect to obesity. The inverse relationship between all three measures of SES and obesity among women in high HDI countries might be due to differences according to SES in obesity-relevant health behaviours, with women of higher status or socioeconomic position eating diets of lower energy content, taking more exercise and being more likely to control their body weight through dieting (Molarius 2003; Ulijaszek and Lofink 2006). The difficulties of controlling body weight have been related to a perceived lack of control over time at both collective and individual levels (Felt et al. 2014), something that is felt more strongly among those of low SES. SES is also negatively associated with diet quality and positively with obesity risk in high HDI countries, primarily through the mechanism of cost (Darmon and Drewnowski 2008), in that energy-dense foods are usually the cheapest (Chapter 6). In high HDI nations, women generally have more rigid cultural beauty ideals than men (Striegel-Moore and Franko 2004), and if men of high SES have fewer concerns about body image than their female counterparts, they may also be more relaxed about consuming cheap energy-dense foods and gaining weight. With the credit crunch in the 2000s, overindebtedness has also been shown to be associated with obesity in German adults, to an extent that cannot be explained by traditional definitions of SES (Munster et al. 2009).

The varying relationships of obesity with different measures of SES across countries of different HDI have been explained by Dinsa et al. (2012) in terms of the rich in poor countries being able to afford and demand surplus food and the rich in HICs being able to afford a healthier diet and exercise. Conversely, the poor in low-income countries (LICs) face food shortages while the poor in HICs are particularly exposed to energy-dense foods (Dinsa et al. 2012). These relationships are mediated by educational attainment, employment prestige, differences in the need to conform to body ideals, and the ability to control food intake and personal body size (Chapters 6, 8 and 10). Associations between obesity and occupation may also be influenced by weight bias, as reflected in inequities in employment, often due to widespread negative stereotypes about obese persons (Puhl and Heuer 2009), such that slimmer people in most HDI countries are more likely to have higher status jobs and higher incomes.

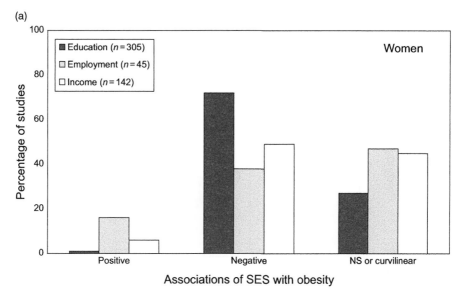

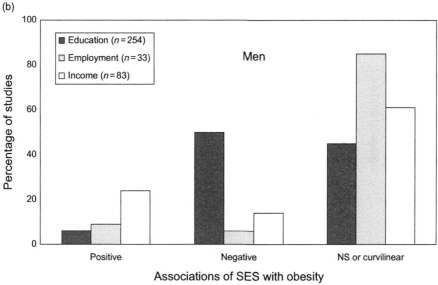

Figure 5.1. Measures of socioeconomic status (SES) and obesity, in high World Bank Human Development Index (2003) nations for women (a) and men (b) (calculated from data given in McLaren 2007). NS, non-significant.

Among children in HICs, the relationships between SES and obesity are generally negative ones (Due et al. 2009), although there are exceptions. In Kuwait and among migrant children in Germany, there are positive relationships between SES and obesity (World Health Organization 2016b), largely because of the continuation of traditionally positive perceptions of body fatness. There is no strong evidence for

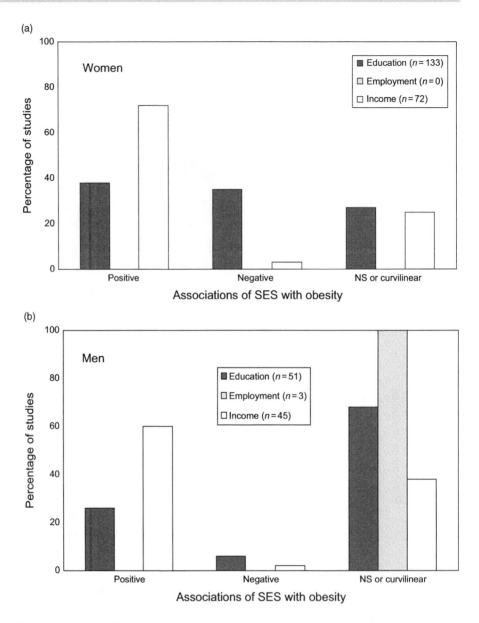

Figure 5.2. Measures of socioeconomic status (SES) and obesity, in medium and low World Bank Human Development Index (2003) nations for women (a) and men (b) (calculated from data given in McLaren 2007). NS, non-significant.

gender differences in SES–obesity relationships in children (World Health Organization 2016b), this being likely to emerge across adolescence with divergent patterns of physical growth, maturation and sexual development. In LMICs, rates of childhood obesity are increasing, the highest rates of overweight and obesity being usually among children of higher SES (World Health Organization 2016b). In both HICs and

LMICs, socioeconomic inequalities experienced by parents can shape childhood rates of overweight and obesity through parental obesity (Lake et al. 1997; Li et al. 2009), most likely from mothers to their offspring (Whitaker 2004; Reilly et al. 2005; Gibson et al. 2007; Rooney et al. 2011) through child development, mediated by a complex reproductive ecology that includes maternal nutrition, pregnancy, childbirth, infant feeding and behavioural upbringing (Chapter 7).

Various models of obesity have been used to describe inequalities in obesity rates. The use of different measures of inequality and of different forces shaping inequality in different nations makes it unlikely that there can be a coordinated and globally uniform description of obesity inequality. Perhaps the most fundamental inequality with respect to obesity is gender inequality, because of the importance of reproductive and early-life history factors on later obesity (Chapter 7). Measuring inequality among women is made difficult by the fact that, in many countries, women do not have occupations or incomes, both standard measures of SES. Relating inequality to obesity rates among women is also more difficult than among men because forms of capital other than income, occupation and education are important in establishing their status.

Gender, Forms of Capital and Obesity

Gender differences in adult obesity rates are global (Wells et al. 2012). When Kanter and Caballero (2012) examined such differences across 105 countries and territories according to the World Bank categories of income (Chapter 1), they found that obesity rates were higher in females of all income groups (Figure 5.3), the greatest

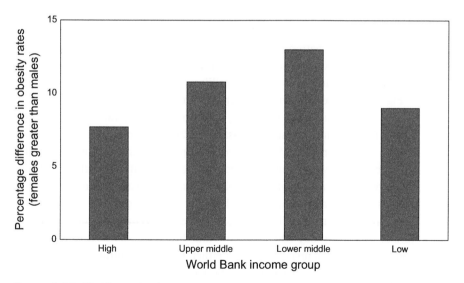

Figure 5.3. Worldwide gender disparities in obesity prevalence according to World Bank income group (data from Kanter and Caballero 2012).

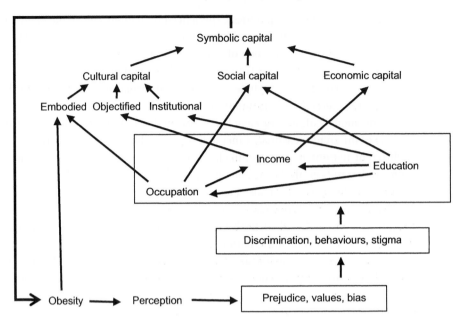

Figure 5.4. Obesity and forms of capital.

differences being in LMICs. Diet and physical activity differences might help explain these differences (Kanter and Cabellaro 2012). For example, in HICs, women consume more foods high in added sugars, including energy-dense processed foods, than men (Wansink et al. 2003; Wardle et al. 2004), while in LMICs and LICs, the shift in physical labour demands from agricultural and subsistence production to wage employment has resulted in larger declines in physical activity in women than in men (McGarvey 1991; Ismail et al. 2002; Aekplakorn et al. 2004; Snodgrass et al. 2006). Divergent patterns in obesity rates by gender and SES (Figures 5.2 and 5.3) might also reflect different forms of capital at play, beyond those captured by income, occupation and education (Ulijaszek 2012).

Figure 5.4 gives a theoretical scheme for relationships among different forms of capital (Bourdieu 1986), including socioeconomic capital (Bourdieu and Boltanski 1976), in relation to obesity (Ulijaszek 2012). Economic capital is easily understood as one component of SES, while social capital is distinct from SES and represents group cohesion, which facilitates cooperation for mutual benefit. The three subtypes of cultural capital – embodied, objectified and institutional – measure different aspects of the same thing. Most broadly, cultural capital is a measure of social position that overlaps with existing measures, but is distinct from them. For example, formal education may teach how to value literature and how to maintain a healthy body, but it is not a precondition for either. Embodied cultural capital involves bodily properties that are either consciously acquired or inherited, such as beauty, bodily symmetry, poise and athleticism. Again, money might help acquire and maintain some of these personal properties, but it is not a prerequisite. Embodied cultural capital is distinct from the embodied capital that is discussed in human evolutionary studies, where, according to Kaplan et al. (2000), it includes strength, immune function, coordination, skill, knowledge and social networks, all of which affect the allocation of time and other resources to resource acquisition, defence from predators and parasites, mating competition, parenting and social dominance. Given the differences in cultural valuation of body size among different groups and populations, obesity may carry greater embodied cultural capital in groups that value greater body weight than among those that do not. In Kuwait, Saudi Arabia and United Arab Emirates, for example, such cultural valuation continues (Al-Kandari 2006; Al-Saeed et al. 2007; Malik and Bakir 2007) as economic prosperity in these nations has continued to rise. Alternatively, objectified cultural capital considers the relationships between people and the objects that confer status upon them. It can include prestigious brands of foods and designer-labelled clothes, as well as more traditional measures of social position obtained through living in the right neighbourhood, living in an expensive house and consumption of high-status food. Again, while economic capital may be helpful in purchasing objectified cultural capital, it is not a requirement. For example, objectified cultural capital can be attained through consuming branded fast foods among those who have little economic capital, and is a potential contributor to obesity among those of low SES (Ulijaszek 2012). Institutional cultural capital consists of recognition of individuals by the state (most usually in terms of academic credentials, qualifications and honours) or by working in a prestigious organization. It overlaps with education as a form of status, but it can further discriminate on the basis of the status of different educational institutions.

In Western HICs, slimness is a form of embodied cultural capital that is sought by the vast majority of women. Discourses in the media and literature in Western societies have largely privileged and validated the slender female body for over 100 years, with cultural beauty ideals rigidly emphasizing thinness for women (Striegel-Moore and Franko, 2004). In reproductive terms, fatness, within bounds, is advantageous. But in societies in which controlled reproduction predominates (as in most HICs), it has diminished value as embodied cultural capital. However, women may also be more preoccupied with their appearance (of which body size is a component) because attractiveness carries greater evolutionary rationality for women than for men (Wade and Cooper 1999). Idealized images of women in mass media privilege thinness, and are among the most powerful influences on how women view themselves (Paquette and Raine 2004). Although people of higher SES in the UK are more concerned about body shape and engage in more efforts to lose weight than people of low SES (Wardle and Griffith 2001), females show greater weight concern than men (Wardle et al. 2002), regardless of SES. Compliance with thin bodily ideals is a way for women to display Weberian formally rational behaviour in the highly institutionalized settings of Western societies, to signal their appropriateness for prestige employment (a practically rational behaviour) and to find reproductive partners of high quality (which is evolutionarily rational) (Chapter 2).

Weight Bias

In Western nations, pursuit of thinness and bodily perfection contributes to the pathologization and stigmatization of body fatness among women (Carryer 2001). Overweight and obesity have been stigmatized in the US for over 100 years (Dejong 1980; Puhl and Brownell 2001), the prevalence of such stigma almost doubling since the mid-1990s (Andreyeva et al. 2008). Such stigmatization has very little to do with the direct health consequences of body fatness. At any BMI between 20 and 34 kg/m^2, women carry around 10 per cent more fat than males (Deurenberg et al. 2002), but deposit more of it in bodily sites generally associated with lower chronic disease risk (Despres et al. 1990). Weight bias, stigma and discrimination have important economic consequences. In the US, data from a nationally representative sample found women to be 16 times more likely than men to report weight-related employment discrimination (Roehling et al. 2007), with obese women being much more likely than thin women to hold low-paying jobs (Pagan and Davila 1997). As a consequence, obesity hinders social and economic mobility for women to a much greater extent than for men (Venator and Reeves 2015).

While weight bias is common in most HICs, it is increasingly so in economically emerging nations (Brewis et al. 2011). More generally, it translates into inequalities in employment and health care, often due to widespread negative stereotypes about obese persons (Puhl and Heuer 2009). Table 5.2 shows the types of weight stigma associated with different domains of everyday life: in employment, when seeking health care, in interpersonal relations and in the media. In health care, professionals often endorse negative attitudes and stereotypes about obese patients (Chamberlin et al. 2002). Media representations of obesity often individualize it while taking a fatalistic position in relation to its reversibility (Shugart 2014) or, in the US, use it as a means of discussing themes society is uncomfortable with, such as poverty, race and/or ethnicity (Boero 2014; Saguy and Almeling 2014). In addition to weight-related pay, employment and job evaluation discrimination (Klassen et al. 1993; Pagan and Davila 1997; Popovich et al. 1997; Roehling et al. 2007), weight bias in employment carries some social mobility penalty. Figure 5.5 shows the extent of economic mobility according to the measure of intergenerational earnings elasticity (the higher the value, the lower the cross-generational economic mobility) among males in 12 HICs (D'Addio 2007). This shows that, in countries like the US and the UK, where a son's earnings strongly match those of their father, there are low levels of such mobility, while in countries like Denmark and Austria there are high levels of economic mobility. Figure 5.6 shows there to be a weak relationship between intergenerational earnings elasticity and obesity in adolescence across the same countries shown in Figure 5.5, those with lower economic mobility having higher levels of obesity in adolescence, regardless of the level of economic inequality as determined by the Gini coefficient.

According to Brewis (2014), there are four interrelated mechanisms whereby stigma can lead to greater body fatness and obesity. First, if fat stigma negatively

Table 5.2. Strong and moderate evidence of stigma and obesity

Evidence	Domain			
	Employment	Health care	Interpersonal relations	Media
Strong	Obese employees perceive weight-based disparities in employment	Health-care professionals endorse stereotypes and negative attitudes about obese patients		Overweight/obese characters are stigmatized in television and film
	Obese employees experience wage penalties			
	Obese applicants face weight bias in job evaluations			
Moderate	Obese employees face disadvantaged employment outcomes due to weight bias	Obese patients perceive biased treatment in health care	Obese individuals perceive weight bias from family members and friends	Overweight/obese characters are stereotyped in children's media (TV, videos, cartoons)
				Weight bias in news media

Adapted from Puhl and Heuer (2009).

affects people's exercise, diet and health-seeking behaviours, then this can lead to weight gain or impede weight loss. Second, weight stigma is usually associated with psychosocial stress that promotes overeating and weight gain. Third, stigma can lead to weight gain through changing social networks, if it leads to people associating with each other according to body weight, physical activity norms and/or habitual dietary intake. For example, Christakis and Fowler (2007) demonstrated in a US sample observed between 1993 and 1999 that individuals in a social network clustered according to their body weight. The fourth mechanism linking stigma to body fatness is through softening the psychological effects of discrimination by comfort eating. Brewis (2014) views there to be good theoretical rationale for possible intergenerational weight gain or weight retention effects of these mechanisms, through stress, insecurity and/or low SES. This model of obesity, inequality and stigma employs generality, is clearly representational and provides a framework for hypothesis production (Chapter 2). For children in HICs, inequalities in childhood and adolescent overweight and obesity are perpetuated through SES and stigma (Puhl and Latner 2007; Hansson et al. 2009). There is considerable stigma surrounding childhood obesity in the US (Greenleaf et al. 2006), which produces social

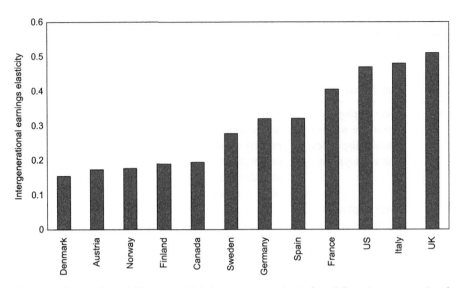

Figure 5.5. Economic mobility in 12 high-income countries, inferred from intergenerational earnings elasticity, showing the extent to which sons' earnings reflect those of their fathers (adapted from D'Addio 2007).

disadvantages in employment, education, health care and interpersonal relationships (Puhl and Brownell 2001; Brownell et al. 2005). There is no significant weight stigma within the US education system (Puhl and Heuer 2009), although inequality in educational provision can institutionalize varying body size norms in different schools and geographical locations.

Both slim-body ideals and fat-stigmatizing beliefs have spread globally in the last few decades, including among societies that have previously had positive perceptions of large body size (Brewis et al. 2011). Where, among migrants, slimmer body size ideals emerge, as among Pacific Islander peoples in New Zealand (Brewis et al. 1998), young Mexican American girls (Hall et al. 1991) and South Asian migrants in Oslo (Raberg et al. 2010), this may reflect a realignment of body size and shape preferences to local norms to minimize rejection, ostracism and negative social relations at school and in the workplace. There are exceptions to the adoption of thin ideals in some HICs, especially in the Middle East. For example, in Kuwait, where adult obesity rates exceed 35 per cent for both males and females (Al-Kandari 2006), obesity in adolescence is not associated with reduced health-related quality of life, either physical or psychosocial (Boodai and Reilly 2013). This may reflect the continuation of positive attitudes towards large body size as a measure of embodied cultural capital, at a time when Kuwaiti society is rapidly modernizing and obesity rates are rising. The traditional role of food in social relations remains very strong in Kuwait, and the plentiful availability of energy-dense foods makes the practice of sociality through food easy to follow. Rising obesity rates are facilitated by the wide availability and

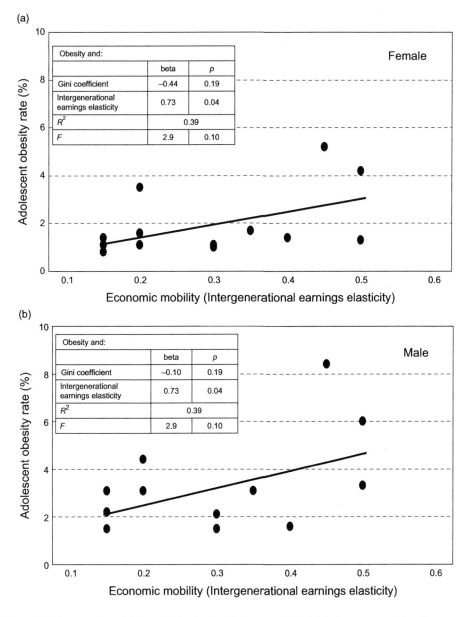

Figure 5.6. Economic mobility and obesity in adolescents in 12 high-income countries for females (a) and males (b) (calculated from data in Due et al. 2009; D'Addio 2007).

convenience of fast food and eating out more generally there. Maintaining an adequate level of physical activity is largely impossible in everyday life in Kuwait (with the exception of migrant labour), because habitual activity is structured by the built environment, which, because of the high temperatures at most times of year, keeps people indoors (Al-Kandari 2006).

Food and Status

The human body is both object and subject for negotiating the material world in all its physicality, and as social identity within that world. If obesity carries cultural capital in a group of people of low SES, it is often one of the few forms of capital available to them. If people of low SES share their urban geographical space with branded fast-food outlets, then the selection, purchase and consumption of fast food may be another achievable form of cultural capital within an obesogenic environment (Chapter 3). Although the data are inconsistent (Cummins and Macintyre 2006), there are associations between levels of urban deprivation and the density of fast-food outlets, indicating that the political ecology of obesity is to some extent structured by obesogenic environments. In Melbourne, Australia, poorer neighbourhoods have two and a half times as many such outlets as wealthier ones (Reidpath et al. 2002), while in New Orleans, there are more fast-food outlets in predominately black census tracts (Block et al. 2004). In England, fast-food outlets are concentrated in local authorities with the highest levels of deprivation (National Obesity Observatory 2012) (Figure 5.7).

Consumption of fast food may be a default behaviour when the urban ecology makes it more available than fruit or vegetables. Fast food may also be consumed in

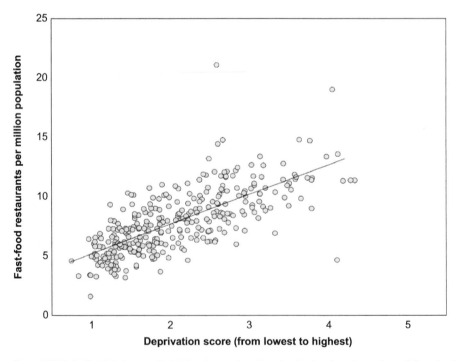

Figure 5.7. Relationship between deprivation at local authority level and number of fast-food restaurants in England (National Obesity Observatory 2012). Contains public sector information licensed under the Open Government Licence v3.0 www.nationalarchives.gov.uk/doc/open-government-licence/version/3/.

greater amounts because it is palatable, secure and predictable in meeting the projected mental expectations from it (Chapter 6). Well before buying a branded burger, for example, the feel, taste, smell and mouth sensation associated with its consumption are unconsciously rehearsed. Fast food may also be consumed because, if branded (as with the global major fast-food products), it allows status, as well as food, to be consumed. Food is the most primary of symbolic goods because it is used to mark status in all societies (Bourdieu 1984). Taste and preference in food can indicate social position, and people of low SES can acquire cultural capital through food by purchasing recognized global brands that are affordable to them (Ulijaszek et al. 2012). The symbolic coding of food has been elaborated to a high degree across history, a process that continued in the twentieth century at great pace, with the development of a global food ecology and the growth of systems of supermarkets and restaurants that deliver often globally sourced foods. The strength of food as a symbol of status or identity is not lost on food manufacturers (Ulijaszek et al. 2012), and the use of such knowledge in branding and marketing has helped the growth of fast-food sales in the US and other HICs. Consumption of fast food has grown to make up a significant proportion of daily intake in the US: a nationally representative dietary survey showed that 42 per cent of children and adolescents and 37 per cent of adults eat fast food daily (Paeratakul et al. 2003). Furthermore, between 2007 and 2010, adults in the US consumed over 11 per cent of their total daily energy intake as fast food (Fryar and Ervin 2013). Fast-food manufacturers have developed product lines that carry images of originality, exoticism and often global power. These attain value as objectified cultural capital (through branding and advertising) among people who consume these food products.

Although the use of food in the quest for status is universal, high-status foods vary enormously across societies (Weissner and Schiefenhovel 1996). Bourdieu (1984) suggests that class distinction and preferences are most marked in ordinary choices of everyday life, with cooking and tastes in food, and are primarily learned in childhood. In HICs, children can identify the symbolic value of foods from an early age. For example, preschool children in the US are aware of and can identify advertised food brands; by the age of 7 years, they can shop independently, find information about what they want to buy and show what they have bought to other children (Nestle 2002). The building of objectified cultural capital through branded foods therefore starts in childhood, and contributes to inequalities in obesity rates through the differential quest for status.

Inequality, Insecurity and Obesity

While inequalities in obesity rates can be measured epidemiologically through the categories of gender, ethnicity, income, education and occupation, the relationships between obesity and insecurity are less easy to demonstrate. Economic inequality is characterized as the variation between people or populations in their incomes and assets, while economic insecurity can be characterized by uncertainty of continued economic solvency of a person or population into the future. Economic insecurity varies according to likelihood of continued employment, welfare provision, savings and pension, among other factors. Hacker et al. (2013) note that, even before the economic recession of 2007–2009, many citizens of the US were concerned about economic risks. Data from the *Survey of Economic Risk Perceptions and Insecurity in the US* (Hacker et al. 2013) show that insecurity, whether expressed as worry or as economic shock, is far greater for households with limited education and with lower income (Table 5.3), with the exception of wealth shock. Worries are more stratified by SES than are shocks themselves, indicating that the psychosocial stress of everyday life that associates with weight gain (Block et al. 2009) and obesity (Goodman and Whitaker 2002; Brunner et al. 2007) is likely to be mediated through inequality.

Insecurity in the form of anxiety about body weight may be social, or deeply personal (Shugart 2016), and there are clear links between directly experienced social inequality, anxiety and dietary energy intake. Work by Bratanova et al. (2016) has demonstrated that people experimentally induced to view themselves as poor (as opposed to wealthy) eat more dietary energy than those who view themselves as being wealthy. Furthermore, people who have previously experienced inequality (viewing themselves as being either poorer or wealthier within the same social grouping) are more anxious than those who see themselves as being equal in such contexts. Within the same study, anxiety was shown to lead to increased energy intake among those with a strong need to belong to a group.

Mechanisms by which insecurity and inequality operate in the production of obesity at the level of the individual include stress alleviation through comfort eating (Dallman et al. 2005) and binge eating (Telch and Agras 1994) (Chapter 6). Other forms of insecurity are mostly structured at the level of institutions, corporations and/or the nation state. Structurally created insecurities that are related to obesity include a lack of representation (unionization in the workplace), uncertainty of holding down a job long term and limited protection against the economic costs of illness (Offer et al. 2010). An analysis of obesity rates across nations shows that the extent of social welfare is a powerful predictor of obesity rates at the national level (Offer et al. 2010) although social and cultural factors may be important, in addition to economic factors, in determining health outcomes in different populations within HICs (Hurrelmann et al. 2011). The concept of welfare regimes was put forward by Esping-Andersen (1990), who made a distinction between different models of welfare: Nordic social democratic, continental European family-oriented and English-speaking liberal. Hall and Soskice (2001) conflated the Nordic and continental European models into one group, collectively characterized by having coordinated market economies (which include Germany, Japan, Switzerland, the Netherlands and Belgium, as well as the Nordic nations of Sweden, Norway, Denmark and Finland). This is in contrast to neoliberal market economies, which are mostly English speaking and include the US, the UK, Australia, Canada, New Zealand and Ireland. Adult obesity rates in the Nordic countries do not differ from those in the continental European family-oriented nations, but both have significantly lower rates than the English-speaking neoliberal nations (Offer et al. 2010).

Table 5.3. Inequalities in employment, health and wealth insecurity in the US

		Employment		Health		Wealth	
		Have been unemployed not by choice (per cent)	Very/fairly worried about losing or finding a job (per cent)	Have had major out-of-pocket medical expenses (per cent)	Very/fairly worried about having major out-of-pocket medical expenses (per cent)	Have had retirement benefits at work cut substantially (per cent)	Very/fairly worried about having retirement benefits substantially cut (per cent)
Education	High school diploma	30	46	28	51	18	36
	Bachelor's degree	21	34	24	44	21	32
	Graduate degree	14	26	24	34	20	27
Income	Lowest	41	49	29	55	16	37
	Middle	21	36	25	45	20	31
	Highest	10	29	21	35	24	31

Adapted from Hacker et al. (2013).

Rising obesity rates may be an unplanned outcome of neoliberal reforms that have stimulated competition in both labour and consumption markets in most countries. Neoliberalism is a political model that transfers control of economic factors from the public sector to the private one and opens markets to trade. This took hold in some HICs from the 1980s, with increased economic integration and deregulation of trade and capital flows across the world (Dreher et al. 2008). Foreign direct investment became an increasingly important source of economic growth from this time onwards (Helleiner 1994). A systematic neoliberalization of governments has since taken place across the world, including in countries controlled or dominated by left-leaning parties. Disinvestment of international capital from nations that pursue redistributive monetary policies risks increased unemployment, and most govern-ments seek to avoid this (Cerny 1995). Thus, neoliberalism has become a political norm. Data from the *Economic Freedom of the World Index* (Fraser Institute 2013) (which amalgamates measures of size of government, legal structure and security of property rights, access to finance, freedom to trade internationally, and the regula-tion of credit, labour and business) show neoliberalism to have increased in all HICs, regardless of welfare regime, whether market liberal, conservative or Nordic (Schrecker and Bambra 2015). Neoliberal reforms have undermined personal stability and security to a greater degree among people of lower SES. Forms of insecurity differ between women and men, and are related to obesity production in different ways. An analysis of obesity rates by insecurity measures (International Labour Organization 2016) according to gender in 13 European countries (Belgium, England, Denmark, Finland, France, Germany, Ireland, Italy, the Netherlands, Norway, Portugal, Spain and Sweden) (Roskam et al. 2010) shows obesity rates among men to be greater in countries where union representation is low. In women, obesity rates are greater where greater proportions of women work more than 48 hours per week and the availability of state-provided health care is lower (Table 5.4). Non-standard parental work schedules (working at weekends, at night or during evenings), more common with neoliberalism, have also been shown to be associated with childhood overweight and obesity in an Australian sample, possibly because of the increased stress that comes with disrupted family life (Champion et al. 2012). Insecurity from illness (as expressed by private medical expenses as a per-centage of disposable income, a proxy for risk of incurring private medical costs) has the strongest relationship with obesity among all individual measures of social insecurity (Offer et al. 2010). The risk of serious illness and the high medical costs associated with it gives rise to psychological stress, and in some instances to sustained physical pain and discomfort. In the US, medical costs are the most frequent cause of bankruptcy (Warren and Tyagi 2003).

Neoliberalism is linked to increased inequalities in obesity rates because it carries significant psychological health costs (Moncrieff 2006; Schrecker and Bambra 2015; Sugarman 2015) that vary by SES. Anxiety levels in the US rose greatly between the 1950s and the late 1990s (Twenge 2000), while in the UK, levels of distress increased between 1991 and 2004 (Oswald and Powdthavee 2007). In 2006, 11 per cent of adults in the US had a lifetime diagnosis of anxiety (Strine et al. 2008); such

Table 5.4. Ordinary least squares regression of obesity rates by insecurity measures for 13 European nations

	B	Beta	t-statistic	B	Beta	t-statistic	B	Beta	t-statistic
Females									
Work >48 hours/week (per cent)	1.33	0.52	2.47*	1.54	0.60	3.20**	1.73	0.67	3.00**
State health care (per cent)	0.33	0.41	2.09	0.37	0.47	2.50*			
Representation	−0.05	−0.19	−0.87						
Constant	−22.59		−1.44	−30.59		−2.43*	−0.03		−0.01
F		6.59*			9.74**			8.96**	
Adjusted R^2		0.58			0.59			0.42	
Males									
Work >48 hours/week (per cent)	0.85	0.41	1.88	0.85	0.41	1.96			
State health care (per cent)	0.05	0.08	0.38						
Representation	−0.10	−0.50	−2.29*	−0.10	−0.53	−2.53*	−0.138	−0.72	−3.42**
Constant	7.68		0.58	12.38		2.64*	20.09		7.02***
F		5.72*			9.30**			11.72**	
Adjusted R^2		0.54			0.58			0.47	

*$p<0.05$, **$p<0.01$, ***$p<0.001$.
Calculated from data in Roskam et al. (2010); International Labour Organization (2016).

individuals are around a third more likely to be obese than those without such a diagnosis (Strine et al. 2008). Feelings of uncertainty and anxiety encourage overeating (Chapter 6), and people put on weight in response to stress, whether due to subordinate status (Marmot, 2004), inequality (Wilkinson and Pickett 2009), work insecurity (Hannerz et al. 2004) or financial insecurity (Gerace and George 1996). Overeating was never cheaper than from the 1980s to the late 2000s, when the US Food and Agriculture Organization extended real food price – a measure of the monthly change in international prices of a basket of food commodities (Food and Agriculture Organization 2017) – was at its lowest ever. Food prices have risen and become less stable since the global financial crisis of 2007–8, and rates of increase in obesity among women in the US have decelerated (Hruschka 2012). However, anxiety rates have not declined (United States Anxiety Disorder Industry 2016), and palatable energy-dense food remains a legal means of self-medication.

In an age when another way of dealing with anxiety through distraction, smoking (Kassel and Unrod 2000), is strongly disincentivized through taxation (Bader et al. 2011), consumption of highly palatable energy-dense food offers an alternative way of managing stress. Figure 5.8 shows the proportion of the US population smoking and the percentage of the US population who are obese, between 1970 and 2014. While the US had more than twice the rate of smoking as obesity before the 1990s, the proportion of the population that is obese has outstripped that of the population that smokes since then (Gruber and Frakes 2006), as the price of food declined in real terms by about a third between 1982 and 2007. While there is no clear and unambiguous evidence that higher cigarette taxes, which lead to lower smoking rates, might also lead to obesity (Gruber and Frakes 2006), smoking cessation is associated

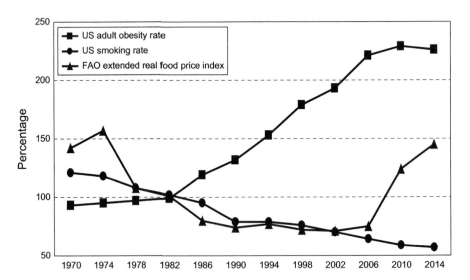

Figure 5.8. Changes in food prices, rates of smoking and obesity in the US, compared with 1982, set at 100 per cent (calculated from data given by Gruber and Frakes 2006; Ogden and Carroll 2010; Centers for Disease Control and Prevention 2011b; Ogden et al. 2015; Food and Agriculture Organization 2017).

with weight gain at the individual level (Klesges and Shumaker 1992; Swan and Carmelli 1995; Filozof et al. 2004).

There are other ways to assuage anxiety than through smoking or comfort eating. Antidepressants are legal, are effective against anxiety disorders (Donovan et al. 2010), and are the third most-prescribed drugs in the US. They may also have contributed to some of the rising obesity rates in the US. The earliest types of antidepressant that went into common usage were the tricyclics, of which amitriptyline and nortriptyline were among the most prescribed. These two are associated with significant individual weight gain (Serretti and Mandelli 2010), and may have contributed to increasing obesity up to the mid-1980s.

These antidepressants were largely displaced by selective serotonin reuptake inhibitors (SSRIs) in the 1980s, the most commonly known of which is fluoxetine (Prozac), which was released in 1987 to popular acclaim. The SSRIs vary in their effects on weight change (Hasnain et al. 2012), and although antidepressant use increased dramatically after 1987, tricyclic use declined, and population weight gain associated with the use of these substances may have also declined.

In childhood, emotional and psychological distress associated with socioeconomic disadvantage may be linked to overweight and obesity in HICs (Hemmingsson 2014). According to Hemmingsson (2014), families of low SES experience higher rates of disharmony, including food insecurity, weak support systems, marital problems and decreased coping skills as a result of parental depression, anxiety, apathy and powerlessness. This may precipitate childhood distress including low self-esteem, anxiety, insecurity, negative emotions and decreased coping, which can lead to physiological responses and maladaptive behaviours that can result in weight gain. A mediating factor in this parent–child relationship is seen by Hemmingsson (2014) to be overall insecurity, as evidenced by the higher rates of childhood overweight and obesity among children whose parents have non-standard work schedules (Champion et al. 2012).

Approaches to parenting may also contribute to this complex set of relationships. Children raised in authoritative homes (where limits are set, children are reasoned with, and parents are responsive to their children's emotional needs) eat more healthily, are more physically active and are less likely to be overweight or obese than children raised in homes where authoritarian, permissive, indulgent, uninvolved and/or neglectful parenting styles are practised (Sleddens et al. 2011). Authoritarian parenting is more common among families of lower SES (Hess 1970; Gecas 1979; Hoff et al. 2002) than among families of higher SES. Inequality also interacts with insecurity in the production of obesity in children through poor maternal nutrition and/or obesity in pregnancy (which can result in low and high birth weight, respectively), and parental patterning of unhealthy behaviour. Although difficult to demonstrate, breastfeeding may be protective against the development of overweight and obesity in children (Beyerlein and von Kris 2011). There are differences in breastfeeding initiation and duration according to SES, with mothers in routine and insecure jobs being at least four times less likely to initiate breastfeeding than women in higher managerial and professional positions (Kelly and Watt 2005).

Inequality, Obesity and Policy

At the national level, governments can regulate environments and food systems, and through taxation and social support can influence the extent of inequality in a nation. But the adoption of neoliberal policies in many countries has led to increased inequality and insecurity (Coburn 2000), and this has contributed to increased obesity rates (Offer et al. 2012). The political economic systems that especially favour neoliberalism have helped create obesogenic environments (Chapter 3), and have helped make cheap energy-dense food an attractive drug of choice among many seeking solace from the stresses of everyday life. Obesity policy, in neoliberal society, has perhaps unsurprisingly placed emphasis on the individual in anti-obesity and health policy, and much less emphasis on societal approaches. This has been the case in the UK, to varying degrees, since the 1980s. Only under the Labour Blair and Brown administrations between 1997 and 2010 was there an emphasis on reducing social inequality and increasing social inclusion, although neither featured strongly in the obesity policy of the time. Societal approaches have been downplayed in obesity-specific policy reports of subsequent administrations since 2010 (Ulijaszek and McLennan 2016), although considerable effort in obesity research and public health has since continued to try to find ways of reducing inequalities in obesity rates. In a recent systematic review of intervention types at the individual, community and societal level for reducing socioeconomic inequalities in childhood obesity, Bambra et al. (2015) concluded that, at best, most interventions do not increase inequalities in rates of overweight and obesity, but nor do they reduce them. These authors claim that reducing inequalities in childhood obesity should be possible at low levels of intervention, but that this would require political commitment to this aim.

While seemingly difficult to shift, inequalities in obesity rates are neither ahistorical nor politically neutral. Public health intervention studies assume a level policy playing field, but this is never the case. Upstream structural interventions have the potential to improve the health and nutrition of national populations, as well as the potential to reduce obesity rates. However, organizations that have a keen interest in their shape and structure include corporations, the world views of which are governed by economic rationality (Chapter 1), not the Weberian substantive rationality (Chapter 2) that underpins health and well-being. Friel et al. (2007) point to the strength of corporate power in structuring inequalities in health through trade agreements, where industry representatives greatly outnumber representatives from public interest groups, giving an imbalance between the goals of trade and consumer protection.

Through their keen involvement in such regulatory activities, corporations help design the structures that influence nutrition and health in favour of their interests (Panjwani and Caraher 2014). Even where corporations are urged to take more ethical responsibility for their actions, they usually shift responsibility onto consumers. For example, an investigation of corporate social responsibility policies of two supermarket retailers in the UK has shown them to use strategies in labelling and promotion that defer their responsibilities for regulating the food choices and intakes of children, to parents (Colls and Evans 2008). The discourse of personal responsibility in public health rhetoric places parents as central to the regulation of their children's weight, and blame for intergenerational patterns of obesity is frequently assigned to mothers (Warin et al. 2012). Parents of overweight or obese children in HICs are given this responsibility against a backdrop of social stigma concerning body fatness, which is concentrated on people of low SES because of the higher prevalence of obesity among them. People of low SES are also more likely to live in obesogenic environments where advertising and promotion of unhealthy foods is targeted at children (Schwartz and Puhl 2003), making it doubly difficult for parents to deliver on this responsibility. Parents of low SES are also less able to regulate the consumption of unhealthy foods of their children than are parents of higher SES, because of generally higher levels of household insecurity, parental anxiety and the relative lack of affordable healthy foods. Herrick (2009) has argued that the food and drink industry has used health as a corporate social responsibility strategy to maintain brand value and consumer goodwill, during a period when governmental and public calls in the US (including the National Governors Association 'Healthy America' task force) and the UK (Chapter 9) to address rising obesity rates demanded higher levels of accountability. The food industry may often use very specific interpretations of health in its view of corporate social responsibility. For example, industry strategies that promote narrow epidemiological understandings of obesity may divert attention away from specific foods (which they produce) to diet (which consumers construct by combining different foods produced by a wide range of companies). Focusing on diets deflects attention away from obesogenic foods that are designed, produced, marketed and sold by food corporations, to diets that are a matter of individual choice. They also dilute any regulatory action a government might take in relation to such foods.

Inequalities in obesity rates are outcomes of processes that are underpinned by economic, evolutionary, Weberian substantive and formal rationalities (Chapter 2). There may be ways in which a number of rationalities might be called upon to help reduce inequalities in obesity rates. Esping-Anderson (2002) called for more child-centred social investment strategies by governments, as life chances, including health, depend increasingly on the cultural, social and cognitive capital that citizens can amass. Following this, Marmot et al. (2010) have offered two policy goals that could help to reduce inequalities in obesity rates of children and adults alike: creating enabling societies that maximize individual and community potential, and ensuring that policies are centred on social justice, health and sustainability. Disadvantage starts before birth and accumulates throughout life, and Marmot et al. (2010) have put forward policy objectives based on these ideals. Giving every child the best start in life, enabling them to maximize their capabilities across life and have control of their lives, would recruit both economic and Weberian substantive rationalities to the regulation of childhood obesity. Furthermore, creating fair employment and good work for all, ensuring a healthy standard of living for all, creating and developing sustainable places and communities, and strengthening the role and impact of ill-health prevention would all recruit Weberian formal rationality to the reduction of inequalities in obesity within an overarching framework of reducing health inequalities.

6 Food and Eating

The global food system is the most significant upstream contributor to human nutrition (Lang and Heasman 2015) in most societies, and food has never been cheaper or as plentiful as in the past few decades. Furthermore, everyday life has never been more automated (Chapter 3). Dietary change, economic growth and public health practice have helped shift disease patterns in the world, from infection and its associations with undernutrition (Ulijaszek 1990, 1996b, 2000), to chronic disease and its associations with overnutrition (Hawkes 2006; Daar et al. 2007). Among the cheapest foods are those based on agricultural commodities, especially cereals, sugars and edible oils, which are easy to overconsume relative to energetic need, and which are produced in great quantity by the global food system. While food consumption is controlled and constrained politically, socially, culturally and personally (Ulijaszek 2002a) (Chapter 10), individual feeding constraints only become important in controlling body weight when there is a plentiful food supply. Where there is not enough to eat, obesity, as a population phenomenon, is unlikely to occur regardless of any genetic or epigenetic predispositions to it (Chapters 3 and 7). Human dietary change has been well investigated, from the transition to agriculture (Ulijaszek 1991), with modernization (Bindon 1982; Ulijaszek et al. 1987; Ulijaszek 2002b) and globalization (Drewnowski and Popkin 1997; Popkin 2009) (Chapter 7). Modernization and the globalization of food supply have affected the eating patterns of populations almost everywhere. Globalization of food has also disrupted, to varying degrees, local cultural and social mechanisms for restraint in food intake, contributing to the rise in obesity rates in many countries.

The global food system is expert and interactive, and is overwhelmingly shaped by large transnational corporations (Clapp and Fuchs 2009). The economic turnover generated by the production, processing, marketing and sale of food is the largest of all industrial sectors in the world (Lang and Heasman 2015). Table 6.1 shows the turnover of the top 20 global food retail companies in 2013 (Deloitte Touche Tohmatsu Ltd 2017), all of which are in the top 30 companies for all retail categories combined, representing in excess of 20 per cent of all retail globally. The food retailers that have greatest overseas penetration are French and German, and while most United States (US) food retail companies have low overseas country penetrance, this is more than made up for by the high penetrance of the world's largest food retailer, Walmart. The extent to which (and ways in which) the food system of a nation is integrated into the global food market depends heavily on history, tradition and the changeability or resilience of existing local and national food systems, as

Table 6.1. Top food retailers in the world in 2013

Rank	Company	Country of origin	No. of countries of operation	Retail revenue (US$ billion)
1	Walmart	US	28	446
2	Costco	US	9	105
3	Carrefour	France	33	99
4	Schwarz	Germany	26	99
5	Tesco	UK	13	99
6	Kroger	US	1	98
7	Metro Ag	Germany	32	86
8	Aldi	Germany	17	81
13	Casino Guichard-Perrachon	France	29	63
14	Groupe Auchan	France	13	62
16	Edeka Zentrale	Germany	1	60
17	Aeon Co	Japan	10	58
18	Woolworths	Australia	2	54
21	Rewe Combine	Germany	11	51
22	Wesfarmers	Australia	2	51
23	E. Leclerc	France	7	48
24	Koninklijke Ahold	Netherlands	7	43
26	J Sainsbury	UK	1	37
27	Intermarche	France	6	37
30	Safeway	US	3	35

Data from Deloitte Touche Tohmatsu Limited (2017).

well as political forces. Local and national food systems often have great time depth, as well as being extremely adaptable. Food is often framed as a consumerist issue, and it is far easier to focus on individual-level factors and place responsibility for obesity on this, as most policy responses have for decades (Chapter 8). The current logic of individualism in obesity prevention and treatment in the United Kingdom (UK), the US and Australia is consumerist, perhaps because the global food system, among other commercially dominated systems, relies on consumption to drive economic demand.

The physiological models that regulate appetite and food intake are complex at the individual level. With respect to eating and the production of obesity, the guiding principle is that palatability, satiation (physiological cues to terminate eating) and satiety (the feeling of fullness that often develops after eating) gained from foods are inversely related to their energy density (Gerstein et al. 2004). Thus, the overconsumption of fat and sugar (both macronutrient commodities that have increased in availability in recent decades) (Chapter 7) have been implicated in the production of obesity (Prentice and Jebb 1995; MacDiarmid et al. 1998; Kuo et al. 2008). At the global level, per capita availability of fat increased by 80 per cent between 1961 and 2011, and of sugar by 20 per cent across the same period (Chapter 7). The desire to eat sugar by individuals is reinforced behaviourally and physiologically, because it induces pleasure through, among other mechanisms, the neuronal release of opioids (Rada et al. 2005).

While fat on its own is not pleasant to consume (Drewnowski and Greenwood 1983), fat is a taste stimulus that does not vary according to mood (Platte et al. 2013), the hedonic response to which is greatly enhanced in complex food combinations, especially with addition of even small amounts of sugar (Drewnowski and Greenwood 1983). The human dietary preference for fat is deep set, since the availability of energy-dense foods rich in fat facilitated the evolution of increased hominin brain size (Navarrete et al. 2011). It is easy to overconsume fat passively, but not so easily sugar, except when the two are combined (Blundell and MacDiarmid 1997), and the combination of sweet high-fat foods in the diet has greater potential for individual weight gain than any other macronutrient combination (Emmett and Heaton 1995). People usually need to consume high-energy-density foods across long periods of time to become obese. The extent of energy imbalance in the production of individual obesity is on average less than 1 per cent of total daily energy intake, and this can happen easily, especially when consuming foods that are high in fat and/or sugar. Overeating on fat and sugar relative to dietary energy need is easy, partly because these two substances elicit minimal satiation and satiety (Blundell and Stubbs 1999).

The global food system has a considerable history, and this chapter describes how it has emerged from individually complex food systems with increasing globalization. It also considers how the global food system structures local food availabilities. It goes on to examine how the complexity of human appetite and the ideology of individualism in neoliberal society work to co-produce obesity, as human evolution-based preferences for energy-dense, palatable foods are exploited by food manufacturers and retailers.

The Structuring of Food Systems

Food systems are comprised of the totalities of processes and infrastructures involved in food production and consumption, including growing, harvesting, processing, packaging, transporting, marketing, preparation, consumption, and the disposal of food waste and food-related waste. These systems have undergone many transformations across prehistory and history (Ulijaszek et al. 2012). With increased population connectedness, technological development and trade, they have globalized and increased in complexity. The global food system is underpinned by the global food regime, which is the international rule-governed structure of food production and consumption. This integrates many different types of technologies and their regulation at many levels, including taxation and international coordination and consolidation of operations and practices (Friedmann 1993). The global food system and regime frame the food choices that people may have in everyday life. While there are very many local variants of diet and of dietary tradition, the global food regime structures the upstream availability of different foods and their relative costs. Price plays a big part in food choice almost everywhere, and is often more important an influence on what is eaten than tradition, especially among poorer people.

As well as being the key evolutionary transformation in the history of humanity (Winterhalder and Kennett 2009), the origin of agriculture had broad-reaching effects on human diet and represents the earliest systematization of food, one that underpins all present-day food systems. Starting from around 10000 years ago (according to location), radical economic, societal and technological change saw agriculture become the dominant mode of provisioning for the majority of the world's populations (Ulijaszek et al. 2012). With this came the dominance of grains and other carbohydrate-rich foods in most human diets. Different grain cultures emerged in different global regions: maize in Mexico, rice in China, and wheat and barley in the Middle East (Bellwood 2005). The ability to produce surpluses of grain set the conditions for the development of religion, government, and social and economic inequality (Ulijaszek et al. 2012), and the formation and growth of institutions that govern food systems to the present day. The emergence of agriculture as an economic system led to the spatial concentration of homogeneous resources, and an intensification of food production, storage and technological development (Lenski and Nolan 1984). The cultural complexity of agricultural food systems displaced the ecological complexity of hunter-gatherer food systems. The emergence, after the origins of agriculture, of city states such as Catal Huyuk in Anatolia and Eridu in Southern Mesopotamia, between 9000 and 7400 years ago (Taylor 2012), further intensified local food production and increased the complexity of the local food systems that serviced their populations. Such early cities were hotbeds of technological and societal innovation (Turok 2009), and required food systems that could generate significant surpluses to feed their populations. The subsequent growth of cities would have required increasingly complex control over food supplies, and would have led to food systems becoming overtly political. Early agricultural and political control of food supply were major factors in the early rise of Chinese civilization between 4600 and 3600 years ago (Dodson et al. 2013). Control of food supply has increased in complexity across millennia, to the point where it now contributes to obesity.

The early expansion of culturally complex food systems across Eurasia was advanced through trade and transport (Beaujard and Fee 2005). Contemporary China has three staple crops, rice, millet and wheat, of which the former two are indigenous. Wheat was an established crop in the Middle East by around 10000 years ago, was introduced into regions where millet was already well established as the dominant crop, from around 4000 years ago, and gradually expanded in importance across Eurasia (Dodson et al. 2013). The introduction of wheat to China and the diversification of agriculture there was coincident with the introduction of metallurgy and domestication of several species of animals (Lee et al. 2007; Dodson et al. 2009). Wheat agriculture in China predated the trade between West and East Asia by at least 2000 years (Dodson et al. 2013), when the Silk Road was established. This traded in goods, and facilitated the expansion and interconnection of local food systems across Europe and Asia. Ideas and people moved along what was a network of trade routes, involving, by around 2000 years ago, present-day China, India, Korea, Vietnam, Malaysia, the central Asian countries of Kazakhstan, Turkmenistan, Kyrgyzstan and Uzbekistan, Syria, Turkey and Italy (Figure 6.1), as well as Portugal and Sweden. While most foods could not easily travel long distance in bulk, ideas associated with growing new types of crop and herding different types of animal could. The Silk Road

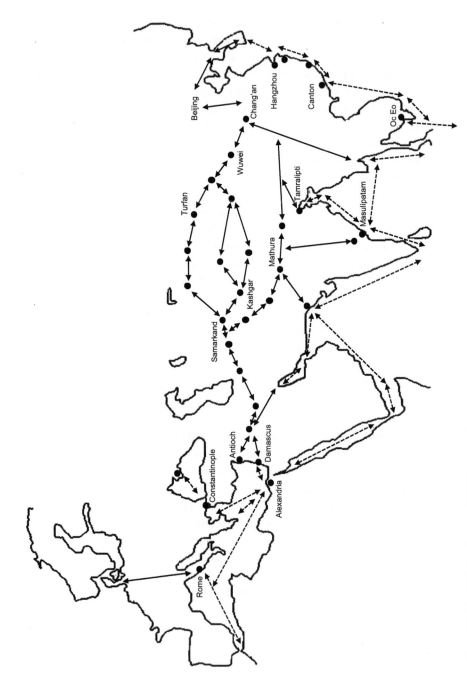

Figure 6.1. The Silk Road, around 2000 years ago.

played a large part in the growth of the civilizations of China, India, Persia, Mesopotamia, Egypt and Rome, and, through trade, speeded the interconnection of Asia and
Europe. As people, cities, politics and economics became connected, so did food
systems. This continued with the rise and fall of many empires: Roman, Gupta,
Sassanian, Byzantine, Bulgar, Pala, Fatimid Caliphate, Ottoman, Serbian and Mughal
among them. Empires put in place political systems and bureaucracies that more or
less unified territories (Eisenstadt 1969) and permitted the flow of goods, including
food, within their boundaries.

More than a millennium later, a number of these empires were to interact with
modern European colonial powers, which included Spain, Portugal, Holland, Great
Britain, Russia and France, extending links between the food systems of earlier empires
and colonizing nations. The European colonial nations went on to link Eurasian food
systems with those of the African and American continents, and to develop the first
global trade in food. From the sixteenth century, food became increasingly commodi-
tized and traded on a large scale. By the seventeenth century, globalization saw
cosmopolitan diets emerge in all places affected by colonialism, among both colonizer
and colonized. The effects of this process persist to the present day, illustrated as
follows with the case of Mexico and its neighbouring nation, the US.

Globalization and Food: The Case of Mexico

Urbanization and agriculture emerged in Mexico between 7000 and 9000 years
ago (Smith 1997), with maize as its dominant staple (Piperno and Flannery 2001).
Many city states had emerged and grown in the Valley of Mexico by the thirteenth
century (Smith 1984), with diverse food systems that incorporated mixed farming
and animal husbandry, underpinned by the dominant cereal crop, maize. The Spanish
conquests of Mexico (1519–1521), and of the Americas more broadly, led to the entry
of New World plants such as tomato, capsicum and potato into European diets, and
of European cereal crops such as wheat, and of livestock such as cattle and sheep,
into American diets. The Spanish introduced European systems of agriculture, along
with new plants and animals (including cattle, poultry, pigs, wheat and rice), which
competed for land and labour with native foods. Haciendas, or large estates, were
granted to Spanish settlers and institutions (including the Catholic Church) in Mexico
from 1529 onwards. These were usually plantations or large farms that intensified the
use of a smaller number of crops and animals for food.

The colonial imposition of the hacienda system marginalized indigenous populations and promoted the welfare of the Spanish colonizers, creating intense social
stratification in rural areas. The dietary consequences of this new type of inequality
were immense (Ulijaszek et al. 2012). The wealthy recreated the gastronomy of
Spain in the New World, based on both local and introduced ingredients. European
styles of food manufacture were also introduced, and from the seventeenth century,
cheese and sausage became part of the Mexican diet. For the upper classes of
colonial Mexico, the fusion of local and introduced foods prepared within the
structure of high European cuisine became the norm, and formed the basis of
present-day Mexican cuisine. The poor, however, reliant on wage labour from

hacienda managers for subsistence, struggled to sustain themselves on diets consisting overwhelmingly of maize and beans.

Similar events took place across the world in the same period. Mercantile trade among the colonies – Spanish, Dutch, British, French, Belgian, American and Russian – created a global food system that linked the food security of the colonial nations (and especially the new mercantile middle classes within them) with that of the colonizers. In the twentieth century, the Mexican food system continued to be shaped by the early colonial geography of social and economic stratification and of the commoditization of agriculture, but was increasingly exposed to foods from the increasingly economically and scientifically dominant US (Morris 1999). In the second half of the twentieth century, the ideology of modernization, open food trade policy and the penetration of heavily advertised transnational food products led to a devaluation of traditional cooking in Mexico. This encouraged poorer Mexicans to incorporate energy-dense foods rich in fats and refined carbohydrates into their diets, as the cheapest source of calories (Ulijaszek et al. 2012). In recent decades, agricultural decline in Mexico has taken place, as food policy there facilitated increased imports from the US and elsewhere (Barkin 1987), with more than 90 per cent of food imports to Mexico coming from the US by the mid-2000s (Pechlaner and Otero 2010). The recent supermarketization of Mexico, much of it under the control of a small number of transnational corporations, has facilitated this process. In Mexico and elsewhere in Latin America, the expansion of retail through supermarkets and large-scale food manufacture has deeply transformed the markets for food (Reardon and Berdegué 2002), local and imported.

Food consumed in Mexico has become increasingly energy dense, containing high proportions of fat and cereal-based refined carbohydrates, overwhelmingly as imports from the US. The most recent dietary trend in Mexico has been the rise of consumption of caloric beverages, including soft drinks, sweetened tea and coffee, sweetened juice and fruit drinks (Barquera et al. 2008, 2010; Stern et al. 2014). By 2012, the daily per capita energy intake from sugar-sweetened beverages (SSBs) in Mexico was the second highest in the world, after Chile but slightly ahead of the US (Stern et al. 2014; Popkin and Hawkes 2016). Together with the increasing mechanization of everyday life (Ulijaszek and Lofink 2006), dietary change has left Mexico with a burden of obesity that is now comparable to that of the US (World Obesity Federation 2017). Mexico now experiences disproportionate exposure to the US food system and its governance, which sets norms for a food regime that is almost universally obesogenic. In an attempt to regulate exceedingly high obesity rates, the Mexican government put in place a policy that imposed an excise tax on SSBs in 2014 (Stern et al. 2014). This resulted in a 6 per cent reduction in volume of SSBs purchased during the first year of the tax, the decline in consumption being greatest in households of lowest socioeconomic status (SES) (Colchero et al. 2016).

Globalization and the US Food System

Both US food policy and the US food system now largely shape the global food system, but the latter emerged and developed from the interaction of particular historical, political and economic circumstances. Mass production of food was an early aspiration of the US in the 1800s, with the agricultural settlement of European migrants across its land mass displacing Native American food systems. The US equivalent of the Silk Road was the railroad, which from the mid-nineteenth century accelerated trade and the movement of commodities, especially food, from the Mid-West to the rapidly expanding and industrializing cities. Developments in agricultural technology and transport brought new ways of food production, processing, distribution and delivery to its consumers (Popkin 2009), including the industrialization of many aspects of the food system. This industrialization included the development of new food technologies that made food safe and free from contamination, and that were used to create new food products and food categories (such as corn flakes and breakfast cereals). The food industry that emerged was engaged in the technological transformation of Mid-Western agriculture into part- or wholly processed food products for consumption overwhelmingly in the urban US, but also internationally. By the late 1800s, cheap food from the US was undermining food economies in Europe (O'Rourke and Williamson 1999), as well as shaping urban diets in Mexico.

Across the twentieth century, increasing standards of living and higher discretionary incomes in Europe, North America and Australia led to changing patterns of food demand and global food trade, which allowed the possibility of selling foods for which there was little or no prior domestic demand. Examples of this include the creation of a market for breakfast cereals (initially corn flakes, invented in the US in 1895) in Britain in the 1920s, the sale of mutton flaps from New Zealand to Pacific Islands nations (Gewertz and Errington 2010), and the sale of white chicken meat to Western national markets and red chicken meat to Eastern ones (Dixon 2002). Globalization in the late twentieth century saw the spread of the dietary cosmopolitanism of fast foods and convenience foods. This was, and continues to be, underpinned by the subsidy of specific agricultural commodities (including wheat, maize and soy), especially by the US government (Franck et al. 2013). The fall in food prices between 1980 and the year 2000 (Figure 6.2), largely in response to overproduction stimulated by agricultural subsidies in the US, helped the spread of fast food made from subsidized agricultural commodities, as well as contributing to obesity rates in high-income countries (HICs) more generally (Swinburn et al. 2009; Offer et al. 2010). According to Franck et al. (2013), while the first agricultural assistance programmes in the US were implemented in the 1920s to address the overproduction of commodities resulting from World War I support efforts, attempts to stabilize prices resulting from overproduction by introducing grain to open markets paradoxically encouraged farmers to grow even more. This trend continued well after World War II, when industrialization and specialization gave rise to increasingly large companies, traders, manufacturers and processors whose competitive interest was rooted in oversupply (Franck et al. 2013). By promoting quantity of production and sale, the US food system facilitated the emergence and growth of obesity across the second half of the twentieth century within its own borders (Ulijaszek et al. 2012; Franck et al. 2013) and in many of the nations that it trades with, especially Mexico (Popkin 2009).

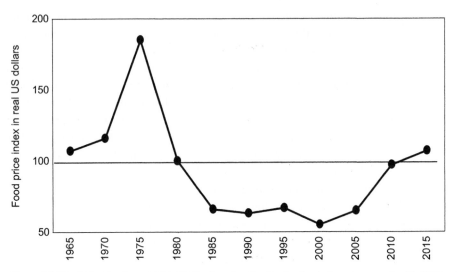

Figure 6.2. World food prices, 1965–2015, showing the food price index compared with 1980 set at US$100 (data from World Health Organization 2015b).

The Elaboration of Food Systems

Since the 1990s, increased gross domestic product (GDP) per capita in most nations (World Bank 2016a) has allowed the expansion of more diverse markets for foods and food products. With increased prosperity, there has been increased expression of status through material goods, including food (Bennett et al. 2009) (Chapter 5). Changing occupational structure in the US (less labouring work, more clerical and office-based work) and the continued rise of both secular society (Grossmann and Varnum 2015) and of consumerism (Veblen 1994) after World War II have favoured consumption (including that of food) increasingly to serve the reproduction of social class (Holt 1998). In recent years, increasing valorization of foods on the basis of both authenticity and exoticism has helped to resolve a tension in the US between the inclusionary ideology of democratic cultural consumption (for example, going to the ball game and eating a hot dog), and an exclusionary ideology of taste and distinction (dining out on French cuisine, for example) among those of high SES (Johnston and Baumann 2007). Globally, there has been extensive consolidation of science-supported food production, processing, marketing and retail, creating a complex food system that responds to, and creates markets for, novelty and status (Ulijaszek et al. 2012). As part of this process, a number of extremely palatable products high in sugar and/or energy density have become brand icons. These pander to individual taste preferences for sweetness and sensory stimulation, but need persistent marketing to uphold their status (Jones and Morgan 1994).

The retail of food in the second half of the twentieth century has increasingly involved branding, with many variants of similar foods competing for the attention of consumers. A brand is a set of associations that people make with a company or product, and usually not the product itself. While the material costs of Coca-Cola, for example, are small (primarily involving carbonation of water and of adding sugar and/ or high-fructose corn syrup to that water), its brand value (and status) lies with typical perceptions of it – that it is the original cola drink, its recipe is secret and unsurpassed, and it represents all things American or global, and youthful and energetic. Visual perceptions are key to its brand value, and include the unmistakable red and white logo, corporate colours, and the unique shape and tint of the original glass bottles (Design Council 2017). In the 2010s, Coca-Cola was the world's largest buyer of sugar, the biggest global brand of drink, and the most bought fast-moving consumer good (Kantar Worldpanel 2013). The power of this brand in conferring status upon its consumers is so high that it is not affected by strong evidence that links the consumption of sugar and high-fructose corn syrup-sweetened drinks to obesity and Type 2 diabetes (Ludwig et al. 2001; Bray 2004; Malik et al. 2006), and the dietary availability of high-fructose corn syrup with Type 2 diabetes (Goran et al. 2012).

Coca-Cola and other similar brand icons have helped spread the consumption of sugar throughout the world because of the power of brands, and not just because of the human desire to eat sweet things. Mintz (1985) argues that the rapid incorporation of sugar into the English diet in the nineteenth century reflected much more than the human dietary preference for sweetness. Sugar was implicated in slave labour and colonial domination, industrialization and urbanization, and was, according to Mintz, not merely a bearer of sweetness but a profoundly social substance (McLennan et al. 2014). In the time since Mintz's (1985) writing, the 'social' in sugar has, with the help of the Coca-Cola Corporation and others like it, extended with globalization. SSBs are centrally placed consumer items in the present era of global food corporations, mass consumption and the near-ubiquity of food marketing (McLennan et al. 2014). Choice and individualism are linked in the production of social status through consumption (Triandis 2001), and the global food system has accelerated the pace at which new food products are generated, dramatically changing what people can eat. Because food products are placed in competitive marketplaces in most countries, they must maximize some combination of novelty, status, price and palatability to ensure their economic success. The cheapest raw ingredients are overwhelmingly cereal-based commodities and fats, and it is unsurprising that the majority of food products on the market carry some palatable combination of these ingredients (Ulijaszek et al. 2012). Where palatability leads, increased consumption follows. The creation of highly palatable high-fat and/or high-sugar food products by transnational companies has had profound effects on human food consumption patterns, as well as creating ambivalence about eating (Maio et al. 2007) and facilitating disordered eating (Ifland et al. 2009) among many. Human appetites are evolutionarily rational and there is no surprise that such appetites are large. Constraints to the desire for sweetness are few, especially in individualist societies.

Appetite and Individualism in the Co-production of Obesity

Individualism, as a form of thought within political philosophy, has a deep history. Individualist societies are those in which people work to further their own interests without taking broader interests into consideration. Individualists are chiefly concerned about protecting individual autonomy against obligations imposed by social institutions (such as the state or religion). Individualism and self-governmentality are easier among those with greater control of their own lives, but more difficult when the physical, and mental resources for self-control are fewer, as among the poorer members of HICs (Chapter 4). From the late 2000s, individualism has been wed to the ideology of neoliberalism, a reassertion of liberal economic beliefs of the nineteenth century, which rose quickly in the 1980s (Haymes et al. 2015) under the legislations of Margaret Thatcher (1925–2013) in the UK and Ronald Reagan (1911–2004) in the US. The neoliberal turn in the UK changed workplace policy with respect to equality and diversity (Ozbilgin and Tatli 2011), public health approaches to illness (Evans et al. 2011) and politics more generally. The growth of consumerism that came with both neoliberalism and increased individualism helped create new, more fluid notions of society, which hollowed out the shared public domain, transcended territorial identities and eroded often solid identities based in work and locality (Bauman 2001, 2003). In the US, commercialism and consumerism has grown at the expense of political participation, and shrinking civil society has helped to fragment social life (Cross 2000). Along with cheap energy-dense food, the rise of neoliberalism and individualism across most societies set the conditions for the dramatic increases in obesity rates.

Individualism is linked to the production of obesity via the reduced need for people to recruit psychological feedback on personal actions and behaviour, thus reducing checks and balances on potentially socially unacceptable behaviour. Eating patterns have long been recognized as being linked to obesity (Stunkard 1959), and in the absence of socially calibrating checks and balances, cheap, palatable, energy-dense food can easily be overconsumed – for stress alleviation, pleasure or both (Sinha and Jastreboff 2013; Kringelbach 2015). In the absence of other forms of emotional support, consumption of cheap, energy-dense food can also provide comfort (Adam and Epel 2007; Groesz et al. 2012) (Chapter 5). Comfort eating usually involves the consumption of energy-dense foods in large amounts to reduce negative emotions, such as anger, loneliness, boredom and depression (Ganley 1989; Zivkovic et al. 2015). Eating high-fat diets also reduces sensitivity to stress as well as reducing stress itself, although there are withdrawal symptoms associated with reducing fat intake, which result in elevated stress and increased desire to return to a high-fat diet (Teegarden and Bale 2007).

In societies promoting individualist values, the regulation of obesity is often synonymous with individual self-control, and models for obesity regulation over-whelmingly focus on responsibilization and self-management: for eating healthily, maintaining a healthy body weight and undertaking adequate physical activity (Brownell et al. 2010; Ulijaszek 2014). Where self-management is difficult or impossible, as among young children, there is considerable responsibilization of parents and schools for the prevention and reduction of childhood obesity (Share and Strain 2008; Maher et al. 2010; Evans et al. 2011) (Chapter 5). The extent to which children can be morally responsible agents is limited, however (Ochs and Izquierdo 2009), and it is usually left to schools (Razer et al. 2013) and teachers (Bergem 1990) to provide moral guidance, when and where parents are generally not able to set consistent standards and expectations for their children (Ochs and Izquierdo 2009). In public health terms, schools are institutionalized risk environments where young people are most exposed to governmental strategies (Kelly 2003), including those of obesity prevention.

Models of obesity regulation in the age of individualism are made complicated by social inequality (Chapter 5). It has been argued in the UK that individualism has fragmented social class distinctions (Savage 2000). Government policy towards inequality during the Labour administration of 1997–2010 encouraged such fragmentation by focusing heavily on parenting as a means of encouraging children to become individualized agentic selves, rather than class-based social selves (Gillies 2005). This favoured the soft individualism of upper-middle-class communities above the hard individualism of working-class communities (Ochs and Izquierdo 2009). With respect to childhood, hard individualism encourages children to be tough enough to handle obstacles, while soft individualism encourages them to realize and express their full potential in the broader world (Kuserow 2004). Parents of lower SES more often practice authoritarian rather than authoritative parenting (Chapter 5), and often lack the skills to practise soft individualism (Gillies 2005), let alone have the desire or ability to teach it to their children. Many types of advertising and branding target soft individualism; this is particularly true for the marketing of high-fat, high-sugar food products. According to McLennan et al. (2014), consumption of specific brands has become a major form of meaning-making in the lives of people in HICs since the 1970s. Soft individualism, with the capital resources to support it (as among the established middle classes), may be better able to resist marketing and branding than soft individualism without those resources. For example, in an analysis of adolescent consumer behaviour in the US, Moschis and Churchill (1979) found middle-class adolescents to be better able to manage consumer finances, filter advertising and have stronger motivations for consumption than their lower-class counterparts. In the Labour-administered UK of 1997–2010, state support for the development of soft individualism in families of low SES used discourses of social exclusion, in which poorer parents were framed as lacking in personal skills and moral responsibility, destined to transfer disadvantage to their children in cycles of deprivation. The answer to this was to impose middle-class values at all points of contact with the state (Gillies 2005), be it social services, health centres or schools. The imposition of soft individualism on children of low SES, coupled with their higher susceptibility to branding and advertising and the greater symbolic value of fast foods to them (Chapter 5), may have helped the demand for obesogenic foods among poorer people in the UK.

The ideologies of individualism, in which people of higher SES are more able to self-regulate than those of lower SES (Ochs and Izquierdo 2009), are central to models of food consumption. The biological drives of feeding, hunger and the dietary regulation of macronutrient intake involve shared physiological and behavioural bases with other animals (Ulijaszek 2008), and are evolutionarily rational. Humans and other animals can easily overeat and deposit body fat when presented with diets that are plentiful, palatable and/or high in fat (Widmaier 1999). For humans, both food variety at a meal (Norton et al. 2006) and palatability (Bobroff and Kissileff 1986) play to powerful behavioural responses to food cues, as does the way in which food is consumed across the day. Social regulation of eating is less powerful in individualist societies, where the need for people to check their personal actions and behaviours is less. In countries that place great emphasis on maintaining a strong meal structure, there is less snacking (Fjellstrom 2004), which limits energy intake both socially and culturally (Jahns et al. 2001). By contrast, the highly individualist US has seen increased energy intakes from snacking among children and adolescents, while energy intakes from meals have remained constant (Jahns et al. 2001).

Responsibilized consumer citizenship places the task of resisting palatable, highly energy-dense foods upon the individual. Neoliberal systems and ideology form the discursive basis for many public health interventions (Ayo 2012), which assume that individuals will make rationally 'good' food choices once educated about the health implications of consuming obesogenic diets. These assumptions have been robustly critiqued (Guthman 2011), leaving open to question the idea that weight management should be left to the individual, and obesity control to individualism. While individual appetite control is frequently promoted as a rational way of controlling body weight, it does not come naturally to most people. Across human evolutionary time, uncertain and unstable environments would have made food security precarious at times, and being able to eat energy-dense foods plentifully when available would have favoured survivorship and, by extension, reproductive success (Ulijaszek and Bryant 2016). This would have been helped by heightened responses to visual cues associated with foods of high pleasure value when hungry (Cornier et al. 2007). Humans are predisposed to consume energy-dense, palatable foods quickly, as an evolutionarily based adaptation to food uncertainty. This evolutionary predisposition is a neurophysiological one, and has been retained in late modern times, where in HICs food uncertainty no longer exists and obesity rates are high and rising (Chapter 1). Food intake and energy expenditure are controlled by complex, redundant and distributed neural systems that reflect the fundamental biological importance of adequate nutrient supply and energy balance, and the predisposition of humans to develop obesity can theoretically result from any pathological malfunction or lack of adaptation to changing ecologies of this system (Berthoud and Morrison 2008). Neural feed-forward mechanisms that produce anticipatory responses to known food cues (sight, smell and even discussion of particular foods) dominate in situations where such cues are plentiful, food is easily available (because of low cost and the low amount of effort required to get it), is palatable and energy dense, and its consumption is socially enhanced (Berthoud 2004).

The predisposition to develop obesity may also be a species norm (de Vries 2007). The highly complex system of appetite regulation may not be able to adapt to the changed food ecology, where cheap energy-dense food products are easily generated by the global food system. While appetite regulation may not be able to adapt to such ecological changes, the gut microbiota do, but not necessarily in ways that mitigate against obesity. Modern industrial diets change the selection pressures on gut micro-biota ecology, and altered exposures of infants to bacteria (mostly through food) during early life may contribute to the subsequent development of obesity (Cho and Blaser 2012; Thompson 2012). Gut microbiota can aid nutrition, resist pathogens and promote human adaptive immunity (Dethlefsen et al. 2007). The microbial community composition of any person is inherited from their mother, and there is a core microbiome ecology that most people in a community share (Turnbaugh et al. 2009). In HICs, deviations from the community microbiome ecology are often associ-ated with obesity (Turnbaugh et al. 2009), and obesity in turn affects gut microbiotic ecology (Ley et al. 2005). Individualism may thus influence the likelihood of develop-ing obesity right down to the level of gut microbiota ecology.

Obesity, Consumption and Regulation

Behaviours associated with causes of obesity – eating more dietary energy than is expended, over prolonged periods – involve a range of potential rewards, including pleasure, distraction, and relief from stress and anxiety, which can ultimately lead to obesity. Such behaviours can be seen as being both evolutionarily and psychologic-ally rational. But models for the regulation of obesity are more likely to call on people to be or become economically rational actors. Self-control of appetites and impulses is easier among people who already have a good deal of control over their lives, and it is little surprise that individualist advice, towards economically rational action, is more easily enacted among those of higher SES. In HICs, obesity is usually highest among those of lowest SES (Chapter 4), where psychological and evolutionary rationalities (Chapter 2) predispose to overeating. Without social and environmental checks, enactment of these rationalities allows obesity to flourish.

Many of the ecological factors that are seen as having contributed to obesity across recent decades involve consumption, not only of highly energy-dense food and drinks, but of other goods and services (Ulijaszek 2007b). This includes the consumption of motor cars, personal computers and electronic devices, all of which facilitate increased convenience and physical inactivity (Ulijaszek 2007b). Consump-tion has been fostered by neoliberal approaches in politics since the early 1980s, which have also promoted ideologies of soft individualism (Ochs and Izquierdo 2009). Under the administration of Margaret Thatcher (1979–1990), the key political unit of the UK became the individual, and no longer society (Loughlin 2000). UK governments, of all ideologies, have framed policies overwhelmingly around the construct of the individual consumer as the target for regulation. This formulation of consumer citizenship obliges individuals not merely to be free to choose, but to be obliged to be free, and to understand and enact their lives in terms of choice (Rose 1999). The conflict embedded in this idea is that political theory defines citizens as being willing to serve the common good while consumers are defined by their individualist 'pleasure-seeking' characteristics (Mol 2009). Consumption and citizenship therefore often pull in different directions, perhaps nowhere more than in obesity governance. Obesity is overwhelmingly represented in the UK by the media, medical establishment and the government as an issue for personal responsibility and control, while government policy encourages good citizenship through consumption. For people, bounded and Weberian substantive rationalities (Chapter 2) concerning consumption, the body and citizenship are in constant internal negotiation and open to scrutiny by other people and institutions. This creates stress and anxiety, which can recruit overeating relative to biological need as an alleviation response, especially when energy-dense food is cheap.

In most HICs, food cues are abundantly present in obesogenic environments and in everyday life (Chapter 3), and are easy to respond to in the context of the stresses and psychological insecurities of everyday life. According to Wisman and Capehart (2012), the putting on of weight is a natural response to insecurity. Overeating relative to immediate energetic need is a response to insecurity with deep evolutionary roots (Ulijaszek and Bryant 2016). High reactivity to external cues such as colour, taste and smell (Ulijaszek 2002a), and subsequent disinhibited eating under conditions of food scarcity, and/or high levels of competition, would have favoured survivorship for most people and populations until fairly recent times. Human impulsivity in relation to food is both psychologically and evolutionarily rational, in that such rationalities underpin human decision making (Samuels and Stich 2004), which may be short term, situational, and related to pleasure, sociality and distraction. Binge eating may be a physiological feeding adaptation to food uncertainty (Cornier et al. 2007), which can take place in the absence of a hunger stimulus from the gut, especially when highly palatable foods offer pleasure (Lowe and Butryn 2007). Food consumption under such conditions has been termed hedonic hunger (Witt and Lowe 2014). Binge eating usually involves highly palatable, energy-rich food, typically high in fats, sugars or both (Avena et al. 2009), and might reflect the evolutionary drive for immediate rewards (Davis et al. 2010) in uncertain environments. Hedonic hunger is likely to have an evolutionary basis, and this mechanism has been deliberately hijacked by food corporations whose business is to trade in highly palatable, energy-dense foods.

Checks and balances to overeating include the many social conventions surrounding food and its consumption in all societies (Lupton 1996; Coveney 2000). These mediate the physiological drive to eat, whether for hunger, pleasure or both. Social and cultural mediators of eating are quite easily overridden, however, especially in individualist societies. Eating while listening to the radio or watching television, or eating in the presence of friends and family, increases the amount consumed (de Castro 1994; Bellisle et al. 2004). Both sets of circumstances allow diversion of attention from food consumption, resulting in reduced self-monitoring of intake, allowing food consumption beyond immediate needs (Hetherington et al. 2006). Engaging in other tasks, such as working and playing at the computer, also reduces self-monitoring of food intake. Individualism, modern life and cheap palatable foods make disordered, disregulated and distracted eating easy to practise. Regulating against overconsumption of food is extraordinarily difficult at a time when social and cultural checks and balances have been eroded in many societies, and when consumerism more broadly is celebrated.

Policy that calls upon people to take responsibility for their health through their eating actions is appealing – amounting to minimal political intervention – but has limited impact on obesity rates. Alternatively, the regulation of food systems by governments involves many competing interests and is politically difficult, but is more likely to be effective. There are several competing interests and rationalities in regulating complex food systems – governments seek to have a healthy and economically productive population, food corporations seek profit, and citizens often respond to policies and market forces individualistically. The food corporations are part of an expert system that no single agency controls, but many of them have financial turnovers that exceed those of many nations, and therefore carry economic power to the extent that individual governments may not be able to regulate them. Economic rationality (Chapter 1) is paramount for food corporations, their prime function being profitability. In meeting this aim, the processes of food production, transportation, processing, distribution and sale have been increasingly streamlined and increasingly focused on the production of foods that are highly profitable, which are mostly those that can contribute to obesity. Corporations make more profit if people eat more, and economic rationality in food production does not have to square with optimal nutritional health. In the UK, government policy introduced voluntary codes for self-regulation of food corporations in 2013 with the Food Network Responsibility Deal. While it ostensibly places responsibility on the food industry to drive change, in practice, consumers are framed as being ultimately responsible for their own consumption behaviours (Ulijaszek and McLennan 2016). The ideology of individualism and the rhetoric of choice is embedded in this and other food-related industry-led voluntary codes, as economic rationality is placed centrally to all policy in neoliberal society.

The stresses of everyday life in HICs are quite different from those experienced in the human evolutionary past, but the mechanisms for dealing with them are much the same. Overeating is often a personal response to chronic life stresses, such as those created by neoliberalism, especially in countries such as the US, the UK and Australia, where individual insecurity can cut across social gradients (Wacquant 2009). The amelioration of stress and anxiety through comfort eating helps drive up obesity rates in such countries (Offer et al. 2012). Work-related insecurity, including low income, poor job mobility and the absence of union protection, all of which have increased under neoliberalism, raise the likelihood of ongoing stress and illness. Responses to stress, in turn, include overeating and consumption of highly energy-dense foods, both of which are implicated in the production of obesity. The globalization of neoliberal values has been associated with increasing obesity rates across the world, largely as a consequence of the spread of modernity and of the formally rational systems of food production and delivery (Chapter 7). Expert systems such as those that secure global infrastructure and food operate as ecologies and are often too big and complex to be managed by individual governments. Many of the previously keystone functions of state have been handed over to corporate interests in recent decades, especially where such functions are served by expert systems. Corporate responsibility is secondarily social, and primarily economically rational, and answerable to shareholders. This is unlike state responsibility, in which any democratic government is answerable to the population that elected it. This has deep implications for the production of obesity into the future, and the next chapter considers the relationships between present-day (Pattern Four) nutrition transition as it is shaped by food system globalization, and its relationships with the transgenerational production of obesity.

7 Global Transformations of Diet

Obesity has been modelled in one way as an outcome of population exposure to obesogenic environments in high-income countries (HICs) (Swinburn et al. 2011) (Chapter 2), and in another, with modernization in economically emerging nations (Popkin 2009). The global rise in obesity is linked to the recent dominance of chronic disease over infectious disease in the world (Daar et al. 2007) (Figure 7.1) (Chapter 6). In low-income countries (LICs) and lower middle-income countries (LMICs), this is linked to globalization and the expansion of modernity, both of which are, in Weberian terms, forms of formal rationality dominated by economic, legal and scientific spheres through bureaucracy (Chapter 2). The emergence of obesogenic environments across the world has been described as being a part of nutrition transition in which urbanization, Westernization and economic change are accompanied by major shifts in diets to lower nutrient density and higher energy density (Popkin 1999, 2002). The nutrition transition model describes the changing patterns of diet and nutritional health that have accompanied various types of economic transformation, from hunting and gathering, through agriculture, industrialization and urbanization, to the modern and late modern world (Ulijaszek et al. 2012). It overlaps with other transition models, including those of epidemiological and demographic transition, both of which influence policy thinking (Chapter 8) and econometric modelling of obesity (Chapter 4). The term 'nutrition transition' is used in public health whenever links between newly affluent populations and dietary changes are discussed (Dixon 2009). According to Popkin (2002), this refers to Pattern Four, of five patterns of nutrition transition (Chapter 1), and this term is used throughout this chapter and elsewhere. The ecological changes described by the Pattern Four nutrition transition model are long term and persistent (Schmidhuber and Shetty 2005). Some of the major shifts associated with Pattern Four nutrition transition include falling food prices, rapid urbanization, new and improved marketing and distribution infrastructure, improved roads and ports, improved access to foreign suppliers and food imports, and globalization of food consumption patterns. These changes have resulted in a shift towards higher food energy supplies, as well as greater consumption of fats and oils and more animal-based foodstuffs (Schmidhuber and Shetty 2005).

In Schmidhuber and Shetty's (2005) framing, the expert global food system is dominated by very large corporations that dominate the production, manufacture, distribution and sale of food. Their profitability is linked to their increasingly global presence, there being a positive relationship between the annual retail revenue of the

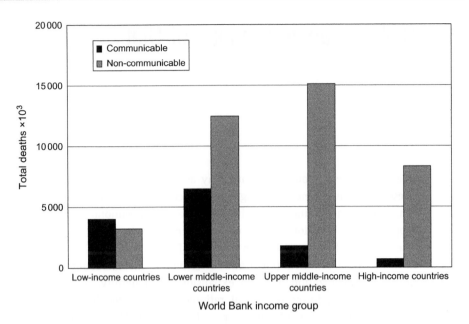

Figure 7.1. Deaths by major cause, by World Bank income group, in 2012 (calculated from data given by World Bank 2016b).

largest food corporations and the number of countries they operate in (Figure 7.2). At the population level, temporal shifts in food consumption patterns have different biological effects at different stages of the life course. According to developmental life-course science, the later in life they come, the less likely they will result in obesity. A number of countries entered Pattern Four of nutrition transition (Chapter 1) in the 1980s. In China, this happened after the major economic transformation of 1985 (Du et al. 2002), while in Mexico, the population shift to increased consumption of diets of higher fat and refined carbohydrate content took place between 1988 and 1999 (Rivera et al. 2002). Brazil entered Pattern Four nutrition transition between 1974 and 1989 (Monteiro et al. 1995). The timing of Pattern Four nutrition transition within a country may condition the extent to which post-natal nutrition contributes to present-day obesity rates. For example, a 50-year-old person in China in 2015 may have experienced lower birth weight and poor nutrition in the first 20 years of life, followed by 30 years of improved nutrition. A 40-year-old in China in 2015 may have experienced low birth weight and 10 years of poorer nutrition in childhood, followed by 30 years of improved nutrition. A 30-year-old in the same year is more likely to have experienced good nutrition, or overnutrition, across their entire life. Despite their ages being only 10 years apart, these three hypothetical individuals would have different predispositions to obesity based on their earlier life history and nutritional experience, in relation to the timing of entry into Pattern Four nutrition transition. In relation to obesity, Pattern Four nutrition transition is incomplete without being related to early life or development origins models.

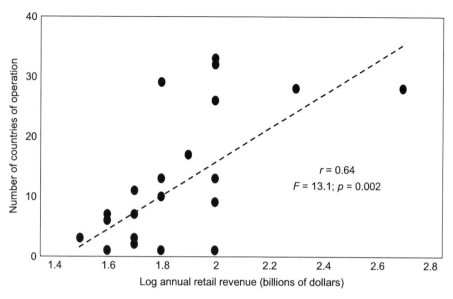

Figure 7.2. Number of countries of operation of top food retailers globally, according to annual retail revenue, in 2013 (billions of dollars) (from Deloitte Touche Tohmatsu Ltd 2017).

The most important developmental life-course periods related to obesity are early: in fetal growth, and in infant development soon after birth (van Dijk et al. 2015). At both times of life, nutritional predispositions to later-life obesity operate through developmental plasticity and epigenetics. Being born before Pattern Four nutrition transition and then experiencing greater availability of dietary energy subsequently has profound implications for population obesity rates. Low birth weight and subsequent catch-up growth are associated with hypertension, Type 2 diabetes and obesity in later life, as a consequence of persisting physiological and metabolic changes that accompany slow growth in utero and compensatory growth in early post-natal life (Gluckman et al. 2011). This chapter examines the relationships between population obesity and models of Pattern Four nutrition transition as experienced at early stages of the life course, and considers how models of developmental plasticity and epigenetics (Burdge and Lillycrop 2010) may be related to nutrition transition models in helping to shape globally complex patterns of obesity. The chapter starts, however, with a description of the Pattern Four nutrition transition model, which structures the political ecology of obesity.

Nutrition Transition and Obesity

Pattern Four of nutrition transition usually involves shifts away from plant-based diets towards higher per capita consumption of animal-based foods, oils and fats, processed sugars and processed carbohydrates (Popkin 1999). Dietary energy availability has increased in all global regions in the past 50 years or so (Figure 7.3), but to

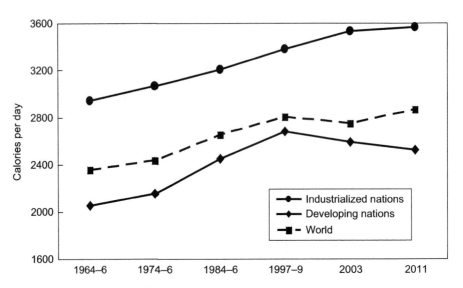

Figure 7.3. Global per capita food availability (data from World Health Organization 2015b; Food and Agriculture Organization 2017a).

a greater extent in upper middle-income countries (UMICs), LMICs and LICs than in HICs. There has been some convergence in daily per capita calorie availability in all regions of the world apart from South Asia and sub-Saharan Africa (Figure 7.4). The regions with the highest daily energy availability per capita over the longest period since the 1960s (Europe, North and Central America) subsequently developed the highest obesity rates, supporting, at a macro-level, the view that time depth and cross-generational factors are important in the production of population obesity. Populations in the Near East and North Africa, Latin America and the Caribbean have the next highest rates of obesity, among the highest rates of increase in obesity rates since the 1980s (Stevens et al. 2012), and among the greatest increases in per capita dietary energy availability between the 1960s and 1980s. Figures 7.5 and 7.6 show global averages of per capita dietary energy availabilities from cereals, fats, meat and sugar between 1961 and 2011. Cereals contribute most to dietary energy availability, per capita availability increasing slightly to the late 2000s. The per capita daily availabilities of sugar, fats and meat have all increased steadily across the second half of the twentieth century and beyond. The increases have been most striking in fat and meat availability, the latter of which has more than doubled. Among HICs and increasingly among UMICs, national food supplies have become more plentiful and diverse, broadly enhancing food security to all but those living in poverty (Dixon 2009). Globally, total energy availability per capita increased by 30 per cent between 1961 and 2011, with energy availability from carbohydrate increasing by 22 per cent. Populations around the world now obtain on average 57 per cent of their daily energy intake from carbohydrate, with intake from sugar being around 7 per cent of total energy availability (Food and Agriculture Organization 2017a). As rates of

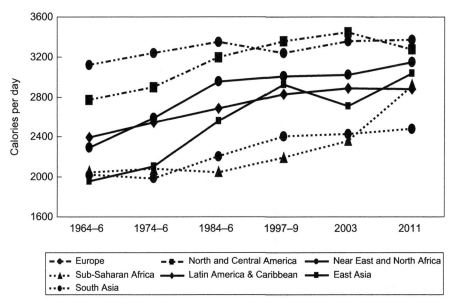

Figure 7.4. Per capita food availability by global region (data from World Health Organization 2015b; Food and Agriculture Organization 2017a).

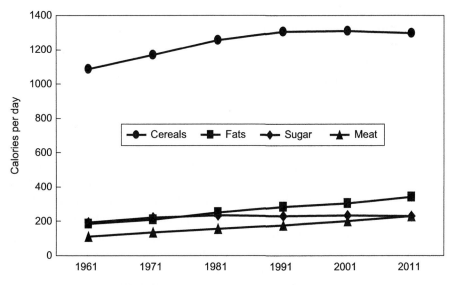

Figure 7.5. Global per capita dietary energy availability from food types characterized by Popkin (2002) as increasing with Pattern Four nutrition transition (data from Food and Agriculture Organization 2017a, b).

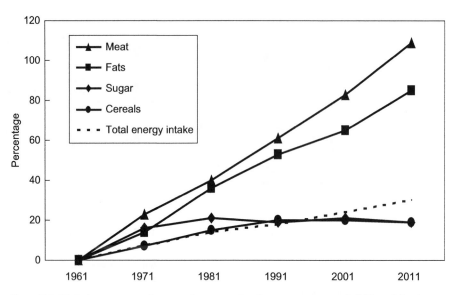

Figure 7.6. Global percentage increase in per capita dietary energy availability of food types characterized by Popkin (2002) as increasing with Pattern Four nutrition transition, with 1961 set to zero (calculated using data from Food and Agriculture Organization 2017a, b).

obesity in most countries have increased (Stevens et al. 2012), so too have the rates of Type 2 diabetes, brought about by hyperinsulinaemia and insulin resistance from high levels of consumption of refined carbohydrates across many years, superimposed on physiological developmental, epigenetic and genetic predispositions (Chapter 3).

Pattern Four nutrition transition is one outcome of recent globalization, a process that has resulted in increased mobility of goods, services, labour, technology and capital throughout the world (Chapter 10). Globalization has accelerated across recent decades, as economic integration and deregulation of trade and flows of capital have increased among the vast majority of nations (Dreher et al. 2008) (Chapter 8). The timing and extent of this process since the mid-1980s (Quinn et al. 2011) is illustrated in Figure 7.7. The two measures of global financial integration shown, capital account (CAPITAL) and financial current account (FIN_CURRENT), are from the International Monetary Fund's *Annual Report on Exchange Arrangements and Exchange Restrictions* (AREAER), the primary source for most indicators of global financial integration. They have been calculated from data given in AREAER reports for 122 countries, using six categories of global trade: payment for imports; receipts from exports; payment for invisibles (non-tangible goods and services, including banking, intellectual property and patents); receipts from invisibles; capital flows (movement of money for investment, trade or business) by residents; and capital flows by non-residents (Quinn et al. 2011). Both CAPITAL and FIN_CURRENT give similar values for levels of integration and openness of world finance, both rising rapidly from the mid-1980s. Integration took place faster and earlier in some countries and regions than others, and the countries that engaged in this process earliest

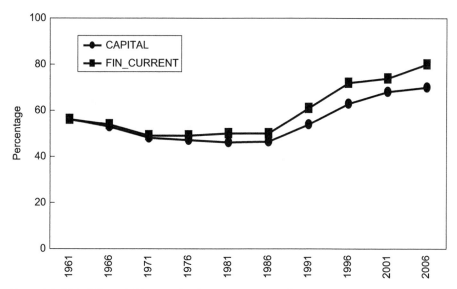

Figure 7.7. Global financial integration by two measures, from 1961 to 2006, on a scale from zero (no integration) to 100 (total integration) (adapted from Quinn et al. 2011).

saw their average economic output rise almost threefold from the late 1970s onwards (Prasad et al. 2005). Integration of trade has greatly contributed to economic growth, and globalization has enhanced the economies of many countries (Huneault et al. 2011). However, the worldwide proliferation of transnational corporations (transnational food companies among them) that has accompanied globalization may have played a key role in influencing rising rates of obesity (Huneault et al. 2011; Costa-Font et al. 2013), especially through the marketing and sale of ultraprocessed foods, soft drinks and fast food from this time onwards (Hawkes 2005; Thow and Hawkes 2009; de Vogli et al. 2011; Monteiro et al. 2015). Global economic integration and the deregulation of trade and of flows of capital (Dreher et al. 2008) provided the conditions for this to happen.

The greatest increases in obesity rates (Stevens et al. 2012) are in the world's regions that have experienced the greatest extent and longest period of economic integration and trade liberalization (Figure 7.8). The wealthy North American subregion and the Central Latin American subregion currently have the highest rates, and rates of increase, in obesity among large nations. The North American Free Trade Agreement (NAFTA) was brought into operation in 1994, eliminating nearly all barriers to trade and investment between the United States (US), Canada and Mexico within a decade of its initiation. NAFTA opened the door to food commodities (including prepared foods, usually of high energy density) from the US to Mexico (Chapter 6) at a time when Mexico was unable to meet demand for food by its own production (Pechlaner and Otero 2010). Across the period of trade liberalization (between 1988 and 1999), the contribution of fat to per capita energy availability in Mexico increased from 23 to 30 per cent (Rivera et al. 2004), as the purchase of

(a)

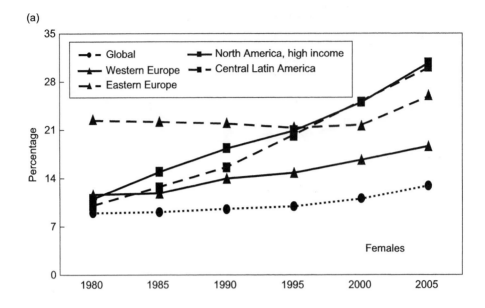

(b)

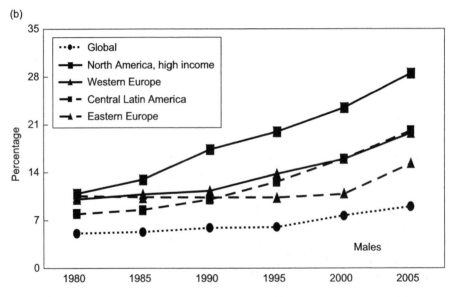

Figure 7.8. Global and regional trends in adult obesity rates between 1980 and 2005 for females (a) and males (b) (calculated from Stevens et al. 2012).

ultraprocessed foods, high in refined carbohydrates and sugar, increased. At the same time, the purchase of more nutrient-rich foods such as fruit and vegetables and milk and dairy products declined (Figures 7.9 and 7.10) (Rivera et al. 2004). Both changes contributed significantly to the rapid increases in rates of obesity (Rivera et al. 2004) and Type 2 diabetes there. Mexico is the most populous and economically most

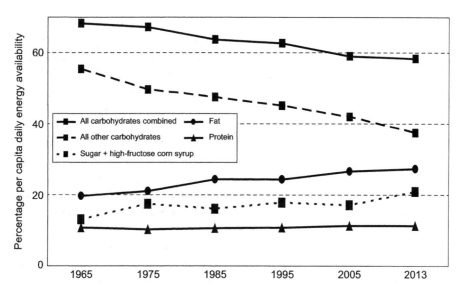

Figure 7.9. Changes in the proportion of daily per capita energy availability from different macronutrient types in Mexico, from 1965 to 2013 (data from Food and Agriculture Organization 2017a, b).

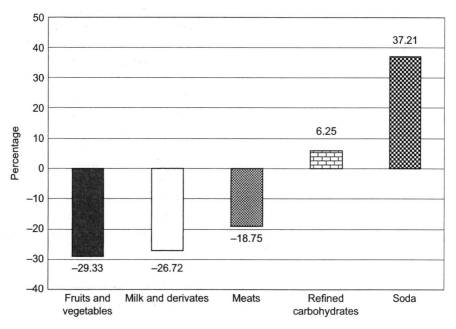

Figure 7.10. Percentage changes in mean food purchases in 1998 relative to 1984 by food group in Mexico (data from Rivera et al. 2004).

powerful of the Central Latin American countries, and the obesity rates there dominate the rates presented in Figure 7.8 for that subregion, increasing at around 10 per cent per decade between 1980 and 2008 (Stevens et al. 2012). Mortality from Type 2 diabetes increased threefold between 1990 and 2010 (Davila-Cervantes and Pardo 2014), making it the dominant disease issue in Mexico as the principal cause of death in women and the second most common cause of death among men since the year 2000 (Rull et al. 2005).

In Western Europe, obesity rates have risen steadily since the expansion of financial integration in the mid-1980s, while in Eastern Europe they remained relatively constant until the 2000s, when they accelerated. The difference in patterns of obesity between Western and Eastern Europe reflect one of the major events in twentieth-century history, the collapse of Soviet-styled communism. Eastern European countries were part of the Soviet Bloc until 1990, but undertook financial integration with the rest of the world rapidly after independence (Lane and Milesi-Ferretti 2007). The financial integration of the Eastern European countries had an important influence on the production of obesity in those countries, due largely, but not solely, to changing diets and increased dietary energy availability (Ulijaszek and Koziel 2007). Other contributors to the increased obesity rates in Eastern Europe after the transition from communism to free-market economics include general declines in physical activity levels, increased real income and increased economic inequality. With respect to physical activity, political liberalization meant a relaxation of the physical fitness expectations of the communist state (Arnaud and Riordan 1998). Data from the *International Health and Behaviour Survey* carried out among university students in 23 countries between 1999 and 2001 showed female youth in Eastern European countries to be much less physically active than their counterparts in Western European and North American nations (Haase et al. 2004). Most Eastern European nations experienced a decline in real gross domestic product (GDP) after the collapse of communism, but this rebounded in the 2000s. For females, who had much higher rates of obesity than men prior to the collapse of communism, obesity showed little decline with economic decline, largely because the cheapest foods were energy dense, and because physical activity levels also declined. Open markets in Eastern Europe also increased the exposure of women to Western ideals of beauty and bodily thinness through the media (Vignerova et al. 2007). Such exposure was much greater in urban than in rural areas (Hoek and van Hoeken, 1996), and this may have contributed to increased urban–rural inequalities in obesity rates among women in Eastern European countries after the collapse of communism.

The transition from communism to free-market economic systems favoured the wealthier nations of Eastern Europe (Poland, the Czech Republic and Hungary) with greater dietary energy availability than the poorer ones (Ulijaszek and Koziel 2007). Although the rise in obesity rates in the Eastern European countries is associated with higher GDP, it also is also associated with increased income inequality since the collapse of communism (Figure 7.11). Economic inequality increased sharply in the Eastern European nations after 1990, soon after the end of communist rule (Rosser

(a)

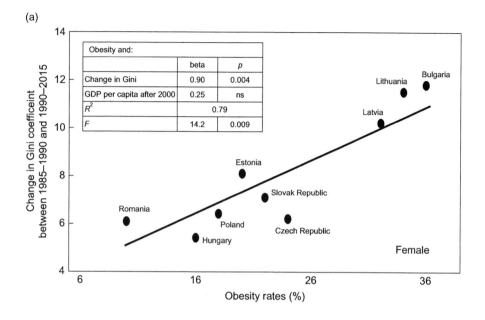

(b)

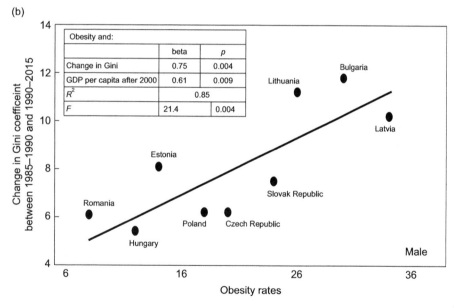

Figure 7.11. Relationships between increased economic inequality after the collapse of communism in Eastern Europe (between 1985–90 and 1990–2015) and adult obesity in the 2000s in females (a) and males (b) (data from World Bank 2016a; World Obesity Federation 2017).

et al. 2000). It continued to increase into the 2000s, fluctuating thereafter at higher levels than before 1990, with much greater between-nation variation in income inequality than under communist rule (Figure 7.12). In contrast to Eastern Europe, Western Europe has experienced a steady rise in obesity rates associated with both

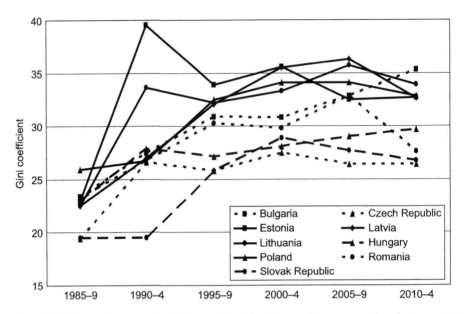

Figure 7.12. Economic inequality (Gini coefficients) of Eastern European nations between 1985 and 2014 (data from World Bank 2016a).

economic inequality (Pickett et al. 2005) and increasing insecurity (Offer et al. 2010), again from the mid-1980s.

Although globalization and the integration of trade have enhanced the economies of many countries (Huneault et al. 2011), they have also have generated imbalances of wealth and power between rich and poor countries (Schrecker et al. 2008), and have contributed to global increases in obesity rates (de Vogli et al. 2014). An analysis of the effects of economic globalization on population-level body mass index (BMI) of adults using aggregate data from 127 countries confirms this effect, after adjustment for GDP per capita, urbanization and population size, in both longitudinal cross-national panel data analyses and in time-series analyses (de Vogli et al. 2014) (Figure 7.13). The mechanisms that connect economic globalization, inequality between countries and BMI remain unknown, but it might be that the liberalization of capital and trade facilitated the rise in obesity rates by promoting the growth of transnational corporations and their greater mobility across borders (Tausch 2012), especially of transnational food corporations (de Vogli et al. 2014). Only a minority of such corporations have a commitment to health improvement or, in the case of transnational food companies, in mitigating the possible risk of obesity from consumption of their products.

Economic and Weberian formal rationalities (Chapters 1 and 2) underpin the processes just described, with global acceptance by governments of economic growth as a measure of progress. This yardstick of progress can be challenged, however. The substantive and psychological rationalities (Chapter 2) that reflect human desires

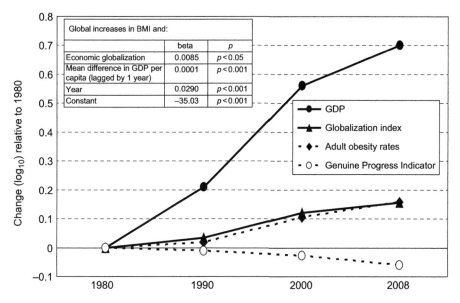

Figure 7.13. Global increases in body mass index (BMI), globalization index and gross domestic product (GDP) (calculated from de Vogli et al. 2014), global adult obesity rates (data from Stevens et al. 2012) and Genuine Progress Indicator (data from Kubiszewski et al. 2013), on a logarithmic scale, with 1980 set as the baseline.

beyond the pursuit of profit have mental health consequences, and the extent to which money can buy happiness is limited (Dolan et al. 2008). Measures of societal progress have been developed that include social and environmental factors, the Genuine Progress Indicator (GPI) being a measure that incorporates both (Lawn 2003). The GPI is a measure of GDP (value of all goods and services produced), minus the environmental and social costs of attaining that level of GDP (Kubiszewski et al. 2013), which include the environmental and social costs of economic development (Costanza et al. 2014). It is an economic measure that takes account of some of the negative aspects of economic growth: environmental degradation, which remains controversial (Farhani et al. 2014), inequality (Atkinson 2015) and unhappiness (Easterlin 2001). The GPI incorporates income inequality and stress-related insecurity due to underemployment, changes in family structure and loss of leisure time, all factors that are associated with obesity (Dallman et al. 2003; Pickett et al. 2005; Offer et al. 2010, 2012) (Chapter 5). The global rise in adult obesity rates since 1980 (Stevens et al. 2012) is positively associated with increasing GDP and globalization (de Vogli et al. 2014). However, it is also associated with declining GPI (Figure 7.13), supporting the view that the negative aspects of economic growth (especially inequality and insecurity) are important in the production of population obesity (Chapter 4).

Nutrition transition theory describes changing patterns of food availability and nutritional disorder associated with economic transformation (Chapter 1). The systems that drive Pattern Four nutrition transition are underpinned by economic and Weberian formal rationalities, involving large bureaucracies, technical orientations to problem solving, and an orientation to economic approaches in government and business. But in everyday life, Pattern Four nutrition transition is negotiated by people using Weberian practical and substantive rationalities. Human engagement with food, including its purchase, consumption and negotiation of its social and symbolic value, involves Weberian substantive rationality, especially when food is thought of as something more than fuel. Described in terms of competing cultural and social norms within and across societies (Lupton 1996; Coveney 2000), the competition for people's attention between international foods and traditional foods in Pattern Four nutrition transition can also be seen as involving conflicting and competing rationalities. In Mexico, for example, the economic and Weberian formal rationalities that naturalize economic growth as desirable also legitimize the sale and consumption of high-energy-density foods and sugar-sweetened beverages as modern (and thus formally rational) forms of consumption. The Weberian substantive rationality that draws on traditional forms with respect to food in Mexico can easily be thought of as being sentimental, and can be ignored by authorities because it impedes modernization. In contrast, in Italy and Austria, the Weberian formal rationality of governments and corporations is challenged by substantive rationalities of trust in discourses about food and other aspects of everyday life (Sassatelli and Scott 2001).

Pattern Four nutrition transition is global and cross-generational, and often invokes clashes of rationalities at the local level, through considerations of what foods are appropriate for which circumstances, including diet in pregnancy and lactation, foods for infants and young children, and types of meal. Some of the biological factors that influence the development of obesity are also cross-generational, and include developmental programming and child growth (Barker 2004; Rolland-Cachera et al. 2006). The science of epigenetics models gene expression as being both biologically and environmentally heritable, and as possibly influencing future rates of obesity (Chapter 10). The next section considers the relationships between the nutritional changes that accompany modernization and globalization, and the developmental programming and epigenetic factors that can influence the onset and progression of obesity.

Life History, Life Course, Developmental Programming and Epigenetics

Transgenerational effects in the causation of obesity were first identified among survivors of the Dutch famine winter of 1944–5 (Ravelli et al. 1976). Follow-up of offspring from mothers exposed to this famine by epidemiological science (Szyf 2015) showed fetal starvation in early pregnancy to be associated with higher rates of obesity later in life. Epigenetic changes affecting growth, metabolic disease and obesity predisposition were found in the same individuals (Heijmans et al. 2008; Lumey et al. 2012), offering a possible physiological mechanism for these relationships. DNA methylation and demethylation are among several related mechanisms by which genes are regulated epigenetically, and such regulation has been identified as being related to subsequent obesity in this group (Heijmans et al. 2008), persisting into the next generation in males but not in females (Veenendaal et al. 2013). The observation that late-onset chronic diseases are programmed by transient (rather than longer-term) early-life experiences has led to the speculation that developmental programming may have an epigenetic component (Vickers 2014).

Two evolutionary models can help place these observations in a broader ecological context. The first of these, using the life-course perspective, views early-life cues as inducing highly integrated responses in traits associated with energy partitioning, maturation and reproduction, such that the individual phenotype is better adapted to the environment that is anticipated to exist across the rest of life (Charnov 1993). For example, maternal and/or neonatally derived nutritional or endocrine cues signalling a threatening environment might favour early growth and reproduction over investment in tissue reserve and repair capacity. Such a response prioritizes insulin resistance and capacity for fat storage for more immediate survival, both of which increase susceptibility to metabolic dysfunction and obesity (Yajnik and Deshmukh 2008), and neither of which is usually expressed if the nutritional ecology is and remains energy limited. For the fetus, responses to environmental stresses include developmental adaptations that maximize immediate chances for survival. These adaptations may include resetting metabolic homeostasis and/or endocrine systems, and downregulating physical growth and development. While these changes in fetal physiology might be beneficial for short-term survival in utero, they might also be maladaptive in post-natal life, contributing to poor health outcomes when offspring experience catch-up growth, diet-induced obesity and other ecological changes associated with modernization. In this sense, developmental programming of adult health and disease can be considered to be part of a broader life-course framing rather than an independent phenomenon (Skogen and Overland 2012).

The second evolutionary model, that of the predictive adaptive response (Gluckman and Hanson 2004), views fetal physiological and developmental responses to mismatches between pre- and post-natal environments as adaptive preparation for their breeding, or 'mature', environment (Wells et al. 2012). For humans living in transitional ecologies (for example, those entering Pattern Four nutrition transition), developmental adjustments are major determinants of subsequent chronic disease (Vickers et al. 2007). Developmental adjustments to adverse environments in utero may be associated with epigenetic processes, either reversible or irreversible. Epigenetics and developmental plasticity are both evolutionarily rational, inasmuch as parental effects on reproductive fitness can operate through context-dependent transgenerational transmission of adaptive phenotypes (Uller 2008). Although the initial focus of developmental programming of adult health and disease research was on the effects of maternal undernutrition, restricted fetal growth and low birth weight, the issue of maternal and fetal overnutrition has gained prominence more recently in the context of global obesity (McMillen et al. 2008). With Pattern Four nutrition transition, developmental plasticity might be maladaptive in populations that are moving from high to low mortality due to extrinsic factors such as infectious disease, and from low- to high-energy-density diets and caloric plenty, with increased potential for longevity and/or susceptibility to metabolic disease (Sloboda et al. 2009).

In the early 2000s, the idea that pre-natal overnutrition might affect lifelong risk of obesity was used to explain relationships between obese mothers, fat babies and the transmission of obesity across generations (Warin et al. 2012), invoking epigenetic mechanisms (Rokholm et al. 2011). Epigenetics involves the regulation of gene expression by environmental factors, which include nutrition (Jang and Serra 2014), and much of the missing heritability in genetic explanations of obesity (Chapter 2) could be due to epigenetic silencing of obesity susceptibility genes. According to Furrow et al. (2011), variations in epigenetic and environmental states can give highly heritable phenotypes through a combination of epigenetic and environmental inheritance. In combination, these two inheritance processes can produce higher familial covariances than can purely epigenetic inheritance, and similar covariances to those due to genetics alone. Over 100 differentially methylated sites at birth are known to be associated with obesity phenotypes in later life (van Dijk et al. 2015). It was initially thought by epigenetic scientists that the increasing prevalence of obesity in women of reproductive age might create transgenerational amplification of obesity with metabolic consequences in subsequent generations (Ebbeling et al. 2002). This idea was further developed in relation to the role of obesity on fertility, intergenerational tracking of high maternal body weight, and increased risk of metabolic disease and perturbed reproductive functioning in grown-up offspring (Davies 2006). Pregnancy and birth weight are central to the development of predispositions to obesity (Figure 7.14), and while low birthweight is associated with obesity in subsequent life in transitional environments, birth is a period of high maternal and infant mortality. Across societies, infant mortality varies in a J-shaped manner with birth weight, although the exact relationship differs across populations and time. The relationship between neonatal mortality and birthweight is robust, even with large mortality rate declines: Figure 7.15 shows this to be the case for the US population between 1950 and 1998. Low birth weight thus persists in populations that experience modernization, as does the attendant risk of low birth weight-related obesity. The effects of low birth weight often persist into infancy, and are associated with slow growth, small body size and increased mortality, especially in LICs and LMICs; these post-natal effects are reversed in Pattern Four nutrition transition in many populations, with greater likelihood of increased obesity rates.

Convergence of scientific research on developmental programming, epigenetics and the life course has taken place in the last decade or so (Warin et al. 2015), with attempts to understand how the former two sets of biological processes are structured by the latter, but also revealing the biocultural complexity of transgenerational obesity production. Adverse pre-natal and early post-natal environments can increase the likelihood of becoming obese in later life (Heijmans et al. 2008; Reynolds et al. 2013), with pregnancy and lactation influencing these outcomes (Muhlhausler et al. 2013). Pregnancy is a critical period for the establishment of the fetal epigenome (van Dijk et al. 2015), while epigenetic programming is especially active from

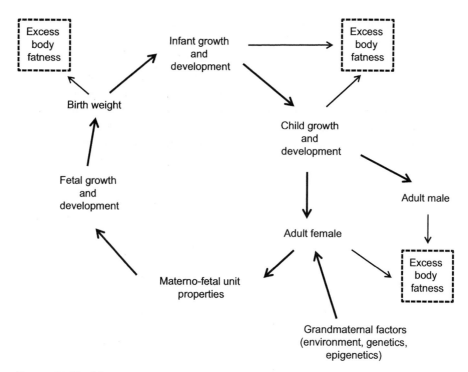

Figure 7.14. The life-course, transgenerational factors and obesity.

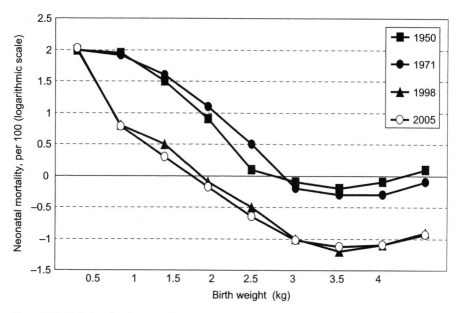

Figure 7.15. Relationship between birth weight and neonatal mortality in the US, from 1950 to 1998 (data from Lubchenco et al. 1972; Wilcoxon and Russell 1983; Lau et al. 2013).

birth to childhood (Wang et al. 2012). Furthermore, the developmental programming associated with living in adverse early-life environments may be epigenetically regulated (Vickers 2014). Pregnancy, lactation and early childhood growth are under intense social and cultural control (Ebrahim 1980; Macadam and Dettwyler 1995; Lancy 2008), and are also likely to influence epigenetic regulation. In turn, there is social epigenetic control of adipose tissue development. For example, exercise, diets and weight-loss surgery each have been shown to alter DNA methylation profiles in different tissue types (van Dijk et al. 2015). Furthermore, DNA methylation in adipose tissue can change after exercise, and differs between high and low responders to weight-loss interventions (Bouchard et al. 2010; Cordero et al. 2011; Rönn et al. 2013). Epigenetic profiling of obese people before and after weight-loss surgery shows DNA methylation profiles to become more similar to those of lean individuals following surgery (Barres et al. 2013), indicating that the epigenome of obese individuals can be modified by reductions in body weight or fat mass. Beyond pregnancy and infancy, other life-course factors implicated in the production of obesity include variable patterns of growth and development in childhood and adolescence according to environmental circumstances, and the secular trend towards increased body size across generations, a measure that is usually taken as a marker of improved diet quality and nutritional well-being (Bogin 1999).

Physiological Plasticity and Obesity

There are different stressors that influence human growth and morphology at various stages of life and across generations, and there are many different pathways to obesity. Humans have an extended period of biological immaturity relative to other mammalian species (Bogin 1998), and this is associated with high ecological sensitivity and growth plasticity (Johnston 1998). Ecological sensitivity is manifest in the processes of stunting and wasting in response to poor nutrition and infection (Waterlow 1988), while growth plasticity is especially demonstrated in the catch-up growth that takes place during periods of environmental improvement following episodes of stress, nutritional and otherwise (Ulijaszek 2006). Both dietary quantity and quality can influence growth and body composition in later childhood, as can infant feeding patterns. Body fatness usually reaches its lowest level postinfancy, between the ages of 5 and 7 years, followed by increased body fatness, a phenomenon that has been termed adiposity rebound by Rolland-Cachera et al. (1984). Early adiposity rebound has been associated with increased relative weight and obesity later in life, including during adolescence (Cameron and Demerath 2002). In the US, low levels of vigorous physical activity and high levels of television viewing have been associated with greater body fatness in children during the adiposity rebound period (Janz et al. 2002).

Catch-up growth is an acceleration of child growth rate following either medical or environmental intervention or ecological improvement, such that body size approaches or reaches normality relative to growth references (Prader et al. 1963). It can take place at all stages of child growth, including adolescence (Golden 1994).

Early growth restriction followed by catch-up growth is associated with the development of abdominal obesity (Dulloo 2006), while higher growth velocity in early childhood, prior to adiposity rebound, has been associated with greater fatness and obesity in subsequent years (Monteiro et al. 2003). Furthermore, low birth weight and catch-up growth predispose to the development of excess body fatness at all stages of life (Oken and Gillman 2003).

The term 'secular trend' is used to describe marked changes in growth and development of successive generations of human populations. Positive secular trends in increased stature and weight, and earlier timing of the adolescent growth spurt, have been documented for many populations (Ulijaszek 2001d). While negative secular trends have been identified among some populations in LICs and LMICs (Ulijaszek 2010), positive secular trends are far more common, and have been largely attributed to improved social, political, nutritional and health conditions (Bogin 1999). Mean heights and weights of adults have increased in most HICs since the mid-nineteenth century, but while increases in height have slowed in the late twentieth century and reached a plateau in some European countries (Schmidt et al. 1995; Larnkjaer et al. 2006), adult obesity rates have only risen (Cole 2003). The rate of secular increase in stature among many modernizing populations in Asia since about 1960 has been almost double that of European populations (Ulijaszek 2001d). In China, the economic reforms of 1978, which were aimed at opening the socialist economy to free markets, led to a very dramatic increase in stature, as well as a subsequent increase in obesity rates (Shen et al. 1996) with Pattern Four nutrition transition. It takes several generations for maximal population stature to be achieved (six by Cole's 2003 estimation), and the emergence of global obesity in the past two generations might include developmental programming and epigenetic effects that go back to the origins of the secular trend and timing of Pattern Four nutrition transition in any population. The secular trend may in turn be associated with both improved nutrition and a reduction in infectious disease mortality in early life (Schmidt et al. 1995). The lower rates of obesity in high- and upper middle-income Asian countries could reflect the more recent and faster secular trends in those countries (Ulijaszek 2001d), as well as their more recent entry into Pattern Four nutrition transition.

Associations between stature and socioeconomic status (SES) are similar in most populations, with height correlating positively with wealth (Bogin 1999). Weight, however, varies socially and culturally in its relationship with wealth, overweight and obesity being more usually associated with low SES in most HICs (McLaren 2007) (Chapter 5), and initially associated with high SES in nations entering Pattern Four nutrition transition (Xu et al. 2005). Growth stunting in association with overweight was first identified in Peruvian children (Trowbridge et al. 1987) and more recently in children in four nations viewed to be undergoing nutrition transition: Russia, Brazil, South Africa and China (Popkin et al. 1996). This population phenomenon may be due to the very rapid onset of Pattern Four nutrition transition, which leads to obesity within a generation but to greater stature across several generations. Constant environmental perturbation was the ecological norm for most past populations, and included seasonality and uncertainty in food supply (de Garine and Harrison 1988; Ulijaszek and Strickland 1993). Human physiology is very responsive to such perturbations, allowing reproductive success and survival under difficult circumstances, and to increased body size and the accumulation of fat when conditions allow (Wells 2010), for future survivorship. It is precisely this set of adaptive features that is expressed in Pattern Four nutrition transition, contributing to the rapid rise of obesity rates in economically emerging countries.

Obesity and Nutrition Transition: A Conflict of Rationalities

Life-course events and practices such as pregnancy, child birth, infant feeding, weaning and supplementation, nutrition and child growth require the deployment of different, and sometimes contradictory, rationalities by people, but, in that they contribute to reproductive success, are underpinned by evolutionary rationality. Nutrition shapes developmental programming and epigenetic regulation differently at different life stages, and is fundamental to survivorship and reproductive success. Obesity can be seen as a perversion of evolutionary rationality when food is abundant, and its use is largely uncoupled from reproduction, as it is in most modern and modernizing societies. Globally, total fertility rates have declined by around a third, while global adult obesity rates almost doubled between 1980 and 2008 (Stevens et al. 2012), a period in which global per capita calorie availability has increased by 14 per cent (Figure 7.16). Ecological decisions about feeding are evolutionarily rational and are geared towards reproductive success, even under conditions of controlled low fertility rates. Pattern Four nutrition transition has generally followed

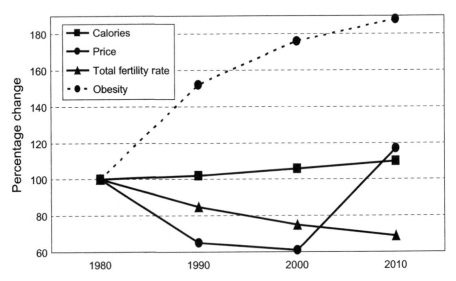

Figure 7.16. Global per capita dietary energy availability, Food and Agriculture Organization Food Price Index and total fertility rates, from 1980 to 2010, with 1980 set to 100, relative to changes in obesity (data from Food and Agriculture Organization 2002, 2017; World Bank 2016c).

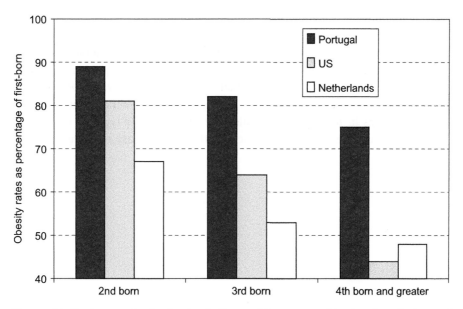

Figure 7.17. Obesity rates by family size, in Portugal (7–19-year-olds; data from Padez et al. 2005), the US (10–11-year-olds; data from Chen and Escarce 2010) and the Netherlands (19-year-old males; data from Ravelli and Belmont 1979); rates for first-born children were set at 100 per cent.

the roll-out of controlled reproduction across the world, and increased availability of dietary energy has not usually translated into increased reproduction. Rather, smaller family size is associated with higher obesity rates among offspring (Figure 7.17), suggesting greater parental energy investment in a smaller number of offspring than is physiologically possible. Planned small family size is an outcome of the practices of Weberian formal rationality in late modernity, and in this situation, evolutionary rationality underpins parental investment in maximizing the quality of offspring. In HICs, it has become costlier in terms of time and physical and mental resources to be thin than to be fat, and biological quality is increasingly signalled through wealth and other forms of capital (Chapter 5), including thinness.

The implications of Pattern Four nutrition transition and developmental programming for obesity and its regulation are long term and transgenerational. How policy deals with early-life predispositions to obesity is a matter of complexity (Chapter 9), however. For policy makers, the past matters, in that history sets precedents and naturalizes cultures of politics and population behaviour. With respect to food, this plays out in ideas of tradition: for example, the 'British diet', 'French cuisine', Italian and French regional food, and American fast food. Other types of history are important too. Maternal and grandmaternal histories shape present-day disease risk, and policy focused on maternal health and child-centred social investment (Esping-Andersen 2002) (Chapter 6) should help to reduce the legacy of obesity and chronic disease created by past political, economic and social environments.

According to Yoshizawa (2012), the hypothesis that developmental programming alters predispositions to chronic disease in adult life does not support solely reductionist, biophysiological paradigms of health and disease, but rather invokes complex understandings that span biology, social positionality, place and generation. The Weberian theoretical rationality that underpins Yoshizawa's (2012) scientific observation does not speak easily to policy and the Weberian formal rationality that underpins it, however. This is also the case for other types of obesity science and policy, and the next chapter describes this often uneasy relationship.

Obesity science has, under one umbrella, various disciplines that often differ in what is taken as acceptable evidence, level of investigation, type of data collected and canonical methods of analysis and interpretation (Table 8.1). Obesity policy similarly brings together disparate interests especially within health, education and economics. Achieving consensus in obesity science and policy is difficult, since fields with often very different world views are required to work together. Even in seemingly straightforward technical areas, such as the regulation of food safety in international trade of agricultural goods, the formation and management of a scientific consensus that can underlie trade-related rule making, standard setting and regulatory activities at the national, regional and international levels presents huge challenges (Vikhlyaev 2005). Difficulties in engaging science with food and nutrition policy generally have been considered by Sanabria and Yates-Doerr (2015) who see food and nutrition as fields with eminently applicable results, where research (and the funding with which to do it) are dependent upon claims to intervention and future policy relevance. Many food and nutrition scientists are therefore in continued conversation with policy makers.

What has been said of nutrition research – its need to deal with applicability and policy, the importance of knowing how nutrition knowledge is achieved and applied – applies equally to the political ecology of obesity. In most countries, adult obesity rates continue to rise, while policies for its abatement continue to accrue. National and international concern about obesity is reflected in the fact that obesity rates are now routinely measured in many nations (Chapter 4), and many nations have policies for its control and regulation. The United States (US) and the United Kingdom (UK) have exceptionally good systems for obesity surveillance, yet also strong histories of failure in obesity policy: obesity rates (using internationally standard metrics) among adults carry on increasing, and while childhood rates of overweight and obesity have stabilized, socioeconomic inequalities in these rates have persisted or grown (Singh et al. 2010; Public Health England 2016). There are many more countries that have high, and usually rising, rates of adult obesity and often rising rates of childhood overweight and obesity with much less experience in obesity policy than the US or the UK. Within Europe, the *European Charter on Counteracting Obesity* (World Health Organization 2006) recognizes the need for an all-encompassing response to obesity, requiring high-level political will, leadership and whole-government commitment to mobilize obesity work across different sectors. The sectoral roles and instruments for dealing with obesity proposed in this Charter are very broad indeed, and there is a

Table 8.1. Some disciplines involved in obesity science and their cultural framings

Discipline	Level of investigation	Types of model	Types of data	Typical types of analysis
Physiology	Individual, bodily organ, cell	Energy balance, experimental (animal, human)	Energetics, endocrinology, body fatness, neuroimaging, obesity phenotypes	Multivariate
Genetics	Gene, genome	Network, phylogenetic, experimental (animal, human)	DNA sequence, obesity phenotypes	Statistical, network, phylogenetic
Microbiome	Gut bacteria	Phylogenetic, network, systems	Species, DNA sequence, obesity phenotypes	Classification, network, multivariate, phylogenetic
Epigenetics	Life course	Developmental, gene expression	DNA sequence, obesity phenotypes, stress measures, fetal and child growth	Multivariate, statistical
Epidemiology	Human populations, population samples	Ecological, descriptive, predictive, variation and stratification, life course, risk factor	Obesity phenotypes, fatness and fat distribution	Statistical, multivariate, mapping
Economics	Population data	Descriptive, experimental	Obesity phenotypes, econometric measures	Statistical, multivariate, mapping
Psychology	Population samples	Descriptive, predictive	Behavioural	Statistical, multivariate
Public health	Human population and population samples	Ecological, interventional (real and modelled)	Obesity phenotypes, intervention measures	Natural experiments, statistical, case–control
Political science	International, national and local human populations	Welfare regimes, inequality	Political structure	Mapping, statistical
Sociology	Society, communities	Inequality, feminism, critical fat studies	Questionnaires, ethnography	Statistical, qualitative
Anthropology	Society, communities	Inequality, insecurity, status and distinction, ecological	Critical approaches, obesity phenotypes, ethnography, questionnaires, life history, narratives	Statistical, narrative, textual
Geography	Region, nation, locality	Mapping, ecological	Frequencies, distributions	Network, topographical, statistical
History	Society	Chronology, genealogy	Historical documents	Text, images, narrative

clear aspiration towards full-scale mobilization of all resources, from the individual to the societal, public and private. The recommended policy tools range from legislation to the development of public/private partnerships, acknowledging the need to demonstrate effectiveness of interventions when designing and implementing policies, where they exist. Similarly, the World Health Organization (2016b) *Consideration of the Evidence on Childhood Obesity for the Commission on Ending Childhood Obesity* sees childhood obesity prevention and treatment as requiring a whole-of-government approach using a comprehensive, integrated package of recommendations. In short, it calls for the political ecology of childhood obesity to be regulated by a complete ecology of politics, akin to the 'joined-up government' approach of the UK Labour administration of 1997 to 2010 (Chapter 9). The World Health Organization (2016b) report also calls for governments to take leadership, and for stakeholders to recognize their moral responsibility to children by reducing the risk of obesity. In addition to these requirements, an all-encompassing response to obesity should recruit evidence from a wide range of sources to inform policy. In obesity policy, the ways in which evidence is harnessed, what is seen as important and what is left out, are all important. This chapter describes the rationalities (Chapters 1 and 2) that frame obesity policy in relation to the ethics of obesity intervention. It goes on to consider how obesity science, with its many models, relates to obesity policy, with an emphasis on how the policy process more generally engages with scientific evidence.

Obesity Policy

The reduction of obesity rates within a country is often not a political aim in itself, but is an object of policy action because it has important economic consequences (Chapter 4). Since obesity has been identified as a complex multifactorial phenomenon with an influence on many issues that are of concern to national governments (Chapter 10), dealing with it has the potential to reduce predispositions to poor labour outputs, sluggish economic growth and low educational attainment, as well as more obvious end points of obesity, which are morbidity and mortality due to chronic diseases (Chapters 6 and 7). As obesity is associated with death and disease, it is usually also the object of medical scrutiny. Obesity in the US was considered a medical issue from the 1940s, when obesity rates were still low. It was then seen principally as a consequence of addiction and an outcome of the psychological defect of oral fixation, a dominant psychodynamic theory of the time (Rasmussen 2015). Both constructions of obesity (addiction and oral fixation) were taken up in popular discourse and clinical practice, and contributed to increased weight stigma and an intervention focus that emphasized correction of individual eating behaviour among obese people through self-help in lay groups modelled, in part, on Alcoholics Anonymous (Rasmussen 2015). The shift to public health approaches in obesity intervention came with the emergence of obesity as a growing population phenomenon in the 1980s (Chapter 7). These approaches were and continue to be state-led. They are now the most broadly applied, and usually invoke individual responsibility towards maintaining a healthy body (Chapter 6), especially in the US (Brownell et al. 2010).

Vallgarda et al. (2015) distinguish between backward- and forward-looking responsibility for obesity – who is responsible for the rise in obesity prevalence, and who is responsible for its reduction, respectively. Exactly how these two types of responsibility are modelled by different governments and agencies is related to the role that different authorities take in framing obesity policy. In the UK, governmental responsibility to the economy as well as for health has resulted in both backward and forward responsibility for obesity being firmly placed on the individual (Vallgarda et al. 2015).

Some UK and US policy has depicted obesity as being a growing threat to the overall health of the population (Department of Health 1992; US Department of Health and Human Services 2000; House of Commons Health Committee 2004). Obesity has also been compellingly depicted as a drag on the economy, both in terms of lost productivity and in terms of costs to state-provided health-care provision (House of Commons Health Committee 2004; Butland et al. 2007; Wisman and Capehart 2012) (Chapter 4), although health departments usually bear most responsibility (and cost) for the regulation of obesity. The categorization of obesity as a disease in the US and by the World Health Organization (WHO) has aimed to raise the profile of obesity for medical intervention (Chapters 1 and 10), but this categorization continues to be contested (Jutel 2005; Campos et al. 2006; Rich 2011; Rich et al. 2011). Obesity as risk factor (Chapter 4) also has traction in the framing of health policy, because it sits among other risk categories, such as smoking, unhealthy diet and physical inactivity, for chronic disease onset and progression (Erlichman et al. 2002). Such categories of risk have ambivalent status in policy making, however. For example, smoking damages health and human productivity, but taxation of it gives a steady stream of reliable income to governments (Chaloupka and Warner 2000). Similarly, an unhealthy diet is damaging, but the food industry supplies uncontaminated and affordable food to large populations and primarily seeks to continue its operations without undue regulation (Ulijaszek and McLennan 2016), if profit is to be made.

The rationalities that underpin obesity intervention usually involve economic, psychological and Weberian practical and formal rationalities (Chapters 1 and 2). They offer no moral guidance as to what approaches might best be taken. If obesity is taken to be a public health problem, medical ethics are important to the framing of interventions. The ethics of medical interventions are seemingly straightforward – to save the patient – while the ethics of public health interventions are more complex. The Nuffield Council on Bioethics (2007) argues for simplicity of intent for public health intervention more broadly. Public health intervention needs to balance individual choice, preservation of autonomy, reduction of inequalities, protection of vulnerable groups and the targeting of at-risk groups (Nuffield Council on Bioethics 2007). The Nuffield intervention ladder (Table 8.2) is a 'proportionality device' that can be used to consider the balance between influencing behaviour and direct regulation. There are many possibilities for public health anti-obesity intervention, at different levels of the Nuffield intervention ladder. It is not a formulaic device, but something that can help identify the ethical

Table 8.2. The intervention ladder for public health policies

Possible policy	Action
Eliminate choice	Regulating in a way to entirely eliminate choice
Restrict choice	Regulating in a way to restrict options available to people with the aim of protecting them, for example through compulsory isolation of patients with infectious diseases
Guide choice through disincentives	Fiscal and other disincentives, which can be put in place to influence people not to pursue certain activities, for example through taxes on cigarettes
Guide choice through incentives	Regulation that guides choice by fiscal and other incentives, for example by offering tax breaks to reward health-producing behaviour
Guide choices through changing the default policy	Regulation through establishing healthy norms, for example by making non-smoking the norm in public buildings and on public transport
Enable choice	Enabling individuals to change their behaviour, for example by offering participation in a smoking cessation programme
Provide information	Informing and educating the public
Do nothing or monitor the current situation	Surveillance and monitoring, for example with governmental health data collection

Adapted from Nuffield Council on Bioethics (2007).

appropriateness of one intervention as compared with another. The Nuffield Council on Bioethics (2007) frames the range of options available to government and policy makers as a ladder of interventions, with progressive steps from individual freedom and responsibility towards state intervention as one moves up the ladder. In considering which 'rung' is appropriate for a particular public health goal, they place importance on weighing the benefits to individuals and society against the erosion of individual freedom, while taking into account economic costs and benefits alongside health and societal benefits. The Nuffield intervention ladder can be applied to the regulation of obesity (Table 8.3), allowing the costs and benefits of a range of existing approaches to be evaluated. The least intrusive step on the ladder is to do nothing, or at most undertake surveillance, while the most intrusive is to legislate in such a way as to restrict freedoms significantly. In many countries, obesity policy is restricted to data collection and reporting to the national health department. At the early stages of population obesity emergence in the US, obesity policy was limited to such collection and reporting. In 1985, only around half of all the states of the US reported their obesity rates, because many of them did not yet view obesity to be a problem worth monitoring or reporting. Most nations did not have obesity policies until after 1997, when the WHO Consultation on Obesity (World Health Organization 2000) took place. At this time, most countries pledged to undertake systematic reporting of adult obesity rates using internationally agreed cut-offs for body mass index (Chapter 3).

Table 8.3. Examples of the intervention ladder as might be applied to obesity

Possible policy	Action	Examples
Eliminate choice	Regulating in a way to entirely eliminate choice	Excluding vending machines selling sugar-sweetened beverages from schools
Restrict choice	Regulate in a way to restrict the options available to people with the aim of protecting them	Setting limits on the energy content of specific foods; reducing the availability of sugar-sweetened beverages in schools
Guide choice through disincentives	Fiscal and other disincentives put in place to influence people not to pursue certain activities	Discouraging the use of cars in inner cities through charging schemes or limitation of parking spaces
Guide choice through incentives	Regulation that guides choice by fiscal and other incentives	Offering tax breaks for the purchase of bicycles for commuting to work
Guide choices through changing the default policy	Regulation through establishing healthy norms	Building safe cycle lanes in cities; setting healthy food options as standard in restaurants
Enable choice	Enabling individuals to change their behaviour	Building cycle lanes; providing free or cheap fruit in schools and/or at the work place
Provide (or withhold) information	Informing and educating the public	Campaigns to encourage people to walk more or eat five portions of fruit and vegetables daily
Do nothing or monitor the current situation	Surveillance and monitoring	Measuring children, as in the UK National Child Measurement Programme; reporting rates of overweight and obesity

The next level of intervention, providing individualized anti-obesity information, is a low-level intrusion into people's lives. Education through practice is also framed at this level, especially among school children and their families. This includes multicomponent family-based programmes for children (American Dietetic Association 2006; Hoelscher et al. 2013) and school programmes for adolescents (American Dietetic Association 2006). Another intervention at this level might be the development and marketing of probiotic foods. With evidence that certain types of human gut microbiotic ecology are associated with obesity (Tsai and Coyle 2009) (Chapter 6), and with arguments for the therapeutic value of manipulating gut microbiota ecology for obesity reduction (Kootte et al. 2012), probiotic foods have been recruited to the cause of obesity reduction as well as for their other health-related qualities (Shah 2007). Probiotic foods are developed and sold by food corporations, their use is widespread, and the role of government in this domain is to regulate their appropriate use (Klein and Dwyer 2008). Yet another intervention at this level is the use of dietary guidelines. In Brazil, for example, recently published sustainable national dietary guidelines emphasize a preference for dietary intake based on a variety of natural or minimally processed foods, mostly plant based, and on freshly prepared meals eaten in company, for health, well-being and sustainability (Monteiro et al. 2015). Here, obesity is indirectly targeted via many components of the Brazilian food system. At the next level of the Nuffield intervention ladder, structuring environments in ways that make obesity control easier by enabling choice is a common approach in most high-income countries (HICs). For example, nutritional information on food packaging is widespread, while active transport policies proliferate. The next level of intervention involves guiding choices by changing default policies. While a powerful approach, this is rarely used, largely because it usually involves difficult decisions by governments and other agencies about how to structure individual choice in ways that might inhibit obesity. Given the complexity of obesity (Chapter 9), it is very difficult to show that any such intervention would lead to declines in obesity rates. Intervention at the next level up might involve incentivizing choice through price subsidy. This rarely happens: in the US and the European Union, farming subsidies are more targeted to support existing food production systems than to incentivize change in production towards better nutritional health.

Higher again on the Nuffield intervention ladder, obesity control through guiding choice with disincentives such as taxation has gained momentum in recent years, especially in relation to sugar-sweetened beverages (SSBs) (Landon and Graff 2012; Public Health England 2015b). The effectiveness of such taxation has been argued to vary according to baseline taxation rate. Taxation of SSBs is more likely to be effective where overall taxation rates are low and where existing obesity prevalence and soft drink consumption levels are high (Jou and Techakehakij 2012). Taxation of unhealthy aspects of diet may be regressive, however, if poorer people have no economically viable food purchasing alternative. In 2015, Public Health England (2015b) advocated a price increase of a minimum of between 10 and 20 per cent on high-sugar products such as SSBs through the use of a tax or levy. In 2016, the UK government proposed a tax at the highest level proposed by Public Health England (2015b) for such products, intended to come into effect in 2018. In modelling the effects of such taxation, Briggs et al. (2013) have indicated that it would be financially regressive. However, Brownell et al. (2009a) suggest that such a tax at the same level in the US might be progressive in terms of health outcomes, because the medical costs of treating diseases associated with obesity are disproportionately greater among those of low socioeconomic status, and outweigh the financial burden associated with the purchase of SSBs. Moving yet higher on the Nuffield intervention ladder, restricting choice through regulation is the most resisted by commercial interests, because this also restricts the market. Promises of increasing governmental regulation of potentially obesogenic foods in the UK have resulted in the food industry making highly visible pledges to curtail children's food marketing, to sell fewer unhealthy products in schools, and to label foods in responsible ways (Sharma et al. 2010). Voluntary self-regulation of the food industry is currently the dominant mechanism in the UK (Ulijaszek and McLennan 2016). Sharma et al. (2010) examined

Table 8.4. Nine standards that should be met if self-regulation of the food industry is to be effective

Aim	Standard
Transparency	Transparent self-regulatory standards created by a combination of scientists (not paid by industry) and representatives of leading non-governmental organizations and parties involved in global governance (such as the World Health Organization, United Nations Food and Agriculture Organization) and industry
	No one party given disproportionate power or voting authority
Meaningful objectives and benchmarks	Specific codes of acceptable behaviours based on scientifically justified criteria
	Predefined benchmarks to ensure the success of self-regulation
Accountability and objective evaluation	Mandatory public reporting of adherence to codes, including progress towards achievement of full compliance with pledges and attainment of key benchmarks
	Built-in and transparent procedures for outside parties to register objections to self-regulatory standards and the enforcement thereof
	Objective evaluation of self-regulatory benchmarks by credible outside groups not funded by industry to assess health, economic and social outcomes
	Periodic assessments or audits to determine compliance and outcomes
Oversight	Possible oversight by an appropriate global regulatory or health body, such as the World Health Organization

Adapted from Sharma et al. (2010).

corporate self-regulatory successes and failures and identified nine standards that should be met if self-regulation of the food industry is to be effective (Table 8.4). The aims of these standards – transparency, meaningful objectives and benchmarks, accountability and objective evaluation, and oversight – are only partially met in the UK. Given that the UK has one of the most comprehensive approaches to food system regulation in the world (Swinburn et al. 2015), the only very partial observance of self-regulation standards by food companies there suggests that this approach to obesity has too few teeth with which to bite properly.

At the second highest level of the Nuffield intervention ladder there is the possibility of eliminating choice, for example by excluding vending machines that sell high-energy-density food products from schools. This has been carried out in a number of HICs including the US, Australia, France and the UK. At the highest level of the intervention ladder, there is the possibility of state intervention by isolation or imprisonment. One form of isolation, quarantine, is a mechanism sometimes invoked by governments in times of medical crisis. To date, nobody has been imprisoned or isolated because of their obesity, although in the UK, obese children may be taken into care. Child abuse laws have been invoked for the parents of severely obese children, using the rationale that such children face imminent health risks that their parents have repeatedly failed to address (Viner et al. 2010; Murtagh and Ludwig 2011).

The Nuffield intervention ladder is useful for framing obesity regulation in relation to a set of ethical principles, offering guidance in relation to values that particular governments might hold to. For example, governments might differ in the extent to which they are concerned with inequality and protection of vulnerable groups, or promoting individualism and autonomy. Science can offer little to discussions of what constitutes ethical intervention, since models of obesity more generally cannot help in identifying what should be done, among a range of options. With respect to diet, for example, scientific notions of the healthiness of diets and of individual foods can be, and are, contested by food producers and manufacturers (Chapter 6). Evidence that the geographical distribution of obesogenic environments (Chapter 3) maps onto epidemiologically measured obesity rates does not lend itself to any particular ethical action or model for obesity intervention, either. The vagueness of the concept of obesogenic environments makes it attractive to policy makers because they can interpret it in a range of different ways, and according to different ethical principles. With respect to governmental policy to increase physical activity in the general population, this is made difficult if most workplaces require or privilege sedentism, and there are politically powerful industries that promote the use of cars (Caterson 2000) and forms of sedentary leisure (Brownson et al. 2004), as there are in both the UK and the US.

Obesity framed as an outcome of long-term positive energy balance (Chapter 3) became an object of governmental concern in both the UK and the US in 2001, with the National Audit Office (2001) report (Chapter 3), and *The Surgeon General's Call to Action to Prevent and Decrease Overweight and Obesity* (US Department of Health and Human Services 2001; Novak and Brownell 2012), respectively. Energy balance models for obesity intervention prioritize individual action and represent an easily made governmental response. Another policy approach to obesity involves the use of epidemiological models to assign risk to different population groups (Chapter 4). The emphasis on geographical, social and economic differentiation in obesity rates in countries such as the US and the UK (Chapters 4 and 5) has been central to the identification of priorities for obesity intervention since the 2000s, but it has also contributed to stigmatization of obesity among poorer members of society in the UK (Flint et al. 2015), the US (Carr and Friedman 2005) and elsewhere (Puhl and Heuer 2009; Spahlholz et al. 2016).

Social, economic, political, technological and environmental factors have been linked in the political ecology of obesity in different countries. The possibility that global economic integration and neoliberalism also contributed to rising obesity rates has also been examined by scientists (Chapters 5–7 and 10). The linkages between these different macro-level explanations have been poorly developed until recently, however. The move to complexity in obesity policy and science (Chapter 9) is one attempt at making these connections. Complex systems often have many levels of organization that may form a hierarchy of subsystems (Simon 1962) that interact within and across levels, exhibiting causal regularities (Ladyman et al. 2013). They are inherently intricate and are rarely completely deterministic. Mathematical models of such systems usually involve non-linear or chaotic behaviour. Such systems are also predisposed to unexpected outcomes, or emergent behaviour (Foote 2007). According to this framing, the emergence of new phenomena (such as population-level obesity since the 1980s) occurs because of order that arises from interactions among parts at a lower level of a system that are robust or detectable, measureable or definable, in a range of interdependent ways (Wimsatt 1994). Obesity ecology as a complex problem involves multiple actors and factors that are connected either directly or indirectly, and it is impossible to anticipate the effect of any single intervention to regulate it (Ulijaszek 2015). This is unlike any simple problem where the outcomes of actions are linear, and where the effect of a single intervention can be predicted; however, many obesity interventions continue to treat obesity as a simple problem, with linear expectations of outcomes. Complexity has been invoked in culturally driven models of obesity causation, with many factors associated with obesity being seen as the mechanical expression of underlying culturally based decisions (Foresight 2007a). Policy discourse has moved away from complexity in the UK since 2010, partly because of the shift in dominant political ideology (Chapter 9), and partly because there do not appear to be any easily applicable instruments for predictably regulating the complexity of obesity.

Obesity Science and Policy

While obesity science is used to inform obesity policy, the models that each of them use often engage different rationalities. The policy response that any particular government might choose involves some balance of pragmatism, evidence and ideology. Ideologies shift and change, and what may be seen as an acceptable obesity intervention by policy makers in one country at one time may not be for another, or at another time. Many aspects of obesity policy have been framed with comparatively little scientific underpinning, and Brownell and Roberto (2015) have argued for a 'strategic science' approach to address this issue. In their model for obesity prevention, Roberto et al. (2015) identify important gaps between obesity science and policy, arguing that, while evidence-based policy making (EBPM) is an important aspirational goal, only a small proportion of research has the policy impact it might have. They go on to say that most researchers are not trained to create policy impact from their work, nor is engagement with policy makers encouraged or rewarded in most settings. In the UK, great efforts have been made to link scholarship and policy making, but competing claims in different sectors of obesity science complicate the process of EBPM on obesity (Ulijaszek 2015). Evidence from obesity science comes from varied sources including government, and corporations involved variously in food production, food retail and weight management, as well as state-funded organizations, including universities. The latter are ambiguously placed when privately funded, as are individual researchers and research groups when they accept corporate funding to carry out research (Gornall 2015). The diversity of agencies that offer advice on obesity contributes to the obesity policy cacophony described by Lang and Rayner (2007), where many and varied policy analyses and solutions compete for attention.

In the UK, the report of the National Audit Office (2001) noted that obesity interventions by the National Health Service and Department of Health were largely either local strategies, or involved care (including screening, personal advice, drug therapy and referrals) delivered through general practice. While the report spoke to the significant amount of joined-up cross-governmental work on obesity prevention that was already in place by 2001, the existence of eight different strategies for promoting activity and healthy eating among children and adults undermines this assertion (Ulijaszek and McLennan 2016) and testifies to the cacophony of effort in obesity policy (Lang and Rayner 2007). To address this issue, Swinburn et al. (2005) proposed a framework for translating evidence into action. They broadly grouped evidence into a number of categories: observational, experimental, extrapolated and experience based (Table 8.5). The authors offered no hierarchy of quality for these types of evidence, because their intrinsic strengths and weaknesses play out differently for each of the questions posed for obesity prevention. Evidence from randomized control trials was not privileged, perhaps recognizing that such trials do not offer superior forms of evidence (Grossman and MacKenzie 2005) outside of medicine and public health. The equivalence given to different forms of evidence in the scheme of Swinburn et al. (2005) reflects the process of policy making more generally, where scientific evidence is on a similar footing to evidence from marketing, industry and lobby groups, as well as from arm's-length bodies and non-governmental organizations, which may have their own obesity policies. Table 8.6 gives a list of arm's-length bodies sponsored by the UK Department of Health and of non-governmental organizations producing obesity and obesity-related policy documents between 2000 and 2010 (Association for the Study of Obesity 2011). These organizations are numerous, represent a diversity of interests and vary in the extent to which obesity is a central issue for them.

Filling gaps in knowledge between obesity science and policy may help in formulating more strategic questions, such as the projected impacts of competing policy approaches to obesity, costs of implementation and likely public support for different policies (Brownell and Roberto 2015). There are, however, significant intervention biases, including variation in the extent to which primacy is given to responsibilized individual citizenship by policy makers (Vallgarda et al. 2015). Responsibilized citizenship as obesity intervention is often supported by health-promotion messaging, brief interventions from general practitioners, and governmental nudge tactics across areas of daily life, especially in the UK and the US. Politically, individualism may be best for the regulation of everyday practices, and collectivism best in response to crisis (Triandis 1995). Policy approaches that target individuals implicitly frame obesity as a matter of mundane governance (Woolgar and Neyland 2013) and not one of crisis, despite some media (Rich 2011; Eli and Ulijaszek 2014) and public health (Lobstein et al. 2004) rhetoric to the contrary. Lang and Rayner (2014) have argued for an ecological public health that both downplays individualism and embraces complexity (Chapter 9).

Table 8.5. Description of types of evidence and information relevant to obesity prevention

Type	Method	Outputs
Observational	Observational epidemiology	Rates and comparisons of obesity and obesity risk factors in populations and risk groups, using (for example) cross-sectional, case–control or cohort studies
	Monitoring and surveillance	Population-level data collected regularly to provide time-series information
Experimental	Experimental studies	Intervention studies where investigators have control, such as with randomized controlled trials, or with non-randomized trials in individuals, settings or whole communities
	Programme/policy evaluation	Assessment of whether a programme or policy meets both its overall aims (outcome) and specific objectives (impacts), and how the inputs and implementation experiences result in these changes (process)
Extrapolated	Effectiveness analyses	Modelled estimates of likely effectiveness of an intervention that incorporate data or estimates of programme efficacy, programme uptake and (for population effectiveness) population reach
	Economic analyses	Modelled estimates that incorporate costs and/or benefits, including intervention costs, cost-effectiveness and/or cost–utility
	Indirect (or assumed) evidence	Information that strongly suggests that evidence exists. For example, high and continued investment in food advertising is indirect evidence that there is positive evidence that food advertising increases the sales of those products and/or product categories
Experience	Parallel evidence	Evidence of intervention effectiveness for another public health issue using similar strategies. Examples of this include the role of social marketing, policies, curriculum programmes or financial factors on changing health-related behaviours such as smoking, speeding or dietary intake. This includes evidence of the effectiveness of multiple strategies to influence behaviours in a sustainable way, such as health promotion in schools, and comprehensive tobacco control programmes
	Theory and programme logic	Rationale of effect and described pathways of effect, based on theory and experience, such as linking changes in policy to changes in behaviours and energy balance, or ascribing higher levels of certainty of effect to policy strategies such as regulation and pricing, compared with other strategies such as education
	Informed opinion	Considered opinion of experts, practitioners, stakeholders and policy makers able to inform judgements on implementation issues and modelling assumptions

Adapted from Swinburn et al. (2005).

Table 8.6. Arm's-length bodies sponsored by the Department of Health and non-governmental organizations producing obesity and obesity-related policy documents in the UK between 2000 and 2010

Arm's-length bodies	Non-governmental organizations
Cycling England	Royal College of Obstetricians and Gynaecologists
Commission for Architecture and the Built Environment	Royal College of Paediatrics and Child Health
	Faculty of Public Health
Food Standards Agency	British Dietetic Association
Care Quality Commission (formerly the Healthcare Commission)	Diabetes UK
	Association of Chief Executives of Voluntary Organisations
Local Government Improvement and Development	Caroline Walker Trust (promotes public health improvement through good food)
National Institute for Health and Care Excellence	
Natural England	National Heart Forum
Ofcom (regulatory authority for communications industries)	National Obesity Forum
	Sustrans (promotes active transport)
Ofsted (Office for Standards in Education, Children's Services and Skills)	
School Food Trust	
Sport England	
Sustainable Development Commission	

Adapted from Association for the Study of Obesity (2011).

Evidence in Obesity Policy

The relationship between evidence and policy is far from straightforward, and researchers who are asked to contribute to policy making are often frustrated because their evidence is rarely directly acted upon. At its simplest, policy is the outcome of policy making, a social and political process. The process of policy making includes the identification of problems that need to be addressed, the development of policy ideas by researchers and public servants, and the shaping of these ideas in the political environment by politicians, interest groups, lobbies and public opinion (Kingdon 1984). Policy makers use, ignore or downplay research in response to the pressures of politics, timing, advocacy by special interest groups, changing tides of public opinion (Haynes et al. 2011) and/or changing priorities of governments. Obesity policy relies on processes that are saturated by ideology and which are intolerant to certain types of evidence, alternative discourses and non-normative knowledge (Rail et al. 2010). Policy-making outputs include documentation issued by a government's legislative body, reports published by governmental departments and agencies, and documents published by non-governmental organizations such as think tanks. Policies usually contain normative and prescriptive assumptions, which can be used to shape regional, national and international rhetoric agendas. Belshaw (1976) sees public policy as being based on an implicit or explicit theory of the way society works, and obesity policy is no different in this regard. Policy approaches to obesity control and prevention reflect how obesity is viewed in society, how the various agencies and actors that are seen as potential regulators of obesity are politically disposed, what type of problem obesity is seen to be by policy makers and politicians, and what types of opportunities its regulation might offer. Policies also actively create new categories of individuals to be governed (Wedel et al. 2005), and obese persons are a recently created category.

Public policy instrumentation and its modes of operation are part of the governmental rationality of methods (Lascoumes and le Gales 2007). Through the use of carefully constructed language and rational–legal frameworks, policy presents assumptions that may be taken for granted, and neutralizes potentially contested topics. With respect to obesity, policy emerging from the UK Foresight Obesities process (Chapter 9) did not examine values and norms surrounding large body size, including blame and stigma, while more recent policy documents on obesity in the UK do not consider inequality. In the US, the 'facts about obesity' (Casazza et al. 2013) (Chapter 1) largely support the American Medical Association's recommendation of 2013 that obesity be classified as a disease. The World Health Organization's (2014) 'ten facts about obesity' (Chapter 1) limits the number of viewpoints that can be used to regulate obesity by excluding from its frame economic inequality, biomedical intervention and taxation of obesogenic foods. Fact one is an instrumentalization of obesity, defining the metric. Fact two sets up obesity as a global problem, based on fact one. Fact three is an extension of fact two, applied to children. Fact four sets up obesity as the dominant nutritionally related cause of mortality, while fact five states that the energy balance logic of obesity production places responsibility on individuals rather than political or societal structures for regulating obesity. Facts six through nine invoke public health action, by mobilizing individuals and the communities in which they are situated, while fact ten supports the World Health Organization's (2009b) *Action Plan for the Global Strategy for the Prevention and Control of Noncommunicable Diseases* to establish and strengthen initiatives for the surveillance, prevention and management of non-communicable diseases, including obesity. Obesity policy framed by the WHO reflects its strong public health focus. It also takes into account the resources available to, and the socioeconomic conditions of, individual nations that it anticipates will comply with it (Vallgarda et al. 2015).

Obesity policy at the national level is diverse, often developed in relation to earlier policy and in relation to various interested lobbies, actors and activists, as well as showing some compliance with WHO policy. For example, the UK government's *Childhood Obesity: A Plan for Action* (Department of Health, Prime Minister's Office, Her Majesty's Treasury and Cabinet Office 2016) accepts and acts on many of the recommendations in the World Health Organization's (2016b) report *Consideration of the Evidence on Childhood Obesity for the Commission on Ending Childhood Obesity*. Important recommendations concerning structural processes are ignored, however, in relation to competing interests – within government, and between government, corporations and interest groups. The World Health Organization (2016b) report recommends there to be regular high-level policy dialogues in government on childhood obesity, and clear mechanisms for the management of conflicts of interest in policy making, both of which are absent from the UK government's policy

Childhood Obesity: A Plan for Action (Department of Health, Prime Minister's Office, Her Majesty's Treasury and Cabinet Office 2016).

Lang and Rayner (2007) note that many obesity policy initiatives have been framed in terms of the personalization of health choice, with strong incentives for governments to present obesity policies based on individual choice and economic rationality. The use of metaphors for obesity in policy rhetoric (Cosgel 1992) – such as it being sinful behaviour (gluttony or sloth), a disability, a form of eating disorder, a food addiction, a reflection of time limitation, a consequence of manipulation by commercial interests or a result of a toxic food environment – are independent and powerful predictors of support for public policies to control it (Barry et al. 2009). Policy presentation utilizes storytelling, a rhetorical device that advertisers know well (Cosgel 1992). Most metaphors for obesity (Barry et al. 2009) are grounded in the idea that responses to obesity should be individualist. While seemingly harmless, they help to naturalize the narratives that organizations or governments use to discuss obesity and frame appropriate responses to it.

Most HICs are, or are fast becoming, consumer societies, in which consumption is an active form of relationship. Consumption and citizenship have become inextricably linked since the 1990s, prior to which time they were located in opposing private and public domains, and associated with competing inner- and outer-regarding norms and actions (Trentmann 2007). Baudrillard (1970) anticipated the importance of consumption in late modern society by saying that, in the same way that medieval society was balanced on God and the Devil, so modern society is balanced on consumption and its denunciation. The rhetoric of choice has penetrated most aspects of policy formation and implementation since the 1980s, and obesity is not exempt from this. Governments may use models of rational choice in constructing obesity as an economics issue, but use the rhetoric of choice in models for obesity regulation. In recent times, the rhetoric of choice has been employed by governments in their use of nudge tactics in framing how people make decisions in everyday life (Thaler and Sunstein 2008), while recognizing that food corporations also employ the rhetoric of choice, often in quite different ways, in marketing and branding their products (Hansen and Christensen 2007).

As a way of dealing with the expanding range of interest groups and evidence providers, the UK Labour administration of 1997–2010 adopted a process of EBPM (Banks 2009). This was seen as a way of anchoring policy making to delivering 'what works', unsullied by political position or the consideration of values, within a bounded rationality framework (Botterill and Hindmoor 2012) (Chapter 1). EBPM involves the systematization of scientific evidence by policy makers and the distillation of bodies of research into summaries that provide an overall picture of the scientific consensus on a particular issue, with the assumption that flaws in the policy process can be overcome by accessing and using the best possible evidence (Botterill and Hindmoor 2012). Inevitably, this ideal cannot be met, as decision making and policy formation are usually carried out under conditions of bounded rationality (Simon 1956), that is, with lack of complete information, a limited ability to assimilate information if not accessibly packaged, and limited time in which to formulate policy. Roberto et al.'s (2015) call to bridge obesity science and policy would improve evidence assimilation through accessible summaries of scientific evidence, but would have no impact on how, or if, that evidence would be used.

While the interface between research and policy is often overwhelmingly complicated, many researchers and policy makers share the belief that research can, does and should have some influence on the policy process (Haynes et al. 2011). The idea of EBPM has been challenged as being unable to develop models that reflect messier social processes, however (Haynes et al. 2011). There are often systematic distortions in the choice of evidence used in policy making, such that assumptions and world views that reflect the dominant political ideology are more likely to be supported (Stevens 2011). When obesity is framed as a medical issue, for example, it is potentially more amenable to solution by reference to scientific advice than when it is framed as a social issue, when deeply held values are often invoked by politicians (Botterill and Hindmoor 2012). To be acceptable, a policy must cohere with the dominant governmental narrative to minimize uncertainty in the facilitation of action (Stevens 2011). EBPM can be undertaken in different ways, however, with different underlying assumptions. It can combine policy-making models in knowledge-driven, problem-solving, interactive, political, enlightenment and tactical models (Bowen and Zwi 2005). The knowledge-driven model expects that new research about an issue will result in direct application in policy, while the problem-solving model charges research with providing useful evidence that can be applied to policy. The interactive model incorporates the influence of politics and of special interests in the research process, while the political model describes policy makers as being solely interested in research with potential political applications and as seeking evidence to justify a particular course of action. The enlightenment model emphasizes the influence of bodies of research across time on thinking about social issues and other perspectives, while the tactical model views evidence (or the lack thereof) as being something that can be used to justify governmental inaction. According to model, EBPM varies in the extent to which it is affected by the dominant political position and/or the consideration of values. Most usually, obesity policy takes up evidence from obesity science in ways that do not necessarily make sense to scientists. This is because the practical craft of policy development involves weaving strands of information and values according to the values and assumptions of different key stakeholder groups (Head 2008) of which science may be one of several. Obesity science itself represents a range of world views, and the scientific evidence chosen usually reflects the political position of those in power. Disparate bodies of knowledge become multiple sets of evidence that often reflect political norms, and which can only inform and influence policy rather than determine it (Head 2008).

The sometimes terse relationships between obesity research and obesity policy reflect tensions between the production and delivery of evidence, practical constraints and ideology. Greener et al. (2010) found that, among UK governmental policy makers, most considered large-scale environmental and social policy changes to be the most effective obesity interventions. These policy makers also noted, however, that structural policies of this type could not be implemented without popular support and political will (Greener et al. 2010). Scientific models of obesity are varied (Grundy 1998; Finkelstein et al. 2005; Anderson and Butcher 2006; Rolland-Cachera et al. 2006; Ulijaszek 2007a; Wright and Aronne 2012), and may be individually persuasive. When recruited to policy, they collectively contribute to the policy cacophony described by Lang and Rayner (2007), especially when the science is weighed against the practicality and effectiveness of intervention, in relation to the dominant political ideology of the time. Making obesity mundane makes obesity policy more resilient to changes in ideology, but also places it lower in the hierarchy of issues for political action. Obesity science has not yet identified interventions that can provide quick positive outcomes that could be used by politicians to gain popular support for intrusive anti-obesity regulation, high up on the Nuffield intervention ladder (Table 8.3). Governments are usually reluctant to adopt policies that might be perceived as intruding on the rights and free choices of individuals (Lang and Rayner 2007), and usually require compelling evidence for the efficaciousness (and cost-effectiveness) of anti-obesity interventions for them to be adopted. Public views about obesity in the US have shifted towards considering it more as involving systemic ecological and environmental risk (Lawrence 2004), however, while in the UK, belief that obesity is outside individual control is associated with greater support for government policies to regulate it (Beeken and Wardle 2013).

The ways in which obesity is framed and modelled by any research discipline influence what is important to know about it, how the research is done, and what types of policy options and interventions might best be viable. Equally important is the flow-back from policy making to obesity research, in priority setting and structuring research agendas through funding. A good example of such two-way communication in obesity science and policy is framed in the UK governmental policy document *Tackling Obesity: Future Choices* (Foresight 2007a, b). Among the various anti-obesity policies in the UK in recent decades, this was unique in its attempt to reframe obesity as a problem of complexity, requiring multiple sites of intervention, well beyond the range of personal responsibility. In addition to attempting to 'de-individualize' obesity policy, it has had important implications for obesity science, and the next chapter describes the development and attempted implementation of Foresight Obesities.

9 Complexity

Among the various policy objects of anti-obesity activity in the United Kingdom (UK) in recent decades, the Foresight (2007a, b) Report *Tackling Obesity: Future Choices* (henceforth, Foresight Obesities) was unique in attempting to reframe obesity as a complex problem. Foresight Obesities deserves much credit for stimulating the increase in integrated and interdisciplinary approaches to obesity research since then (Chapter 1). Although obesity had been described as being complex prior to 2007, the vast majority of scholarly literature considered its complexity within the domains of physiology, psychology, genetics and medical treatment (Chapters 2 and 5). A Google Scholar search carried out in January 2016 for the period between 1950 and the end of 2015 using the keywords 'obesity' and 'complexity' in association with each of the domains of 'psychology', 'physiology', 'systems, prevention and control', 'genetics', 'treatment' and 'epidemiology' showed 61 per cent of all 181 articles to have been published in the 9 years since the start of 2007, the other 39 per cent in the 56 years prior to then (Table 9.1). Unlike articles published prior to 2007, nearly two-thirds published since then were on systems, prevention and control. The obesity research discourse thus tipped towards complexity in 2007, as a complement to more 'classic' foci such as energy balance, genetics, psychology and medical treatment (Hamid 2009; Frood et al. 2013). Prior to 2007, much obesity science (and epidemiology especially) was largely driven by a risk factor approach, which rapidly accreted over 100 such factors for, and predispositions to, obesity (Chapter 4). The new task in the 2000s was to identify how this large number of predispositions and risk factors might operate together. This concern was not unlike the one that is central to the field of metabolomics (German et al. 2005), alternatively known as metabonomics (Nicholson and Lindon 2008), which also emerged across this period. Metabolomics/metabonomics is concerned with making statistical and mathematical sense of large numbers of biological variables and biomarkers in an age of big data, where both have proliferated. Typical approaches include the mapping of the complexity of biological systems and identifying how risk factors cluster in relation to chronic disease markers and phenotypes. Metabolomics/metabonomics was made possible with systems, networks and complexity approaches in biology from this time (Ideker et al. 2001; Kitano 2002; Hood et al. 2004; Aderem 2005; Nicholson and Lindon 2008; Palsson 2015), and Foresight Obesities very much engaged with the spirit of this new era.

The turn to complexity in obesity science and policy in 2007 came as other scientific fields and policy areas, including natural resource management and

Table 9.1. Framings of obesity complexity in the academic literature, from 1950 to the end of 2015

Domain	Number of articles			
	1950 to the end of 2006		2007 to the end of 2015	
	n	Percentage	*n*	Percentage
Psychology	8	11	9	8
Physiology	15	21	10	9
Systems, prevention and control	6	9	63	57
Genetics	22	31	9	8
Treatment	15	21	11	10
Epidemiology	4	6	9	8
Total	70		111	

governmental planning, started to embrace this approach (Allison and Hobbs 2006; Mitchell 2009; Innes and Booher 2010). Since then, many theorists have treated obesity as a system problem, with failures at many points being seen as leading to obesity, with a corresponding conclusion that system-wide solutions are required for intervention (Hamid 2009; Huang et al. 2009; Hendrie et al. 2012). Various types of complex systems approaches to obesity have been attempted, including the development of political ecological, multilevel and complex adaptive frameworks and models (Lang and Rayner 2007; Hammond 2009; Huang et al. 2009). Foresight Obesities aimed to link obesity science and policy within a single framework of systems complexity (Ulijaszek 2015), and this chapter describes how this process was undertaken. It opens with consideration of how obesity ecology came to be framed as an issue of complexity by policy makers in the first place.

Towards Obesity Complexity

Foresight Obesities, launched in 2005, was the first obesity policy project in the world to engage with complexity. It was part of a much larger programme of projects undertaken by the UK government think-tank Foresight (Table 9.2). The overall Foresight programme was initiated in 1994, during the Conservative administration of John Major, explicitly to harness scientific evidence for the making of policy, independently of party-political ideology. The use of complexity approaches in the Foresight programme and in government more broadly came in 1997, with the Labour Blair administration. The ethos of dealing with complexity in the formulation of policy by this administration was influenced by Geoff Mulgan's (1997) book, *Connexity: How to Live in a Connected World*. In this, the utility of using complexity and self-organizing systems in guiding policy is described. The Blair administration placed globality central to its approach to international relations and in its domestic politics of reform (Johnson 2007). It engaged with complexity, because the high degree of interconnectedness of global systems and processes was increasingly

Table 9.2. Foresight projects, from 2002 until 2016

Project	Date completed	Themes	Systems focus
Cognitive systems	2003	Opportunity	Yes
Flood and coastal defence	2004	Risk	No
Exploiting the electromagnetic spectrum	2004	Opportunity	No
Cybertrust and crime prevention	2004	Threat	Yes
Brain science, addiction and drugs	2005	Social benefits, ethics	Yes
Intelligent infrastructure systems	2006	Opportunity	Yes
Detection and identification of infectious diseases	2006	Threat	Yes
Tackling obesity: future choices	2007	Threat	Yes
Powering our lives: sustainable energy management and the built environment	2008	Uncertainty, opportunity	Yes
Mental capital and well-being	2008	Opportunity	Yes
Land use futures	2010	Opportunity	Yes
Technology and innovation futures	2010	Opportunity	Yes
Global food and farming futures	2011	Threat	Yes
International dimensions of climate change	2011	Threat	Yes
Migration and global environmental change	2011	Threat	Yes
Reducing risks of future disasters	2012	Threat	Yes
The future of computer trading in financial markets	2012	Opportunity	Yes
The future of identity	2013	Opportunity	No
The future of manufacturing	2013	Opportunity	No
The future of cities	2016	Opportunity	Yes
The future of an ageing population	2016	Risk, opportunity	No
Technology and innovation futures	2017	Opportunity	No

Adapted from Foresight (2017).

understood in this way (Law 2004a, b), while understanding complexity both internationally and at home was seen as a key to effective governance. Although complex systems imply self-organization, Mulgan (1997) called for a tempering of this with some strategic guidance, because according to him, people of low socioeconomic status (SES) have a poor capacity to watch for threats, avert disaster or take responsibility for the future (Parsons 2002). This view pertained to all aspects of governance, including inequalities in health and obesity (Chapter 5).

Mulgan was an influential figure for Labour party policy orientation. He was appointed Chief Advisor to future Prime Minister Gordon Brown in 1990 when Brown was Shadow Secretary of State for Trade, and founded the think-tank Demos in 1993, which he also led. From 1997, he was appointed Director of Policy directly under the Prime Minister, Director of the Prime Minister's Performance and Innovation Unit in 2000, and Head of the Government Strategy Unit in 2002. By 2005, when Foresight Obesities was initiated, the application of complexity approaches to difficult policy issues was already common. Obesity joined cognitive systems (Taylor 2003), intelligent infrastructure systems (Curry et al. 2006) and climate change (Foresight International Dimensions of Climate Change 2011) as problems that the Blair administration viewed as requiring complexity approaches. In making obesity a Foresight project, the importance with which obesity was taken by Prime Minister Tony Blair in the early 2000s was made clear. The purpose of the overall Foresight programme is to help government think systematically about future risks, challenges and opportunities, by combining the best evidence with futures analysis for tackling complex issues (Foresight 2016). The Foresight programme continues to be responsible to the Prime Minister, signalling its importance in the policy-making process. Futures analysis, Foresight-style, is designed to influence policy, and includes elements of forecasting, forward thinking, strategic analysis, priority setting, and networking of experts, ideas and strategies. Using this approach, Foresight Obesities would bring 'different government departments together to stimulate and inform the development of strategies, policies and priorities, which are more resilient and robust across a range of possible futures' (Foresight 2016).

Discerning complexity in objects for governance by the Blair administration was seen as the first step to resolving them. The second was to use the instruments of governance in a joined-up way. Much government activity runs on short timescales usually associated with electoral cycles and ministerial tenure (Exworthy and Hunter 2011), and joined-up policy was an approach to so-called 'wicked problems' that would require long-term approaches to change them (Bogdanor 2005). Joined-up government has been defined by 6 (2004) as showing consistency between the organizational arrangements of programmes, policies or agencies that may enable them to collaborate, with mutually consistent objectives, mutually consistent means, and means to support objectives consistently. A characteristic of wicked problems is that each is unique and resists resolution (Rittel and Webber 1973), often, but not always, because of its complex nature. It was precisely with the need to problematize complex systems, and to identify potential futures and potential policies to mitigate risk emerging from such systems, that most of the projects launched with the second wave of Foresight projects (from 2002) were designed.

The overarching aim of Foresight Obesities was to examine how the UK could respond sustainably to the increasing prevalence of obesity by the year 2050. Sustainable responses to obesity were seen in government circles as being policy interventions that were effective, while promoting economic growth and being permissive of environmental and food production viability. Foresight Obesities harnessed scientific evidence from a wide range of disciplines including biological, medical and social sciences, in identifying influences on, and risk factors for, obesity. It went beyond epidemiology and economics (Chapter 4) in the totality of its approach and its acceptance of some qualitative evidence. It also identified the relative importance of factors influencing obesity rates, and attempted to create a shared understanding of obesity complexity between policy makers in different arms of government, policy makers and researchers in cognate areas, and researchers in different streams of obesity research. Of central importance to the project was the development of cross-talk between government departments (joined-up government), and after that, joined-up policy advice and joined-up research. The priority placed on governmental cross-talk on obesity was made concrete with the formation of the Cross-Government Obesity Unit in 2008 (Cross-Government Obesity Unit, Department of Health and Department of Children, Schools and Families 2008), which was responsible for the initiation of the report *Healthy Lives, Healthy People* (Department of Health 2010), and the Change4Life programme. Both of these outputs met the Foresight Obesities objective of building on evidence gathered, and identifying effective solutions for change. Another objective was to analyse how future rates of obesity might change and what might be the most effective future responses to them.

The use of the term 'obesities' rather than 'obesity' in the framing of Foresight Obesities acknowledged that there are multiple paths to obesity, and that it may be impossible to come to a generalization about its causation that can apply to all circumstances (Ulijaszek 2015). Foresight Obesities had a major ambition to reorient approaches to obesity. By problematizing obesity as being complex, policy makers sought to move obesity science away from more discrete and siloed ways of practice towards more joined-up ways, and to increase the extent to which obesity science could produce evidence that is useful for policy making (Chapters 1 and 8). In treating obesity as a complex problem, Foresight Obesities placed the biological aspects of weight gain and the different logics of medical intervention and treatment for obesity within a broader ecological framework. The low emphasis given to medical and physiological intervention was notable, given that there had been nearly 30 years of world-leading research into the nutritional physiology of human energy balance in the UK (Chapter 3) by the time Foresight Obesities was initiated. By de-emphasizing medical aspects of obesity (Ulijaszek 2015), Foresight Obesities advanced thinking about relationships between biological and social models of obesity, although not comprehensively so.

Making Obesity Complex, with Foresight

From the start, Foresight Obesities involved a wide range of UK-based evidence producers (mostly scientific), policy makers (UK government officials who had been university educated in a range of disciplines including the humanities and sciences), and public and private organizations with interests in promoting health, healthy food consumption and physical activity. While the breadth of disciplines and organizations engaged in this process was far greater than in any other scoping exercise in the past, there were some notable omissions. Foresight Obesities did not engage with social critiques of framings of obesity (Gard and Wright 2005), nor did it examine values and norms surrounding large body size, including blame and stigma (Puhl and Heuer 2009) (Chapters 1 and 5). Nor did it question or evaluate existing or previous obesity policy as part of its process (Bluford et al. 2007) (Chapter 8). It also excluded any examination of relationships between power, knowledge and the citizen, or of social structure, in the production of obesity (Holm and Fruhbeck 2013) (Chapter 5).

The idea of framing obesity production as a system was implicit to the process, as was the systems modelling approach used to characterize the drivers of obesity. A causal loop, soft systems model was chosen, of the type commonly used in ecological systems energetics (Ulijaszek 1995). There are many different ways of representing a system, many of which could have served Foresight Obesities well. Functional, business processing, econometric, operational research, enterprise and soft systems models (Pidd 2004) each bring their own assumptions and rationalities (Chapters 1 and 2). Alternatives to a soft systems model would have started with different aims and would have given different outputs. The outputs from a business process model might include reductions in obesity rates of dietary energy intakes, while an enterprise model could explore the linkages of the different agencies – governmental, non-governmental and private – implicated in the production or amelioration of obesity. Such an approach had been previously taken in 2001 (National Audit Office 2001) in an examination of feedback between formally rational cross-institutional responses to obesity. Soft systems models are most frequently used for the understanding of problems that have psychological, social and cultural elements (Flood 2010), and the idea that obesity was a social issue (Chapter 5) that was politically tractable was implicit in this model.

With a design specification that obesity production in the UK was best delineated as a soft system, the primary aim was to map it (Ulijaszek 2015) as fully as possible. This involved gathering and reviewing evidence that was seen to underpin obesity as a system, and exploring future scenarios of obesity production, based on this model. The scoping process for both experts and evidence was wide-ranging, iterative, and involved many obesity, obesity-related and obesity-interested fields (Table 9.3). It identified scientific experts and stakeholders within academia, government, non-governmental organizations and major corporations (whose operations might be affected by policy recommendations) who could inform the development of a qualitative model of complexity (Table 9.4). In-depth interviews were held with stakeholders and chosen experts about how to map obesity and the issues related to it. Policy approaches that might have challenged government, non-governmental organizations or corporations were not advanced. The type of complexity accorded to this mapping was romantic, or upward looking, one that could be susceptible to regulation at the macro-level. According to Kwa (2002), romantic complexity favours stable metaphors, such as the self-correcting cybernetic machine. In the case of Foresight Obesities, the self-correcting cybernetic machine was energy balance (Chapter 3), placed at the centre of the qualitative model. An alternative approach to obesity, which would have allowed deeper scientific understanding to be gained, could have involved baroque, or micro-level, complexity (Kwa 2002; Law 2004a). This would have given governmental permission for obesity science to delve more deeply into existing research areas. If Foresight Obesities had chosen a baroque complexity approach to obesity, it could have considered any, or all, of the following as discrete complex systems: genetics; gene–environment interactions; obesogenic environments; early-life programming of physiology and body composition; appetite behaviour; food production and distribution; and macro-economic factors

Table 9.3. Expert areas and organizations engaged in the process of drawing up the Foresight Obesities Systems Map

	Expert areas	Expert organizations
Biological and medical sciences	Epidemiology, public health, genetics, biochemistry, physiology, nutrition, endocrinology, pharmacology	Medical Research Council
Medicine	Psychiatry, paediatrics	Department of Health (DoH), British Medical Association (BMA), Bupa (private health-care association)
Social sciences	Anthropology, psychology, sociology, social care	
Food production	Food science, chemical engineering, catering, marketing, chemical engineering	Department for Environment, Food, and Rural Affairs (DEFRA), Tesco (grocery and general merchandising retailer)
Media	Journalism, media studies	Department for Culture, Media and Sport (DCMS), Ofcom (independent telecommunications regulator and communications authority for the UK)
Political and economic advice		DoH, DEFRA, DCMS, food policy experts, Her Majesty's Government Treasury, the Local Government Association, Association of British Insurers
Additional expertise	History, ethics, visual art and design	

Data from Foresight (2007a).

influencing food choice and physical activity patterns. Epigenetics had yet to become implicated in human obesity by 2007 (Campion et al. 2009) (Chapter 7), so was not made part of the obesity complexity landscape of that time. With baroque complexity, there is no limit to potential internal complexity and there is no overview, nor is there any assumption of coherence to any system under investigation (Law 2004a). Such discrete baroque-complex systems would not have been amenable to joined-up government, however. Foresight Obesities was charged with producing a coherent view of obesity production, which made the case for a joined-up government approach to its regulation, and an approach that risked offering a non-coherent model of obesity could not be used to make such a case.

The mapping of the obesity system was coordinated by public servants in consultation with scientists, initially by establishing domains representing factors that influence energy balance at the individual level (food intake, physical activity, biology and psychology) and upstream of the individual (societal factors, the food supply system and the physical activity environment), then by establishing linkages between factors within and across domains. Visualizations were commissioned from the design company shift[n], and from speculative designer Jessica Charlesworth who

Table 9.4. Experts and stakeholders within academia, government and non-governmental organizations who informed the development of a model of complexity for obesity in the UK

Group	Chair	Membership
High-level stakeholder group	Dawn Primarolo, Minister of State at the Department of Health	Parliamentary Under Secretary of State at the Department for Culture, Media and Sport Head of the Health Team at Her Majesty's Treasury Parliamentary Under Secretary of State at the Department for Children, Schools and Families Chief Scientific Adviser at the Government Office for Science Deputy Chief Medical Officer at the Department of Health Chief Executive of the Medical Research Council Chief Executive of the Economic and Social Research Council Chair of the Board of Science at the British Medical Association Chair of the Food Standards Agency Director of Corporate and Legal Affairs of Tesco Corporation Chairman of Sport England Representatives from the Office of Communications Representatives from the Food and Drink Federation Representatives from Weight Watchers Representatives from Business in Sport and Leisure
Food, physical activity and obesity experts	Peter Kopelman (chronic disease medicine, University of London)	Phillip James (obesity policy, International Obesity Task Force) Susan Jebb (diet and population health, Medical Research Council) Edmund Rolls (psychology, University of Oxford) Ken Fox (physical activity and health, University of Bristol)

Data from Foresight (2007a).

worked in collaboration with artist Michael Burton (Charlesworth 2006). The final modelling of the Foresight Obesity Systems Map (FOSM) was undertaken by the WS systems design team in Brussels in the first half of 2007. The shift[n] map, designed by Vandenbroeck et al. (2007a), formed the basis of all forms of the FOSM. In all, 108 variables were linked in various ways, with solid or dashed lines to indicate positive or negative influences (Finegood et al. 2010). There are 34 versions of the FOSM (Foresight 2007b), from the full overview, to segmented ones and those that illustrate possible policy implications of different types of intervention (Vandenbroeck et al. 2007b). All versions subsequent to map zero were based upon it (Foresight 2007b). The earlier subsequent versions are layered, such that the first few show the core drivers of obesity, while the ones that follow them show the thematic clusters that influence them. These thematic clusters were defined as belonging to four major areas – human physiology, physical activity patterns, human psychology and the food environment. The latter three major areas were subdivided into two clusters, one group of factors linked to the individual, and another to the societal and environmental context of obesity production. The maps that follow show linkages between clusters, the interactions between expert-identified key variables, relationships among leverage points for obesity interventions, and weighted causal linkages among factors and predispositions as determined by expert opinion. The final seven versions of the FOSM show relationships among variables according to different policy scenarios and responses.

The mapping of relationships among factors moved beyond the listing of risk factors influencing the development, prevention and management of overweight and obesity, as presented in the *World Health Organization Consultation on Obesity* (World Health Organization 2000). In 2001, the International Obesity Task Force introduced the idea of a causal web model of factors that influence increasing obesity rates (Kumanyika et al. 2002), although they did not consider feedback among these factors, but, rather, black-boxed them (Finegood et al. 2010). Feedback loops are central to the energy balance model (Chapter 3), and such loops were additionally used by Foresight Obesities to enhance the core energy balance model by incorporating factors seen to influence it either directly or indirectly (Finegood et al. 2010).

The key drivers of obesity remained elusive across the entire period of the Foresight Obesities modelling process, in that the importance of any factor seen as being important could be related to other factors within causal loops. For example, while the plentiful availability of cheap, palatable, energy-dense foods can be seen as being important to the production of obesity, in the FOSM it is in a causal loop with factors including dietary habits, pressure of food companies to cater for acquired tastes, the desire of food companies to maximize volumes of food production, the purchasing power of consumers, exposure to advertising, the nutritional quality of food and drink, the dominance of motorized transport, exposure to advertising, the achievement of satiety and appetite control. In the FOSM, it is nigh-on impossible to assign primacy even to such a powerful factor in obesity causation as the plentiful availability of cheap, palatable, energy-dense food (Chapter 6). It is not surprising, therefore, that the generation of driver-based scenarios of the future of obesity in the UK (in effect, models for obesity regulation) was undertaken in a very tentative way.

Obesity Complexity in Policy

As a policy-producing process, Foresight Obesities was conducted to offer tools for national policy planning looking forward to 2050, and such tools needed to be adaptable to changes in political ideology across time. In order to future-proof the approach, public servants filtered the many policy options offered by the Foresight process with a version of Schwarz and Thompson's (1990) 'grid–group

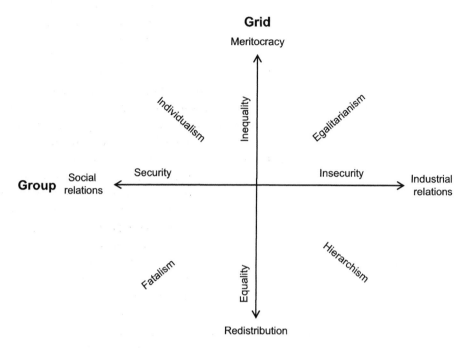

Figure 9.1. Grid–group typology of social solidarities (adapted from Schwarz and Thompson 1990). Grid: constraint by rules; group: constraint by incorporation into a bounded social unit (Douglas 1978).

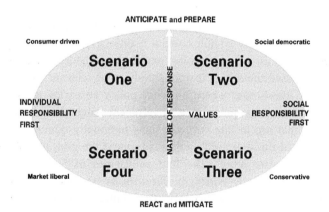

Figure 9.2. Policy scenario framework developed by Foresight Obesities, using the Schwarz and Thompson (1990) grid–group typology (adapted from Foresight 2007a). Contains public sector information licensed under the Open Government Licence v3.0 www.nationalarchives.gov.uk/doc/open-government-licence/version/3/

typology of social solidarities' (Figure 9.1). Foresight Obesities had four types of policy future scenarios, along a grid–group typology of social solidarities in a two-by-two grid (Figure 9.2), an approach that had been used in previous Foresight projects.

The Schwarz and Thompson (1990) typology co-opted a framework first advanced by Douglas (1986), who theorized there to be four distinct cultural biases (or social solidarities) that coexist in any society at all times, and to different degrees, each possessing a world view that forms the basis for its viability. According to Schwarz and Thompson (1990), conflict and contention between solidarities can destabilize other solidarities in a political system conceptualized as being in self-organizing disequilibrium, 'in which each of the solidarities is acting so as to undermine the others while, at the same time, needing them to define itself against' (Grendstad et al. 2003). One axis of Schwarz and Thompson's (1990) typology articulates the power of different formal modes of control, and the degree to which the social roles, behaviours and interactions of people are governed, irrespective of membership of any group (Douglas 1978, 1996; Gross and Rayner 1985). These formal modes of control include overarching mechanisms such as the law, the economy and governmental regulation. The other axis registers the strength of commitment of individuals to other members of a social solidarity, and the extent to which that social solidarity standardizes the thoughts and actions of its members. Examples of groups as social solidarities, in this framing, might be local communities, neighbourhoods or families. This form of analysis contends that different organizations, should they exhibit similarities in social structure, would also present some consistencies in cultural patterns, biases and values – social constructions that generate norms and narratives through which to view reality and world views (Schwarz and Thompson 1990; Thompson et al. 1990). Summaries of the four social solidarities are given in Table 9.5.

The grid–group taxonomy generates a dimensional framework that can be used to decode and classify complex social realities (Wildavsky et al. 1997), either instrumentally, or as an overarching explanatory theory (Mamadouh 1999). Foresight Obesities used the device instrumentally to be relevant to differing political ideologies into the future, where different policy scenarios would apply depending on which ideological quadrant a government might largely adhere to (Figure 9.2). Policies that are in line with any new nationally dominant political ideology can be recruited through a different quadrant of the grid, potentially making Foresight Obesities 'future proof'. The four solidarities of Schwarz and Thompson (1990) were redescribed by Foresight Obesities as 'scenarios' according to the ideology underpinning them. In Scenario One, enlightened consumers would respond to obesity by driving the market towards offering healthy options. In Scenario Two, social democratic governments would anticipate the future, and plan obesity away through upstream levers such as taxation. In Scenario Three, conservative approaches would rely on tradition to find responses to obesity, locally and nationally. And in Scenario Four, market-liberal approaches would seek individualist responses to obesity. These scenarios can only be mapped onto political party ideology very loosely, however, because ideologies within any political party can change considerably over time, often in relation to future electability (Adams et al. 2004). Furthermore, governmental ideologies almost everywhere have increasingly functioned within neoliberal frameworks since the 1980s. Above all, the grid–group

Table 9.5. Description of Schwarz and Thompson's (1990) grid–group typology of social solidarities

Solidarity	Grid/group	Nature	Description
Individualist	Low/low	Competitive	Characterized by weak restrictions on individual behaviour, and strong respect for individual rights. Members of this solidarity are responsible for themselves. Boundaries are subject to negotiation, and individuals maintain a high spatial and social mobility. The free market is a prototypical structure
Hierarchical	High/high	Bureaucratic	Defined by rules, restrictions to mobility and inequality, this solidarity functions on the basis of security through process, duty and accountability. This solidarity is characterized by social structures that value tradition and social role differentiation
Fatalistic	High/low	Isolated	This solidarity depicts a social environment in which the individual's station is socially assigned and restricted, often excluded from any group and decision making, implying coercion into this category
Egalitarian	Low/high	Sectarian	A social context in which the external group boundary is typically the dominant consideration. Individual behaviour is subject to controls exercised in the name of the group. There are formal internal divisions. Segregating, delegating and specializing roles are absent

Grid: constraint by rules; group: constraint by incorporation into a bounded social unit (Douglas 1978). Adapted from Gross and Rayner (1985).

approach to obesity gives insight into how the UK Labour administration of 1997–2010 imagined the future.

Foresight Obesities was also charged with developing a quantitative model to predict how future rates of obesity might change. This involved cross-sectional analysis and microsimulation of different intervention strategies on obesity rates to the year 2050 (including: no interventions, and intervening with a universal strategy of reducing average body mass index (BMI) across the population, and of reducing BMI among potentially overweight or obese people), using two types of modelling procedure. The first involved a longitudinal analysis, which predicted BMI into the future, and the second involved an assessment of disease-related costs of obesity (McPherson et al. 2007). Both analyses used epidemiological and health economics data (Chapter 4) to project the rates of obesity and their costs to the economy into the future (McPherson et al. 2007). Annual datasets for adult heights and weights, collected by the Health Survey for England (HSE) between 1993 and 2004, were used. These datasets typically included between 10 000 and 20 000 records per year for weights and heights, from which BMI was calculated. The use of HSE data on weight and heights of adults in the predictive model assured the Weberian theoretically rational instrumentalization of this survey for obesity surveillance into the future.

The year 2007 also saw the introduction of the National Child Measurement Programme (NCMP), set up to monitor childhood obesity by the National Obesity Observatory. The NCMP continues as an annual programme of measurement of heights and weights of the vast majority of children in the first and final years of state-funded primary schools in England. Both HSE and NCMP obesity monitoring are on the lowest rung of intervention of the Nuffield Council on Bioethics public health intervention ladder (Chapter 8), and hold UK National Statistics status in the same way that the reporting of births, deaths and marriages does.

Why Obesity Complexity?

Causal loop models were used in this and other Foresight projects, with governmental intent to demonstrate problems as systems, involving complexity. A problem with such models, however, is that they make no distinction between the flow of stocks (for example, energy), risk factors (for example, overeating of palatable foods) and of informational links between factors (for example, that the type of foods available influences what people eat) (Chapter 6). Despite placing energy balance central to the FOSM, Foresight Obesities chose not to study the flow of energy between the different factors that use or consume it within a system, because this would have limited the model to the risk factors and influences that have energy as a currency or stock, and not to the broader range of issues that make obesity structurally complex. Foresight Obesities also chose not to model the extent of scientific writing about obesity and its links across disciplines (for example, physiology, genetics, psychology, nutrition) according to the number and type of articles written within each discipline, and the ways in which they are networked across disciplines. Had it done so, it would have provided knowledge about the extent to which obesity research was siloed, or otherwise. Since initial consultations declared obesity research to be siloed (much in the same way that the leadership in the Blair and Brown administrations viewed UK government departments in the 2000s to be inward-looking), this was already prejudged. There was no material output from the model chosen for use by Foresight Obesities, such as might be the case with an economics-based balance sheet (a possible output from an econometric model), which would have been useful for economic intervention (Chapter 4). Had body size been used as an outcome of interest, an econometric model could have offered observations with very different implications for obesity policy, especially with respect to upstream interventions. This might have suited economists, but would not have easily brought a wide range of scientists with varying research interests to the project. In addition, an econometric approach would have risked demonstrating that free-market economics might carry additional risks for obesity, as was demonstrated subsequently (Offer et al. 2010). This would not have been useful for the Blair administration, nor for the governments that followed it, given the centrality of neoliberalism to UK politics from the 1980s onwards. A medical model would have privileged the treatment of obesity as a disease; medical approaches were excluded from the project design from the beginning. The choice of a causal loop model by Foresight Obesities resulted in a map that purposely fitted existing thinking within the UK government, and introduced the possibility of a new approach for obesity research (Ulijaszek 2015), in line with complexity and systems thinking elsewhere in science.

Why were the scientists engaged in Foresight Obesities amenable to a systems approach to obesity, when such thinking was only nascent in a few obesity scientists' minds (Hamid 2009)? Part of the answer lies with the choice of scientific experts. Of those involved in Foresight Obesities, many were already familiar with systems thinking. Some had used it in their work already, often in related fields. The energy balance model is itself a system, and those working in energy balance have no problem intuiting other kinds of causal loop models. This type of model is commonly used in modelling and illustrating physiological, endocrinological, developmental and psychological processes, and scientists in these fields saw them as natural types even before they came to Foresight Obesities. With respect to other domains within the model, most experts involved in Foresight Obesities working on physical activity, transport, food supply, food consumption and psychology also used causal loop models in some or all aspects of their work.

Foresight Obesities sought to bring obesity science and policy together as never before, and the FOSM was constructed as a boundary object (Fox 2011) that could bring different disciplines, fields and interest groups to work together. The boundary between politics and science is a constantly negotiated one, and boundary objects and boundary organizations help stabilize relationships between the two. The Technology Strategy Board, an advisory body within the former UK Department of Trade and Industry, was set up in 2004 to negotiate the boundaries between research and commercial outcomes by working with major research councils and regional development agencies. It became an independent arm's-length body in 2007, and was renamed 'Innovate UK' in 2014, as it continued to do the same work. Foresight projects such as the one on Intelligent Infrastructure Systems (completed in 2006) and Technology and Innovation Futures (completed in 2010) inform the activities of Innovate UK in their dealings with research councils. The primary mission of the Foresight programme generally was, until the election of the Conservative–Liberal Democrat coalition government in 2010, the production of boundary objects to engage in the work of joined-up government and departmental modernization. Since that time, the boundary work that the Foresight programme does in its various projects has been harnessed for the development and commercialization of research by Innovate UK in its negotiations with research councils and private commercial concerns.

Obesity Science and Policy, from Complexity and Beyond

The model of obesity complexity produced by Foresight Obesities did not translate into meaningful models for obesity intervention, even though this had been the hope. There were early criticisms that the FOSM was unintelligible (Jack 2007), and its sheer complexity may have deterred from its direct use in intervention. There were, however, important consequences of Foresight Obesities for both science and policy.

For policy, these included subsequent attempts to understand the cross-talk between expert systems (Chapters 1 and 10) such as those of food, medicine and transport, and how they might be regulated towards improved health and reduced obesity. The work of Foresight Obesities led to the establishment of the Cross-Government Obesity Unit, and the policy report *Healthy Weight, Healthy Lives* (Cross-Government Obesity Unit, Department of Health and Department of Children, Schools and Families 2008). By connecting very diverse stakeholders and developing directives that facilitated 'joined-up government', this unit became the instrument of joined-up obesity governance. Among stakeholders, the National Institute for Health and Care Excellence has used the Foresight Obesities report as a basis for some of its own publications, while the National Obesity Observatory has pursued complex systems approaches for obesity intervention (Foresight 2010). For obesity research, attempts by Foresight Obesities to integrate approaches in the biosciences and social sciences led to increased interdisciplinarity (Chapter 1). In framing obesity as a problem of complexity, Foresight Obesities placed the biological aspects of weight gain and the different logics of medical intervention and treatment for obesity within a broader ecological frame. Of the 17 options for policy interventions put forward, only three of them involved health: targeted public health interventions for young children and those most at risk of obesity; population-wide public health interventions; and a focus on the health consequences of obesity rather than obesity itself (Foresight 2007b).

The main policy intervention to come from Foresight Obesities and the Cross-Government Obesity Unit was the Change4Life programme. The discourse of complexity promoted by Foresight Obesities was absent from its roll-out, however. Planned as a 3-year-long social marketing campaign initiated in 2009, Change4Life focused on modifying individual behaviour (or nudging) (Chapter 1) as a means of addressing population-level obesity. It used social marketing and advertising techniques with media, public and private sector partners, with the aim of catalysing consumer-driven social change. Private industry was involved only insofar as sponsors were encouraged to support Change4Life and assist in altering consumer behaviour (Chapter 6). This presented opportunities for publicity, product placement and advertising, and permitted industry partners to participate in obesity reduction in ways that did not conflict with their obligations to their shareholders. Where initiatives that were intended to improve food environments were implemented, such as making sure that stores in deprived areas were stocked with fresh foods, emphasis was on the provision of goods rather than communication and collective action towards dietary and health improvement (Adams et al. 2012).

The aim of Change4Life to reframe obesity so that it is not seen as the fault of individuals or families, but as being the result of modern life, came directly from Foresight Obesities (Department of Health 2009). However, this did not translate into practice. Rather, individual consumer behaviour (Chapter 6) was foregrounded in the Change4Life report as the target for change. Change4Life distributed information and tools to help people make better lifestyle choices, and the success of the programme was to be evaluated using NCMP data (Evans and Colls 2011). Change4Life had 'assumed necessity to target particular individuals and families with an ideal, rational consumer-subject remaining at the heart of what is considered healthy' (Evans and Colls 2011) – there was no space for evolutionary or Weberian substantive rationalities in this programme. Implicit social values, assumptions and ideologies in Change4Life doctrine concerning class, race, gender and the role of the individual in society were no different to those underpinning earlier UK government obesity reports (Evans and Colls 2011), despite the elevation of obesity as a target for governmental intervention (Chapter 8) by virtue of the establishment of the NCMP.

Even while obesity science has continued to contest, debate and experiment with complexity models of obesity, the world, and political administrations within it, has changed. The political framing of obesity as a complex phenomenon was downplayed when Foresight Obesities was initially operationalized with Change4Life during the Labour administration of Gordon Brown, and more completely under the subsequent governments after 2010. The Conservative–Liberal Democrat coalition government of 2010–15 promoted corporate social responsibility deals, offering some moral kudos to food corporations that self-regulate in reducing their obesogenic practices. Foresight Obesities continued to inform obesity policy, even with the change in political ideology from 2010 onwards, showing that the grid–group typology of policy scenarios is resilient. The governmental approach to obesity shifted in 2010 from enlightened consumerism to market liberalism (Figure 9.2, from Scenario One to Scenario Four). The UK government's 2010–15 policy paper on obesity and healthy eating, entitled *Helping People Make Healthier Choices*, made this shift clear: the government would offer advice and guidance to improve labelling and consumer information, and encourage businesses to include information on, and with, their food products so that people could make healthier choices.

In keeping with the adoption of Scenario Four, the policy document *Call to Action on Obesity* (Department of Health 2011) placed emphasis on individual-level behaviour change (Jebb et al. 2013), recruiting the Nuffield intervention ladder (Chapter 8) towards nudge-based approaches (Thaler and Sunstein 2008), which rely on bounded rationality (Chapter 1). Also in keeping with Scenario Four, the Public Health Responsibility Deal was initiated in 2011, and within that, the Food Network Responsibility Deal (FNRD), initiated in 2013. By 2013, however, national government funding for Change4Life was reduced to around one-fifth of its opening level in 2009. It was perhaps lucky to be kept active with mostly governmental funding a year after its intended end. Change4Life continues with sponsorship from commercial brands and non-governmental organizations matched with funding from government, on a project-by-project basis. This has led to some ambiguous messages to programme participants about what constitutes 'good' consumption, because consumption that is good for income generation of sponsors and supporters is not necessarily good for health (Chapter 6). While framed as a partnership, most of the work programme of the FNRD was (and still is) guided by the food industry. The FNRD is underpinned by a governmental ideological emphasis on market growth, and while it places responsibility on the food industry to drive change, this is seen by some as being ineffective (Monbiot 2015). In practice, consumers are framed as being ultimately responsible for their own consumption behaviours, again in keeping with Scenario Four of Foresight Obesities' grid–group typology. The framing of obesity as an outcome of individually non-rational behaviours by Conservative governments since 2015 is as easy to understand as the economically rational framing of obesity that led to the Foresight Obesities project in the first place, under a Labour administration; that is, obesity, if not controlled, would become very expensive to the national purse. The activation of the FNRD has significantly added corporate issues of profitability and market competition to governmental concerns about the costs of obesity to the economy.

Foresight Obesities created the possibility of complexity thinking for obesity regulation more generally, but the UK government did not recruit complexity thinking to dealing with the structural and upstream issues that matter for obesity management, especially with respect to the expert systems that regulate food, health and the environment (Chapter 10). Since 2015, the two Conservative governments have had no need for either joined-up government or complexity. Instead, upstream regulation in the form of a tax on sugar-sweetened beverages (SSBs) (Chapter 4) was announced unexpectedly in 2016, on the back of the Public Health England (2015b) report *Sugar Reduction: The Evidence for Action*. SSB taxation is now a central part of the UK government policy for controlling childhood obesity, along with incentivizing approaches to get primary school children to eat more healthily and to be more physically active (Department of Health, Prime Minister's Office, Her Majesty's Treasury and Cabinet Office 2016), while the FNRD continues.

Obesity, Complexity and Power

How can policy regulate the expert systems that interactively and inadvertently produce obesity? While Foresight Obesities recruited the Weberian theoretical rationality of science to the Weberian formal rationality of policy, the objects that require governance in order for obesity to be controlled have become increasingly complex. These include the systems of medicine, transport and communication, food, media and economics, which, while growing across the past century or so, have become expert with the connectivity technologies that computing brought since the 1980s (Chapter 10). Computing (and other technologies that involve and/or are underpinned, aided or enhanced by it) has allowed transport to move faster, food to be cheaper, medicine to offer more fixes for more ailments, and media to communicate knowledge, information and trivia more broadly and frequently than ever before. At the macro-level, the operations of many expert systems have facilitated the decline in global mortality rates and have promoted economic growth. Negative consequences of their activities have also emerged, however, with the rise of neo-liberal political systems. These include: increased economic inequality (Navarro 2007; Jacobs and Myers 2014), increased insecurity (Webster et al. 2008; Wacquant 2009), and rising obesity rates (Guthman and du Puis 2006; Anand and Gray 2009; Offer et al. 2010). Although expert systems are structured by power relations within and across nations, there is generally a lack of discussion of how systems and complexity thinking consider the distribution and use of power (Room 2015).

The absence of concern about power rings true for science and policy work on obesity complexity. The power exercised by the Conservative UK government in announcing a tax on SSBs in 2016 came without any call upon complexity or Foresight Obesities. It also came without significant policy discussion, which reduced the voice of the sugar lobby in the UK and internationally in this policy decision. For the Coca-Cola Corporation, the world's largest buyer of sugar in 2016 (Chapter 6), a tax on SSBs must be seen at worst as being a brand killer, although the corporation is sure to adapt. Of all that has been written about obesity and complexity from 2007, almost nothing has been written about inequality and obesity (Chapter 5), although this was very briefly touched on in Foresight Obesities.

An alternative approach to complexity might involve a focus on understanding expert systems and how they interact (Chapter 10). This could help policy makers steer corporate social responsibility deals and pacts away from possible negative health outcomes associated with corporate activity. The Foresight Obesities planning and consultation process began to shift the framing of obesity from being a problem of individual responsibility to one of collective responsibility (Butland et al. 2007). However, there is no particular systems modelling reason (Ulijaszek 2015) or scientific rationale as to why the individual (as framed by energy balance) should be at the centre of the FOSM (Ulijaszek and McLennan 2016). The final chapter of this book considers the multiple rationalities that are made explicit in attempts to develop models of obesity that involve complexity and the expert systems that structure everyday life in late modern society.

10 Systems and Rationalities

From the rise of neoliberalism in the 1980s, economic rationality has pervaded all aspects of life and the world (Chapter 1), and policy-related understandings of obesity are most easily framed in this way. This book examines how the emergence and persistence of obesity in late modern, neoliberal society is understood by institutions, agencies, corporations and people according to different world views, underpinned by often differing and sometimes conflicting rationalities. While the underlying simplicity of energy balance models (Chapter 3) makes them attractive for policy makers, it is argued that they have poor efficacy when used to support the individualist approaches to obesity control that predominate under neoliberalism (Chapter 8). More broadly, obesity science and policy will continue to contribute to policy cacophony (Lang and Rayner 2007) as long as they, and other constituencies with interests in obesity, operate from differing world views without understanding the rationalities that underpin models of obesity other than their own. The most easily intuited rationality in present-day life is economic (Chapter 1), but this has only become naturalized in framings of obesity since the 1990s (Chapter 8).

Obesity science emerged from concerns about human energetics, heredity and genetics, and physiological and morphological plasticity, and from the sociology and anthropology of the body. Other disciplines have additionally laid claim to being obesity sciences as the obesity phenomenon has grown since the 1980s. Epidemiology, human ecology, economics, epigenetics, microbiology and complexity science all have legitimate reasons for engaging with obesity. Obesity science has informed knowledge of obesity at all levels, from the environmental and ecological (Chapter 3), and the macro-structural levels that inform Pattern Four nutrition transition (Chapter 7), the global food system (Chapter 6), and the political and governmental domains that economics and epidemiology inform (Chapter 4), to the societal, social and familial levels (Chapter 5), and the individual, organ-system and molecular levels (Chapter 3) that inform human life history (Chapter 8) and evolution (Chapter 3). Obesity has also been framed as being more broadly complex and multilevel (Finegood 2011), and many of the structural issues and macro-level factors that governments regulate (or which may be beyond the control of individual governments to regulate) are now under scrutiny by obesity scientists (Chapter 7). The current framing of obesity as a complex scientific problem (Chapter 8) reflects the breadth of disciplines trying to make sense of it (Ulijaszek 2007a) (Chapter 1), and the difficulty of trying to discipline obesity with any singular approach. Rationalities form the disciplinary world views that make implicit how obesity and its contributing factors should be understood, modelled and acted upon by different interests, including scientific, governmental and corporate ones. These rationalities vary according to actor in obesity science, policy and intervention, and incompatibilities in rationality of approach by different agents limit the extent to which effective interdisciplinary work in obesity research and policy can be done.

This final chapter examines how models of obesity differ and/or interrelate with each other, according to rationality. It also examines the extent to which polyrational approaches might help in identifying overlapping and conflicting rationalities in obesity science, policy and intervention. The idea of polyrationality was developed by Hartmann (2010) to examine the relationships among different rationalities in negotiating the complex interactions of different agents and interests in flood control and urban planning (Hartmann 2012; Hartmann and Spit 2012). What works in urban planning might also work for obesity, and this is also considered here.

Multiple Rationalities

The way in which obesity is framed by any research discipline influences what is important to know about it, how the research is done and types of evidence that are deemed important. The model that has formed the basis of most obesity policy and intervention across decades is that of energy balance (Chapter 3), which is underpinned by Weberian theoretical rationality (Chapter 2). The number of rationalities at play in energy balance increases, however, when individual, cross-generational, environmental and evolutionary perspectives are incorporated. Obesogenic environments are essential to energy balance explanations of obesity (Chapter 3). Without them, and without the widespread availability of cheap energy-dense food, genetic and epigenetic predispositions to obesity would not result in obesity. Obesogenic environments are characterized as being both physical and social, as promoting weight gain and not being conducive to weight loss (Swinburn et al. 1999a). They emerge from the actions of corporations and governments whose Weberian practical and formal rationalities underpin modernity and modernization. Policy that uses the obesogenic environment construct shifts the focus from individual choice to more structural matters, and is explicit about the extent to which the state and other macro-level factors and actors configure the fabric and texture of daily life (Shove 2010). The obesogenic environments model takes as implicit the view that patterns of diet and exercise are socially, institutionally and infrastructurally configured, making such environments also the outcomes of Weberian formal and practical rationalities. Far from limiting the scope of possible intervention, this idea has inspired discussion of the need for societal change not only in eating, but also in patterns of time use and mobility (Shove 2010).

Research into the psychology and neurophysiology of appetite (Chapter 6) seeks to understand energy balance through the regulation of food intake, conscious and otherwise. Appetite, eating, satiety and satiation are physiologically regulated by a complex system of neural pathways and endocrine mechanisms that involve the brain, nervous system and gut. According to Berthoud and Morrison (2008), 'the predisposition to develop obesity can theoretically result from any pathological malfunction or lack of adaptation to changing environments of this highly complex system'. The global food system (Chapter 6), a driver of changing nutritional environments (Chapter 7), is underpinned by economic and Weberian practical rationality, with the food corporations that dominate it taking the most appropriate courses of action to meet their aims, which are ultimately economic. Food corporations make more profit if people eat more and/or eat more expensively, but economic rationality in food production does not automatically square with optimal nutritional health, especially among those of low socioeconomic status (SES) (Chapters 5 and 6).

From individual energy intake and expenditure to the global food system, the drivers of obesity are thus diffuse and global, with many interacting actors and factors, and multiple rationalities. Economics and epidemiology combined have perhaps the only effective macro-level modelling instruments available for the regulation of population obesity (Chapter 3). Epidemiological reporting and modelling provide the basis for understanding the scale of population obesity and its future trajectory, while economists are able to model the inputs of obesity on national and regional economies by incorporating epidemiological data. Global changes in the dietary and nutritional environment, through the operation of expert systems, have led to the emergence of obesity and the chronic diseases associated with it (Chapter 7). These changes have their roots in history and human life history, and are driven by modernization and globalization. Because the global and ecological nature of the expert systems that serve everyday life cannot be regulated by any single agent, however large (Chapter 8), it is difficult to see how obesity might be regulated by singular actions, even by nation states. Even if they could, the relationships between science, policy and ethics remain crucial to determining what such actions might be.

Biology and Society in Obesity Policy

Both the production of obesity (Raymond 1986; Ulijaszek and Lofink 2006) and its policy regulation (Lang and Rayner 2005; Hill et al. 2007) involve discursive relationships between biology and the social sciences, including politics and economics (Meloni 2013, 2014). Obesity may be arrived at by seemingly endless potential pathways, involving countless relationships among predispositions and risk factors. Understanding these relationships and elucidating possible pathways to obesity require interdisciplinary work on relationships between biological and cultural models of obesity and body fatness. The study of these is relatively new (Ulijaszek and Lofink 2006), although the study of biological phenomena with social correlates has a deeper history (Huss-Ashmore et al. 1992; Thomas 1997; Goodman and Leatherman 1998). Any dichotomous positioning of nature versus nurture in interdisciplinary obesity science is problematic (Warin et al. 2015) because any such positioning locates biological human lives (and their social relations) into separate domains according to disciplinary preference (Latour 2004; Landecker 2011; Rose 2013), and continues to silo obesity research.

The social and the biological are entwined in obesity policy, as the following examples show. Biology may help deliver better pharmaceutical interventions for obesity in the future, but the regulation of new drugs falls into social and societal domains (Fox et al. 2005). Biology can also inform improved obesity surgery, but this is not a solution to obesity in itself, because there are both social and biological correlates and consequences of such surgery (Throsby 2007, 2012). Furthermore, social interventions employing energy balance models may vary in success according to SES (Verloigne et al. 2012). While the biology underpinning obesity production at the individual level is indisputable, the construction of obesogenic environments is almost entirely social (Chapter 3), as are the globalizing forces that drive Pattern Four nutrition transition (Chapter 7). Thus, translating obesity science into obesity policy requires an acknowledgement of biocultural relations. According to Shove (2010), the relationship between research and policy is mutual: policy makers fund and legitimize lines of enquiry that generate results that they can handle and which are consequently defined as concrete, achievable and manageable. The result is a self-fulfilling cycle of credibility (Latour and Woolgar 1986), in which evidence of relevance and utility helps in securing additional resources for research and intervention, building capacity in some areas but not in others (Shove 2010). Furthermore, the policy arena is not consistent (Shove 2010). With respect to obesity, the Labour government of Blair and Brown acknowledged this in the call for a Cross-Departmental Committee on Obesity, after foregrounding the complexity of obesity with Foresight Obesities (Ulijaszek and McLennan 2016) (Chapter 8).

Obesity is a late modern phenomenon. Late modernity is characterized by global capitalism, the privatization of services, the spread of individualism and a reliance on the effective functioning of a vast array of expert systems (Unerman and O'Dwyer 2007) that provide and maintain infrastructures such as those of water, transport, communications, health and food. Most individuals, most of the time, think little, if anything, about most of these systems, relying on (often unconscious) trust. Without placing trust in them, individually complex lives would be almost impossible to live, as there would be a need to continually negotiate their operations. The interactions of many of these expert systems may have collectively, if inadvertently, contributed to population obesity, as the following examples illustrate. The easy availability of cheap energy-dense food is a product of the globally expert food system. The sedentariness that is associated with obesity is a product of nationally and locally complex urban planning systems, which prioritize motor car transport above other forms (Frank et al. 2004), and of desk–chair configurations for computer-facilitated work (McCrady and Levine 2009). Just-in-time supply systems (Hines et al. 2004) are facilitated by expert systems that streamline business and work, and make consumerism easy, but lead to individual lives that also operate in a just-in-time way. The outputs of lean thinking and operations in business systems (Hines et al. 2004) are likely to contribute to obesity, through consumerism and stress (Albritton 2009; Dallman 2010).

Complex ecological energetic relationships are fundamental to the function of both nature and society (Smil 2008), and the regulation of obesity requires a fundamental rethinking of humanity's energy relationships (Gortmaker et al. 2011). Such a rethink would require recalibration of many expert systems, which may not be easily retuned without unpredictable consequences elsewhere in society. Calling individuals to control their own body size (and that of their young children, when they have them) using energy balance rhetoric attempts to responsibilize consumer citizens to act in their best non-obesogenic interests, in a marketplace of products and services generated by interactive expert systems. There are several reasons why this does not generally work at societal level. First, trust in individual expert systems (such as the food system) may be misplaced if those systems encourage maladaptive behaviours (such as overeating, in the case of the food system, and over-reliance on the motor car, in the case of the transport system). Second, the body size outcomes of individuals negotiating expert systems in daily life cannot be easily predicted, making the regulation of such systems for obesity control difficult. Third, individuals may insulate some social and consumer practices from the health values they accept and apply most of the time, making obesity an outcome of personally boundaried decisions (using bounded rationality) in a world of personally uncontrollable expert systems.

The success or failure of obesity regulation is as dependent on technical issues as on structural and behavioural ones. To enact obesity policy, it is important to know many things, including: what healthy eating and healthy diets are; what constitutes healthy body size and composition; what types and amounts of physical activity count for obesity control; what constitutes an obesogenic environment; and what aspects of SES and capital are most related to obesity susceptibility. To be able to responsibilize individuals, parents and schools, the answers to such questions have to be translated into guidelines and turned into procedures and practices. The idea of evidence-based policy making (EBPM) is common in government, but its practice is varied (Chapter 8). According to Campbell et al. (2007), evidence can provide the rationale for an initial policy direction, an understanding of the nature and extent of the problem, suggestions for possible solutions, an insight into the likely impacts in the future, and motivation for adjustments to a policy or the way it is to be implemented. This is in contrast to the reality of policy making and delivery, which is also described by Campbell et al. (2007) as being messy and unpredictable, where evidence is one factor among others including the political imperative to act on an issue, and where the response to media and world events is important. There is little surprise that the efficacy of obesity research in EBPM is mixed (Chapter 8).

Complexity, Expert Systems and Policy

High population obesity rates emerge when social, cultural and political processes allow biological predispositions to obesity to be realized. Such processes are complex, integrative and multilevel. Complexity can operate at different levels – Kwa (2002) has framed it as being either romantic or baroque (Chapter 9). Romantic complexity looks at relationships at the macro-level and is upward looking. Baroque complexity is downward-looking (Law 2004a), and in obesity science, different disciplines can represent particular approaches to obesity or obesity predispositions as discrete complex systems in themselves. Baroque-complex systems include obesogenic environments, the genetics of obesity, gene–environment interactions in obesity production, early-life programming of physiology and body composition, epigenetics and body fatness, appetite behaviour, and food production and distribution. Baroque complexity is also involved in economic influences on food availability (Chapter 4), psychological influences on food choice (Chapter 6), the social, societal, political and economic factors that drive inequalities in obesity rates (Chapter 5), and the interplay of forces that shape obesity policy (Chapters 8 and 9).

Baroque-complex systems are often embedded in romantically complex ones. The physiological regulation of food intake in relation to an obesogenic food supply involves complexity at both levels, through the activities of several expert systems and different governmental departments, agentive organizations (including individualist-oriented weight management groups) and corporations (including food and pharmaceutical companies). The search for pharmacological solutions to obesity is another example of baroque-within-romantic complexity. This field is characterized by technical problems over safety, efficacy, abuse and adverse effects (including mortality), marketability and profitability, in the negotiated space between public and private interests within the expert system of medicine. The American Medical Association's (2013) recognition of obesity as a disease (Chapter 1) is an encouragement to continue research towards finding a more targeted and more effective anti-obesity drug by pharmaceutical companies. Such research has a chequered history, however, with many drugs marketed for weight loss subsequently being removed from the market for unintended or undesired consequences (Table 10.1).

Thyroid extract was marketed as an anti-obesity drug in the 1890s (Bray 2008). Its use for body fat reduction was soon discontinued when it was found to result in decreases in muscle and bone mass, as well as in fat, among non-thyroid-deficient obese subjects. In the early twentieth century, dinitrophenol was marketed for weight loss, but with inadequate clinical testing. Skin rash, cataracts and neuropathy followed its use, and it too was discontinued. In the 1930s, amphetamine was identified as a weight-loss-inducing compound (Bray 2008), and was sold as an over-the-counter weight-loss remedy (Rasmussen 2008). In the 1960s, evidence showed that it was addictive, rather than 'habituating' like caffeine (as was asserted when the drug was first introduced) (Rasmussen 2008), leading to its withdrawal for weight-loss purposes by the 1970s. In the 1980s, a combination of fenfluramine and phentermine (Fen/Phen) was shown to be a very effective weight-loss agent, and was very widely used across the United States (US) (Bray 2008). But by 1997, some consumers of this medication began to develop valvular heart disease, and the US Food and Drug Administration (FDA) withdrew it after legal damage payments to consumers exceeded US\$13 billion (Kim et al. 2011). The most commonly used drug that is FDA approved for obesity treatment is orlistat, a lipase inhibitor that can result in sustainable weight loss (Kim et al. 2011; Colon-Gonzalez et al. 2013).

Although corporate rhetoric about weight-loss medication development is inevitably optimistic (economic rationality demands this of the industry), there is

Table 10.1. Unintended or undesired consequences from the use of medications to treat obesity (adapted from Bray 2008)

Drug	Outcome
Thyroid extract	Hyperthyroidism
Dinitrophenol	Cataracts, neuropathy
Fenfluramine/dexfenfluramine	Aortic regurgitation
Phenylpropanolamine	Stroke
Sibutramine	Stroke and myocardial infarction

increasing appreciation by researchers of the difficulty of such development. In large part, this is because of the baroque complexity of the physiological appetite and energy balance systems as they relate to weight loss. Anti-obesity drug discovery lies overwhelmingly in the domain of pharmaceutical corporations, which operate within the expert system of medicine. Governments represent a regulatory component of this system, overseeing the enforcement of safety standards for population use, towards the eventual production and roll-out of safe drugs. This is not a trivial role, especially where there is high demand for anti-obesity medication, as in many high-income countries (HICs), and a corporate thirst for profit.

Food systems are another example of baroque complexity embedded within romantic complexity. At the macro-level, the global food system was well formed, if not yet consolidated, prior to World War II (Chapter 7), and was subsequently manipulated by governments to operate as an instrument of geopolitical influence during the Cold War (George 1977). The governance of food shifted largely from state control into corporate hands with the neoliberal turn of the 1980s. At the micro-level, food production and consumption both lie within the domains of food science and technology, agriculture, plant and animal breeding, the neurophysiology of taste, psychology and physiology, among other disciplines, each with its own set of baroque-complex relationships. At the macro-level, the romantic complexity of the global food system can be described in terms of sets of relationships, but cannot be clearly articulated. In part this is because much of it is in corporate hands, with information that is not openly shared. When combined, the romantic and baroque complexities of the global food system defy understanding, let alone regulation. In the absence of clear understandings of the complexities of food production, processing and consumption, there is but a small number of policy levers that governments can use to make food availability to a national population more healthy. None of these can be evaluated, for example, in the way that a medical intervention can, with randomized controlled trials. In the absence of clear food policy outcomes in relation to obesity at the macro-level, obesity policy easily falls back onto individualized responsibility for consumption. In the United Kingdom (UK), obesity policy has attempted to link individualism with corporate responsibility for the safety of food and the possible health impacts of foods on consumers (Chapter 8). In this case, government offers advice and guidance to improve labelling and consumer information, and encourages businesses to include information on and with their food products so that people can make healthier choices, thus linking public health strategies with market consumerism (Lang and Rayner 2007). This was facilitated, in the Change4Life programme (Chapter 8), 'as a catalyst for this cultural change' (Department of Health 2008) and to 'create a movement in which everyone in society plays their part, helping to create fundamental changes to those behaviours that can lead to people becoming overweight and obese' (Department of Health 2009). Change4Life sought consumer-driven change, using advertising to enlighten consumers and stimulate them to drive change in the market. While an instrument of government, private industry was involved in Change4Life through sponsorship. This presented opportunities for publicity, product placement and advertising, and permitted corporate participation in obesity reduction projects. The Food Network Responsibility Deal (FNRD), which followed it (Chapter 9), sought to place responsibility on the food industry to drive change in food consumption patterns, with the caveat that individual consumers were framed as being ultimately responsible for their own consumption behaviours. In all of these approaches, the UK government avoided macro-level interventions, because there was no clear evidence of their likely effectiveness on reducing obesity rates.

Another example of obesity as baroque-into-romantic complexity lies with the understanding of obesogenic environments and their construction. Obesogenic environments emerged largely since the 1980s, as an unplanned outcome of activities of multiple expert systems, which became increasingly linked and entangled through the use of networked and interactive computing from this time. Such systems are designed to make urban environments stable, clean, safe and efficient to live and/or work in, among other things. Many previously keystone functions of state (such as transport, food, water and sanitation) were increasingly given over to corporate control from the 1980s, with the growth of neoliberalism, at the time when many of these utilities and services were becoming reconfigured within expert systems. Thus, the participation of governments in expert systems declined almost as they ballooned in importance. Policies that aim to regulate aspects of obesogenic environments through the romantic complexity of urban planning, for example, are poorly resourced relative to the corporations and agencies that form significant parts of expert systems that inadvertently created those environments in the first place. Regulating the industries that provide the material basis for obesogenic environments is politically difficult, largely because they are part of the entanglement of expert systems that provide the material infrastructure of late modern society. A characteristic of an expert system is that the outcomes of making a significant change to any part of it are difficult to predict. Expert systems also employ many people and any intervention to such a system may carry important economic costs. One soft policy approach is to tweak or adjust them in ways that do not threaten their stability. This is the basis of the FNRD in the UK, which a minority of food companies and corporations have signed up to some aspect of since 2013. A slightly harder policy undertaking is the taxation of sugar-sweetened beverages (SSBs) (Chapter 8). In most nations, this would involve a relatively small adjustment to the global food system, but even this is strongly resisted by corporations. The regulation of interactive expert systems towards healthy weight for the populations they serve is difficult to negotiate, and it is far easier to focus on individual responsibility. Such approaches to obesity are ones of enablement, education and individualism, set within globally expanding neoliberal frameworks that focus on markets and profit (Swank 2004).

Neoliberalism and globalization set the conditions for Pattern Four of nutrition transition (Popkin 2002), observed in recent decades (Chapters 1 and 7). This is largely driven by the activities of the globally expert food system, and is difficult for nation states to regulate against (although the taxation of SSBs sets an example). There are local oppositions to the development of Pattern Four nutrition transition, especially in Latin America, where indigenous agricultural resistance to the global food system has been successful in feeding people healthily (Desmarais 2012). Furthermore, in Brazil, recently adopted dietary recommendations challenge the production of low-nutrient-density, high-energy-density foods by the global food system (Monteiro et al. 2015). Beyond Latin America, food-based cooperatives in Italy offer alternatives to global food production, manufacture and distribution systems (Tencati and Zsolnai 2009). Such resistance might only be successful in the long term for local and national food producers if they create expert food systems of their own. This might be possible in larger nations such as Brazil (Monteiro et al. 2015), but it would still require infrastructural devices (including computing, the internet and machinery) that are produced within the neoliberal political economic system.

Expert systems are as embedded in society as neoliberalism. They are effective in making the physical aspects of life run smoothly, especially in HICs. Daily engagement with complex systems is conducive to the production of obesity because of the convenience they generate, by making the physical aspects of life run smoothly and making energy-dense foods cheap, but also because of the psychological stress and inequality experienced by many living in the neoliberal societies that have thrived with the growth of such systems. Governments can, however, call upon a range of rationalities in response to increasing obesity rates. One approach might be to consider obesity regulation in the same way as some other locally complex systems. Obesity and urban form have been linked (Sui 2003), and it is not a big stretch to think about the polyrationalities of obesity regulation in similar ways to the regulation of urbanism (Dear and Flusty 1998) and of water systems (Innes and Booher 2010).

Complexity and Rationality

Complexity has left an imprint on obesity science, while obesity policy has struggled to turn complexity analyses of obesity into effective action. This may be at the heart of why complexity approaches to obesity policy are now little talked of. The uncertainty of outcome that is inherent in intervening in complex systems means that even powerful actors and world-renowned experts cannot predict how uncertainty in information, action and perception will manifest as responses to particular obesity-related policies. For wicked problems (Rittel and Webber 1973), no solution may be predictable or optimal (Innes and Booher 2010). Indeed, wicked problems may have no definitive solutions, but may only be managed through settlements that may work only until the problem reasserts itself in a new form (Levin et al. 2012; Rayner 2014). Obesity is situated in a field of competing interests and behaviours, where meanings of the phenomenon are highly contested (Warin et al. 2015), and is the outcome of the actions of interactive expert systems at societal, social and individual levels. The corporations, agencies, governments and institutions that form components of these systems act using a range of different rationalities, incompatibilities in which may contribute to obesity production. Polyrational approaches to the regulation of obesity would require understanding these rationalities, their relationships to each other and the extent to which they predispose to obesity.

Anti-obesity policies to date generally reflect the landscape of policy making, advice, political pressure, values, advocacy and corporate interests as much as, if not more than, the landscape of evidence. The power of corporations, and those supported by them, remains largely unchallenged in obesity policy in the UK. Evidence can, at one extreme, be given strong weight by policy actors or, at another extreme, be ignored (as with Foresight Obesities; Chapter 9). This book is written with a strong conviction that evidence in policy making is essential, but that it is important to consider carefully how evidence is used in the regulation of obesity. It can be used to help improve the understanding of an issue, influence policy thinking, and assist in the communication and defence of decisions. It can be mapped onto different stages of the policy process – in its creation, development, implementation and justification. Robust evidence can give politicians and policy makers confidence in their decisions and an ability to defend these decisions (Campbell et al. 2007). There are many conflicting and competing approaches taken by the disciplines of obesity science, and the obesity science that is directly helpful to policy making is uneven. Brownell and Roberto (2015) have noted that the science to support particular policies may often be non-existent. There is also great inequality in the various types of stakeholders involved in obesity research, policy and intervention. To counter the very unlevel playing field of policy making, Innes and Booher (2010) have proposed a form of planning and policy called collaborative rationality, which departs from Weberian practical or economic rationality for decision making. This requires an equalization of power among all stakeholders, something that is currently impossible in obesity science and policy. With respect to obesity science, some stakeholders do not reach the policy discussion table at all (Chapter 8). With respect to obesity policy, when stakeholders meet, 'dialogues cannot directly change the deep structure of power' (Innes and Booher 2010), and while the wickedness of obesity as a problem can now easily be recognized, there are many different rationalities (Chapter 2) that underpin the interests of the various parties with a stake in mitigating obesity.

As illustrated in Table 10.2, corporations share only some of the rationalities that underpin the work of government, and often challenge regulation if there is a conflict

Table 10.2. Rationalities of organizations, agencies and people in the production of obesity

Rationality	Government	Corporations	Science	Non-governmental organizations	People
Weberian practical	'What works best' policy, evidence-based policy making		The best research for the funds available	The best advocacy for the funds available	Everyday life: whatever works
Economic	Balance of payments, taxation	Making a profit	Funding	Funding	Work
Weberian formal	Bureaucracy and regulation	Corporate practice and production	Running research institutions		
Weberian theoretical	Modelling and policy making		Research	Advocacy, policy making	
Psychological	Consumerism	Consumerism			Individuality, consumption patterns
Evolutionary					Inequality and competition, animal drive to eat
Weberian substantive				Interest group	Family, emotion, loyalty, religion, cultural food choice, affect, sentiment

of world views and they are large enough to do so (van Boom et al. 2014). The embedding of energy balance discourse (Chapter 3) in obesity policy and regulation links it to Weberian formal rationality, although the science approaches that use energy balance models to seek to create commercial outputs for its control are underpinned by Weberian theoretical and practical rationalities. These three rationalities can gel straightforwardly in the translation of science into policy, but are at odds with the evolutionary and Weberian substantive rationalities that predispose people to overeat and put on weight. Obesity genetics is underpinned by Weberian theoretical rationality, but, with commercial investment in gene therapy approaches to obesity, has entered the world of Weberian practical rationality, sometimes at the expense of theoretically rational science. With respect to the global food system – expert, interactive – the rationalities that underpin it are manifold, and involve the coexistence of often widely differing interests. The dominance of economic rationality in this domain, however, is key to the construction of obesogenic environments locally, nationally and internationally (Chapter 3). As obesity is an unplanned outcome of the operations of the global food system (Chapter 6), as well as of the urban and technological correlates of modernity and modernization (Chapter 7), obesogenic environments are also outcomes of enacted Weberian formal rationality.

To regulate obesity at the nation state level, measurement and surveillance are brought in almost as a default option. Many countries, including the UK and the US, engage in constant surveillance of population body size (Chapter 3). This regulatory practice conforms to Weberian practical and formal rationalities. As these two types of rationality are compatible, this practice is easy to instrumentalize. Resistance to such surveillance – as has occurred with parents declining involvement of their children in the National Child Measurement Programme (NCMP) in the UK (Evans and Colls 2009) – is underpinned by the Weberian substantive rationalities of individuals, groups and sometime institutions that find fault with such measurement. Often the most privileged people in society use their status to opt out of obesity surveillance, making resistance to obesity monitoring a matter of social inequality (Chapter 5). In the UK, the vast majority of privately educated children do not take part in the NCMP, while in the US, there are no obesity data on the citizens of Medina, King County, Washington State (where Bill Gates has a residence).

The production of inequalities in obesity rates is an outcome of a mismatch between the Weberian practical and substantive rationalities of people (in, for example, how individuals of low SES balance a budget and feed themselves and their families, as well as find meaning in life beyond just making do), and the economic and Weberian theoretical and formal rationalities of nation states and corporations. The palatable, highly energy-dense foods, affordable especially to those of low SES in HICs (Chapter 5), are products of the economic and Weberian formal rationalities of the global food system that has grown and consolidated since World War II (Chapter 6). Multiple rationalities are enacted when obesity policy attempts to regulate food systems, as there are many competing interests. Governments seek to have a healthy and economically productive population, food corporations seek profit, and citizens respond to policies and market forces with emotion, local logic, tradition and custom, as well as in relation to economic realities. For food corporations, economic rationality is paramount, while governments attempt to balance economic and formal rationalities in their everyday practices.

Individual rationalities concerning consumption, the body and citizenship are in constant negotiation, and it is often evolutionary rationality that underpins the likelihood of overeating relative to biological need. As a late modern phenomenon (Chapter 1), population obesity is in part an outcome of the mismatch between evolutionary rationality and Weberian formal rationality. Pattern Four nutrition transition is global and cross-generational (Chapter 7), and often invokes clashes of rationalities at the local level, through considerations of what foods are appropriate to consume in what circumstances.

Epigenetics and developmental plasticity share evolutionary rationalities, inasmuch as parental effects on reproductive fitness can operate through adaptive and context-dependent transgenerational transmission of adaptive phenotypes (Chapter 7). Obesity is an outcome of such evolutionary rationality, especially when food is abundant, and its use is largely uncoupled from reproduction. Public policy instrumentation, and its choice of models and modes of operation, is part of a governmental rationality of methods (Lodge and Wegrich 2014). EBPM emerged in the past two decades or so as an attempt to anchor policy making in evidence (Chapter 9), unsullied by political position or the consideration of values, within a framework of bounded rationality. If obesity is produced at the individual level through the engagement of bounded rationality in many everyday practices, policy is also made under conditions of bounded rationality, often with incomplete information, a limited ability to assimilate information if not accessibly packaged, and limited time. The dominance of economic rationality in the production of cheap food calories is clear at all levels, as are the psychological and evolutionary rationalities of food consumption and patterns of behaviour that lead to overconsumption. Local food availability in most of the world has become dependent on the globally expert food system, which is beyond the control of any agency, whether governmental or corporate.

The expert interactive systems of the late modern world are ecologies in which any significant change might have unforeseen consequences, particularly on the economy. In recognition of this, governments of whatever persuasion are usually careful in exercising their regulatory powers in relation to them. Polyrational approaches allow minimally applied regulation to work to best effect (Hartmann 2009, 2010), preferably through negotiation to find clumsy solutions (Rayner 2014). Clumsy solutions are inherent to the type of network governance (Innes and Booher 2010) also described for watershed management by rural societies living on Bali, in the Arctic and in the Gran Chaco (Papp and Alcorn 2013). In relation to flood plain management in HICs, human impacts can include disruption of transport and of economic activity, and the flooding of homes and work-related buildings (Hartmann 2010). A number of insurances might protect different stakeholders according to their rationality, protecting landowners against extreme floods but allowing them to sell inundation rights, allowing insurance to be sold, and reducing state intervention in extreme flooding, because landowners have legitimate claims because of their insurance (Hartmann 2009, 2010). However, the state would remain central in its regulation of the obligation to insure, while communities play a key role in local land and river management (Hartmann 2010).

Polyrationality might also be a useful approach to obesity regulation. Like river management, the problem of control of human body fatness in populations is complex, depends on historical and geographical givens, and involves multiple stakeholders (Chapter 1). In relation to river management, Hartmann (2009, 2010) sets out a series of insurances against natural hazards protecting the different stakeholders according to their rationality (Chapter 1). For obesity management, rather than an intervention ladder (Chapter 8), a framework of insurances could be put in place against the worst excesses of existing practices that predispose to obesity. One approach might be to count the full economic, ecological and environmental cost of cheap food, and of particular items such as sugar. Models exist for sugar and fat taxation, and these could be the basis for the development of full economic, ecological and environmental costing models for repricing and reformulation of foods for better population health. This would be nothing new. In 1975/6, the Norwegian government put in place a farm-food-nutrition policy that economically promoted domestic food production and disincentivized food imports to reduce diet-related chronic disease (Milio 1981). Another approach could be to insure against overeating by regulating packaging and portion size in supermarkets and restaurants. Again, this is nothing new. Portion sizes in Polish restaurants under communism were strictly regulated, especially in relation to systemic shortages of supply of meat and meat products across this era (Jarosz and Pasztor 2007). Yet another could be to reduce binge eating and snacking by banning eating in public places, in the same way that smoking is banned in public buildings in many jurisdictions, including the UK and most states of the US.

The forces that produce obesity are far greater than individuals and individualism can resist, and may be greater than most governments. Beyond recognizing the complexity of obesity, it is important to examine the different types of rationality that underpin obesity science, commerce, government, non-governmental organizations, agencies and everyday people (Chapter 2), so that these different societal domains might work together more effectively towards obesity regulation, in a polyrational way. While there are mismatches between many of these domains, there is also striking congruence. For example, in a neoliberal world, economic rationality is important to all actors. Weberian theoretical rationality is invoked by governments to mitigate the worst effects of economic rationality, while Weberian substantive rationality acts as a moral voice in ensuring that economic rationality is regulated. People are possessed of Weberian substantive and evolutionary rationalities in addition to Weberian practical rationality. This is what makes them different from organizations and institutions, which are underpinned by Weberian practical, theoretical, instrumental and formal rationalities (Chapter 2). The extent to which obesity is produced in any population depends more on the extent to which these people-based rationalities differ from those of governments and corporations.

There are many loops within this scheme of rationalities. The theoretical rationality of medical research is underpinned by economic rationality, in funding and in the production of marketable anti-obesity remedies. The Weberian formal, bureaucratic rationality of corporations is underpinned by economic rationality – the need to make a profit. The theoretical rationality of governments is focused largely on balancing the national budget, and is also economically rational. Obesity cannot be fixed by understanding rationalities alone, but they offer a clearer picture of the problem, and why it remains a complex one: we are all implicated in both the problem and the possible solutions to it. By taking a rationalities approach to obesity models, this book has identified a number of gaps that hinder the regulation of obesity. People need to be interested in, and engaged with, good Weberian theoretical rationality to be open to obesity science and its messages, as well as to Weberian formal rationality to better understand obesity interventions. Obesity science needs to be able to engage more effectively in the discourses of Weberian formal rationality that governments and bureaucracies use, to make science more amenable to policy formation and intervention. Governments, obesity science and corporations need a better understanding of the Weberian substantive rationalities of people, beyond influencing them to behave in particular ways through bounded and psychological rationalities. This book hopefully lays bare the rationalities of different types of model that obesity science and regulation use implicitly, towards an improved understanding of both.

References

6, P. (2004). Joined-up government in the Western world in comparative perspective: a preliminary literature review and exploration. *Journal of Public Administration Research and Theory* 14: 103–38.

Adam, T.C. & Epel, E.S. (2007). Stress, eating and the reward system. *Physiology and Behavior* 91: 449–58.

Adams, J., Clark, M., Ezrow, L. & Glasgow, G. (2004). Understanding change and stability in party ideologies: do parties respond to public opinion or to past election results? *British Journal of Political Science* 34: 589–610.

Adams, J., Halligan, J., Watson, D.B. et al. (2012). The Change4Life convenience store programme to increase retail access to fresh fruit and vegetables: a mixed methods process Q6 evaluation. *PLoS One* 7: e39431.

Aderem, A. (2005). Systems biology: its practice and challenges. *Cell* 121: 511–3.

Aekplakorn, W., Chaiyapong, Y., Neal, B. et al. (2004). Prevalence and determinants of overweight and obesity in Thai adults: results of the Second National Health Examination Survey. *Journal of the Medical Association of Thailand* 87: 685–93.

Aiello, L.C. & Wells, J.C.K. (2002). Energetics and the evolution of the genus *Homo*. *Annual Review of Anthropology* 31: 323–38.

Albritton, R. (2009). *Let Them Eat Junk: How Capitalism Creates Hunger and Obesity*. London: Pluto Press.

Albuquerque, D., Stice, E., Manco, L. & Nobrega, C. (2015). Current review of genetics of human obesity: from molecular mechanisms to an evolutionary perspective. *Molecular Genetics and Genomics* 290: 1191–221.

Al-Kandari, Y.Y. (2006). Prevalence of obesity in Kuwait and its relation to sociocultural variables. *Obesity Reviews* 7: 147–54.

Allender, S., Gleeson, E., Crammond, B. et al. (2012). Policy change to create supportive environments for physical activity and healthy eating: which options are the most realistic for local government? *Health Promotion International* 27: 261–74.

Allison, D.B., Kaprio, J., Korkeila, M. et al. (1996). The heritability of body mass index among an international sample of monozygotic twins reared apart. *International Journal of Obesity and Related Metabolic Disorders* 20: 501–6.

Allison, D.B., Zannolli, R. & Narayan, K.M. (1999). The direct health care costs of obesity in the United States. *American Journal of Public Health* 89: 1194–9.

Allison, H.E. & Hobbs, R.J. (2006). *Science and Policy in Natural Resource Management: Understanding System Complexity*. Cambridge: Cambridge University Press.

Al-Saeed, W.Y., Al-Dawood, K.M., Bukhari, I.A. & Bahnassy, A. (2007). Prevalence and socioeconomic risk factors of obesity among urban female students in Al-Khobar city, Eastern Saudi Arabia, 2003. *Obesity Reviews* 8: 93–9.

American Dietetic Association (2006). Position of the American Dietetic Association: individual-, family-, school-, and community-based interventions for pediatric overweight. *Journal of the American Dietetic Association* 106: 925–45.

American Medical Association (2013). House of Delegates Resolution: 420 (A-13). Recognition of obesity as a disease. www.npr.org/documents/2013/jun/ama-resolution-obesity.pdf (accessed 5 November 2016).

Anand, P. & Gray, A. (2009). Obesity as market failure: could a 'deliberative economy' overcome the problems of paternalism? *Kyklos: International Review for Social Sciences* 62: 182–90.

Anderson, P.M. & Butcher, K.F. (2006). Childhood obesity: trends and potential causes. *Future of Children* 16: 19–45.

Andreyeva, T., Puhl, R.M. & Brownell, K.D. (2008). Changes in perceived weight discrimination among Americans, 1995–1996 through 2004–2006. *Obesity* 16: 1129–34.

Aphramor, L. (2005). Is a weight-centred health framework salutogenic? Some thoughts on unhinging certain dietary ideologies. *Social Theory and Health* 3: 315–40.

Arnaud, P. & Riordan, J. (1998). *Sport and International Politics: Impact of Facism and Communism on Sport*. London: Routledge.

Assmann, S.F., Enios, L.E. & Kasten, L.E. (2000). Subgroup analysis and other (mis)uses of baseline data in clinical trials. *Lancet* 355: 1064–9.

Association for the Study of Obesity (2011). *Obesity Policy in England*. Deal, Kent: Association for the Study of Obesity.

Association of Life Insurance Medical Directors and Actuarial Society of America (1912). *Medico-Actuarial Mortality Investigation*. New York: Nabu Press.

Atkinson, A.B. (2015). *Inequality. What can be Done?* Cambridge, MA: Harvard University Press.

Avena, N.M., Rada, P. & Hoebel, B.G. (2009). Sugar and fat bingeing have notable differences in addictive-like behavior. *Journal of Nutrition* 139: 623–8.

Ayo, N. (2012). Understanding health promotion in a neoliberal climate and the making of health conscious citizens. *Critical Public Health* 22: 99–105.

Bader, P., Boisclair, D. & Ferrence, R. (2011). Effects of tobacco taxation and pricing on smoking behavior in high risk populations: a knowledge synthesis. *International Journal of Environmental Research and Public Health* 8: 4118–39.

Bambra, C.L., Hillier, F.C., Cairns, J.-M. et al. (2015). *How Effective are Interventions at Reducing Socioeconomic Inequalities in Obesity Among children And Adults? Two Systematic Reviews*. London: National Institute for Health Research.

Banks, G. (2009). *Evidence-based Policy Making: What Is It? How Do We Get It?* Canberra: ANU Public Lecture Series, Productivity Commission.

Barker, D. (ed.) (2004). *Mothers, Babies and Disease in Later Life*. London: BMJ Publishing Group.

Barkin, D. (1987). The end to food self-sufficiency in Mexico. *Latin American Perspectives* 14: 271–97.

Barquera, S., Hernandez-Barrera, L., Tolentino-Mayo, M.L. et al. (2008). Dynamics of adolescent and adult beverage intake patterns in Mexico. *FASEB Journal* 22: 461.4.

Barquera, S., Campirano, F., Bonvecchio, A. et al. (2010). Caloric beverage consumption patterns in Mexican children. *Nutrition Journal* 9: 47.

Barres, R., Kirchner, H., Rasmussen, M. et al. (2013). Weight loss after gastric bypass surgery in human obesity remodels promoter methylation. *Cell Reports* 3: 1020–7.

Barry, C.L., Brescoll, V.L., Brownell, K.D. & Schlesinger, M. (2009). Obesity metaphors: how beliefs about the causes of obesity affect support for public policy. *Millbank Quarterly* 87: 7–47.

Barsh, G.S. & Schwartz, M.W. (2002). Genetic approaches to studying energy balance: perception and integration. *Nature Reviews Genetics* 3: 589–600.

Basri, H.B. & Stentiford, E.I. (1995). Expert systems in solid waste management. *Waste Management and Research* 13: 67–89.

Basu, S., Vellakkal, S., Agrawal, S. et al. (2014). Averting obesity and type 2 diabetes in India through sugar-sweetened beverage taxation: an economic-epidemiologic modeling study. *PLoS Medicine* 11: e1001582.

Baudrillard (1970). *The Consumer Society: Myths and Structures*. New York, NY: Sage Publications.

Bauman, Z. (2001). Consuming life. *Journal of Consumer Culture* 1: 9–29.

Bauman, Z. (2003). *Liquid Love: On the Frailty of Human Bonds*. Cambridge: Polity Press.

Beaujard, P. & Fee, S. (2005). The Indian Ocean in Eurasian and African world-systems before the sixteenth century. *Journal of World History* 16: 411–65.

Becker, G.S. & Murphy, K.M. (1988). A theory of rational addiction. *Journal of Political Economy* 96: 675–700.

Beeken, R.J. & Wardle, J. (2013). Public beliefs about the causes of obesity and attitudes towards policy initiatives in Great Britain. *Public Health Nutrition* 16: 2132–7.

Bellisle, F., Dalix, A.M. & Slama, G. (2004). Non food-related environmental stimuli induce increased meal intake in healthy women: comparison of television viewing versus listening to a recorded story in laboratory settings. *Appetite* 43: 175–80.

Bellwood, P. (2005). *First Farmers: The Origins of Agricultural Societies.* Malden, MA: Blackwell.

Belshaw, C.S. (1976). *The Sorcerer's Apprentice: An Anthropology of Public Policy.* Elmsford, NY: Pergamon Press.

Bennett, T., Savage, M., Silva, E.B. et al. (2009). *Culture, Class, Distinction.* Abingdon, Oxfordshire: Routledge.

Bergem, T. (1990). The teacher as moral agent. *Journal of Moral Education* 19: 88–100.

Bernard, P., Charafeddine, R., Frohlich, K.L. et al. (2007). Health inequalities and place: a theoretical conception of neighbourhood. *Social Science and Medicine* 65: 1839–52.

Berrington de Gonzalez, A., Hartge, P., Cerhan, J.R., et al. (2010). Body-mass index and mortality among 1.46 million white adults. *New England Journal of Medicine* 363: 2211–9.

Bertakis, K.D., Azari, R., Helms, L.J., Callahan, E.J. & Robbins, J.A. (2000). Gender differences in the utilization of health care services. *Journal of Family Practice* 49: 147–52.

Bertalanffy, L. (1969). *General System Theory.* New York, NY: George Braziller.

Berthoud, H.R. (2004). Mind versus metabolism in the control of food intake and energy balance. *Physiology and Behavior* 81: 781–93.

Berthoud, H.R. & Morrison, C. (2008). The brain, appetite, and obesity. *Annual Review of Psychology* 59: 55–92.

Bevegni, C. & Adami, G.F. (2003). Obesity and obesity surgery in ancient Greece. *Obesity Surgery* 13: 808–9.

Beyerlein, A. & von Kris, R. (2011). Breastfeeding and body composition in children: will there ever be conclusive empirical evidence for a protective effect against overweight? *American Journal of Clinical Nutrition* 94 (Suppl.): 1772S–5S.

Bicchieri, C. (2004). Rationality and game theory. In A.R. Mele & P. Rawling, eds., *The Oxford Handbook of Rationality.* Oxford: Oxford University Press, pp. 182–205.

Billewicz, W.Z., Kemsley, W.F.F. & Thomson, A.M. (1962). Indices of adiposity. *British Journal of Preventive and Social Medicine* 16: 183–8.

Bindon, J.R. (1982). Breadfruit, banana, beef, and beer: modernization of the Samoan diet. *Ecology of Food and Nutrition* 12, 49–60.

Bish, C.L., Blanck, H.M., Serdula, M.K. et al. (2005). Diet and physical activity behaviors among Americans trying to lose weight: 2000 Behavioral Risk Factor Surveillance System. *Obesity Research* 13: 596–607.

Block, J.P., Scribner, R.A. & DeSalvo, K.B. (2004). Fast food, race/ethnicity, and income: a geographic analysis. *American Journal of Preventive Medicine* 27: 211–7.

Block, J.P., He, Y., Zaslavsky, A.M. et al. (2009). Psychosocial stress and change in weight among US adults. *American Journal of Epidemiology* 170: 181–92.

Bluford, D.A.A., Sherry, B. & Scanlon, K.S. (2007). Interventions to prevent or treat obesity in preschool children: a review of evaluated programs. *Obesity* 15: 1356–72.

Blundell, J.E. & MacDiarmid, J.I. (1997). Fat as a risk factor for overconsumption: satiation, satiety, and patterns of eating. *Journal of the American Dietetic Association* 97 (Suppl.): S63–9.

Blundell, J.E. & Stubbs, R.J. (1999). High and low carbohydrate and fat intakes: limits imposed by appetite and palatability and their implications for energy balance. *European Journal of Clinical Nutrition* 53 (Suppl. 1): S148–65.

Bobroff, E.M. & Kissileff, H.R. (1986). Effects of changes in palatability on food intake and the cumulative food intake curve in man. *Appetite* 7: 85–96.

Boe, J., Humerfelt, S. & Wedervang, F. (1957). The blood pressure in a population: blood pressure readings and height and weight determinations in the adult population of the city of Bergen. *Acta Medica Scandinavica* 321: 1–336.

Boero, N.C. (2014). Obesity in the US media, 1990–2011. In K. Eli & S. Ulijaszek, eds., *Obesity, Eating Disorders and the Media*. Farnham, Surrey: Ashgate Publishing, pp. 37–48.

Bogdanor, V. (2005). *Joined-up Government*. Oxford: Oxford University Press.

Bogin, B. (1998). Patterns of human growth. In S.J. Ulijaszek, F.E. Johnston & M.A. Preece, eds., *Encyclopedia of Human Growth and Development*. Cambridge: Cambridge University Press, pp. 91–5.

Bogin, B. (1999). *Patterns of Human Growth*, 2nd edn. Cambridge: Cambridge University Press.

Boodai, S.A. & Reilly, J.J. (2013). Health related quality of life of obese adolescents in Kuwait. *BMC Pediatrics* 13: 105.

Booth, S.L., Sallis, J.F., Ritenbaugh, C. et al. (2001). Environmental and societal factors affect food choice and physical activity: rationale, influences, and leverage points. *Nutrition Reviews* 59: S21–39.

Bosy-Westphal, A., Geisler, C., Onur, S. et al. (2006). Value of body fat mass vs anthropometric obesity indices in the assessment of metabolic risk factors. *International Journal of Obesity* 30: 475–83.

Botterill, L.C. & Hindmoor, A. (2012). Turtles all the way down: bounded rationality in an evidence-based age. *Policy Studies* 33: 367–79.

Bouchard, C. (2008). Gene–environment interactions in the etiology of obesity: defining the fundamentals. *Obesity* 16 (Suppl. 3): S5–10.

Bouchard, L., Rabasa-Lhoret, R., Faraj, M. et al. (2010). Differential epigenomic and transcriptomic responses in subcutaneous adipose tissue between low and high responders to caloric restriction. *American Journal of Clinical Nutrition* 91: 309–21.

Bourdieu, P. (1984). *Distinction: A Social Critique of the Judgment of Taste* (R. Nice, translator). Cambridge, MA: Harvard University Press.

Bourdieu, P. (1986). The forms of capital. In J. Richardson, ed., *Handbook of Theory and Research for the Sociology of Education*. New York, NY: Greenwood Press, pp. 241–58.

Bourdieu, P. & Boltanski, L. (1976). La production de l'idéologie dominante. *Actes de la Recherche en Sciences Sociales* 2–3: 3–73.

Bowen, S. & Zwi, A.B. (2005). Pathways to "evidence-informed" policy and practice: a framework for action. *PLoS Medicine* 2: e166.

Bratanova, B., Loughnan, S., Klein, O., Claassen, A. & Wood, R. (2016). Poverty, inequality, and increased consumption of high calorie food: experimental evidence for a causal link. *Appetite* 100, 162–71.

Braveman, P.A., Cubbin, C., Egerter, S. et al. (2005). Socioeconomic status in health research. One size does not fit all. *Journal of the American Medical Association* 294: 2879–88.

Bray, G. (2004). Medical consequences of obesity. *Journal of Clinical Endocrinology and Metabolism* 89: 2583–9.

Bray, G. (2008). Some historical aspects of drug treatment for obesity. In J.P.H. Wilding, ed., *Pharmacotherapy of Obesity*. Basel: Birkhäuser Verlag, pp. 11–19.

Bray, G.A., Nielsen, S.J. & Popkin, B.M. (2004). Consumption of high-fructose corn syrup in beverages may play a role in the epidemic of obesity. *American Journal of Clinical Nutrition* 79: 537–43.

Brennan, S.L., Henry, M.J., Nicholson, G.C., Kotowicz, M.A. & Pasco, J.A. (2010). Socioeconomic status, obesity and lifestyle in men: The Geelong Osteoporosis Study. *Journal of Men's Health* 7: 31–41.

Brewis, A.A. (2014). Stigma and the perpetuation of obesity. *Social Science and Medicine* 118, 152–8.

Brewis, A.A., McGarvey, S.T., Jones, J. & Swinburn, B.A. (1998). Perceptions of body size in Pacific Islanders. *International Journal of Obesity* 22: 185–9.

Brewis, A.A., Wutich, A., Falletta-Cowden, A. & Rodriguez-Soto, I. (2011). Body norms and fat stigma in global perspective. *Current Anthropology* 52: 269–76.

Briggs, A.D.M., Mytton, O.T., Kehlbacher, A. et al. (2013). Overall and income specific effect on prevalence of overweight and obesity of 20% sugar sweetened drink tax in UK: econometric and comparative risk assessment modelling study. *British Medical Journal* 347: f6189.

Brown, P.J. & Konner, M. (1987). An anthropological perspective of obesity. *Annals of the New York Academy of Science* 499: 29–46.

Brownell, K. & Roberto, C.A. (2015). Strategic science with policy impact. *Lancet* 385: 2445–6.

Brownell, K.D., Puhl, R., Schwartz, M.B. & Rudd, L. (2005). *Weight Bias: Nature, Consequences, and Remedies.* New York, NY: Guilford Press.

Brownell, K.D., Farley, T., Willett, W.C. et al. (2009a). The public health and economic benefits of taxing sugar-sweetened beverages. *New England Journal of Medicine* 361: 1599–605.

Brownell, K.D., Schwartz, M.B., Puhl, R.M., Henderson, K.E. & Harris, J.L. (2009b). The need for bold action to prevent adolescent obesity. *Journal of Adolescent Health* 45 (Suppl.): S8–17.

Brownell, K.D., Kersh, R., Ludwig, D.S. et al. (2010). Personal responsibility and obesity: a constructive approach to a controversial issue. *Health Affairs* 29: 379–87.

Browning, L.M., Hsieh, S.D. & Ashwell, M. (2010). A systematic review of waist-to-height ratio as a screening tool for the prediction of cardiovascular disease and diabetes: 0.5 could be a suitable global boundary value. *Nutrition Research Reviews* 23: 247–69.

Brownson, R.C., Boehmer, T.K. & Luke, D.A. (2004). Declining rates of physical activity in the United States: what are the contributors? *Annual Review of Public Health* 26: 421–43.

Brunner, E.J., Chandola, T. & Marmot, M.G. (2007). Prospective effect of job strain on general and central obesity in the Whitehall II Study. *American Journal of Epidemiology* 165: 828–37.

Burdge, G. & Lillycrop, K. (2010). Nutrition, epigenetics, and developmental plasticity: implications for understanding human disease. *Annual Review of Nutrition* 30: 315–39.

Butland, B., Jebb, S., Kopelman, P. et al. (2007). *Tackling Obesities: Future Choices – Project Report,* 2nd edn. London: Foresight Programme of the Government Office for Science.

Calle, E.E., Thun, M.J., Petrelli, J.M., Rodriguez, C. & Heath, C.W. Jr. (1999). Body-mass index and mortality in a prospective cohort of US adults. *New England Journal of Medicine* 341: 1097–105.

Cameron, N. & Demerath, E.W. (2002). Critical periods in human growth and their relationship to diseases of aging. *Yearbook of Physical Anthropology* 45: 159–84.

Campbell, P. & Ulijaszek, S.J. (1994). Relationships between anthropometry and retrospective morbidity in poor men in Calcutta, India. *European Journal of Clinical Nutrition* 48: 507–12.

Campbell, S., Benita, S., Coates, E., Davies, P. & Penn, G. (2007). *Analysis for Policy: Evidence-based Policy in Practice.* London: Government Social Research Unit, HM Treasury.

Campion, J., Milagro, F.I. & Martinez, J.A. (2009). Individuality and epigenetics in obesity. *Obesity Reviews* 10: 383–92.

Campos, P., Saguy, A., Ernsberger, P. & Oliver, E. (2006). The epidemiology of overweight and obesity: public health crisis or moral panic? *International Journal of Epidemiology* 35: 55–60.

Canoy, D., Boekholdt, S.M., Wareham, N. et al. (2007). Body fat distribution and risk of coronary heart disease in men and women in the European prospective investigation into cancer and nutrition in Norfolk cohort: a population-based prospective study. *Circulation* 116: 2933–43.

Carmichael, C.M. & McGue, M. (1995). A cross-sectional examination of height, weight, and body mass index in adult twins. *Journal of Gerontology, Series A: Biological Sciences* 50A: B237–44.

Carr, D. & Friedman, M.A. (2005). Is obesity stigmatizing? Body weight, perceived discrimination, and psychological well-being in the United States. *Journal of Health and Social Behavior* 46: 244–59.

Carroll, J.F., Chiapa, A.L., Rodriquez, M. et al. (2008). Visceral fat, waist circumference, and BMI: impact of race/ethnicity. *Obesity* 16: 600–7.

Carryer, J. (2001). Embodied largeness: a significant women's health issue. *Nursing Inquiry* 8: 90–7.

Casazza, K., Fontaine, K.R., Astrup, A. et al. (2013). Myths, presumptions, and facts about obesity. *New England Journal of Medicine* 368: 446–54.

Caterson, M. (2000). Car culture and global environmental politics. *Review of International Studies* 26: 253–70.

Cawley, J. (2010). The economics of childhood obesity. *Health Affairs* 29: 364–71.

Cawley, J. & Meyerhoefer, C. (2012). The medical care costs of obesity: an instrumental variables approach. *Journal of Health Economics* 31: 219–230.

Centers for Disease Control and Prevention (2011a). National Diabetes Fact Sheet, 2011. www.cdc.gov/diabetes/pubs/pdf/ndfs_2011.pdf (accessed 11 May 2017).

Centers for Disease Control and Prevention (2011b). *Smoking and Tobacco Use: Trends in Current Cigarette Smoking Among High School Students and Adults, United States, 1965–2010.* Atlanta, GA: US Department of Health and Human Services, Centers for Disease Control and Prevention.

Centers for Disease Control and Prevention (2016). Obesity prevalence maps. www.cdc.gov/obesity/data/prevalence-maps.html (accessed 25 April 2016).

Cerny, P. (1995). Globalization and the changing logic of collective action. *International Organization* 49: 595–626.

Chaloupka, F.J. & Warner, K.E. (2000). The economics of smoking. In A.J. Culyer & J.P. Newhouse, eds., *Handbook of Health Economics, Volume 1, Part B.* Amsterdam: Elsevier Science, pp. 1539–627.

Chamberlin, L.A., Sherman, S.N., Jain, A. et al. (2002). The challenge of preventing and treating obesity in low-income, preschool children: perceptions of WIC health care professionals. *Archives of Pediatrics and Adolescent Medicine* 156: 662–8.

Champion, S.L., Rumbold, A.R., Steele, E.J. et al. (2012). Parental work schedules and child overweight and obesity. *International Journal of Obesity* 36: 573–80.

Chan, J.M., Rimm, E.B., Colditz, G.A., Stampfer, M.J. & Willett, W.C. (1994). Obesity, fat distribution, and weight gain as risk factors for clinical diabetes in men. *Diabetes Care* 17: 961–9.

Charlesworth, J. (2006). Tackling obesities: the future of obesity over the next 50 years. http://jessicacharlesworth.com/2006/tacklingobesities/ (accessed 13 June 2014).

Charnov, E.L. (1993). *Life History Invariants.* Oxford: Oxford University Press.

Chen, A.Y. & Escarce, J.J. (2010). Family structure and childhood obesity, early childhood longitudinal study – kindergarten cohort. *Preventing Chronic Disease* 7: A50.

Chen, J.-L., Tsai, R., Tzeng, H.-W. & Hong, C.-M. (1993). A distributed expert system for distribution planning. In *IEA/AIE '93 Proceedings of the 6th International Conference on Industrial and Engineering Applications of Artificial Intelligence and Expert Systems.* London: Gordon and Breach Science Publishers, pp. 117–22.

Cho, I., & Blaser, M.J. (2012). The human microbiome: at the interface of health and disease. *Nature Reviews Genetics* 13: 260–70.

Christakis, N.A. & Fowler, J.H. (2007). The spread of obesity in a large social network over 32 years. *New England Journal of Medicine* 357: 370–9.

Chung, W.K. & Leibel, R.L. (2005). Molecular physiology of syndromic obesities in humans. *Trends in Endocrinology and Metabolism* 16: 267–72.

Clapp, J. & Fuchs, D. (eds.) (2009). *Corporate Power in Global Agrifood Governance.* Cambridge, MA: MIT Press.

Clarke, S.F. & Foster, J.R. (2012). A history of blood glucose meters and their role in self-monitoring of diabetes mellitus. *British Journal of Biomedical Science* 69: 83–93.

Coburn, D. (2000). Income inequality, social cohesion and the health status of populations: the role of neo-liberalism. *Social Science and Medicine* 51: 135–46.

Colchero, M.A., Popkin, B.M., Rivera, J.A. & Ng, S.W. (2016). Beverage purchases from stores in Mexico under the excise tax on sugar sweetened beverages: observational study. *British Medical Journal* 352: h6704.

Colditz, G.A. (1999). Economic costs of obesity and inactivity. *Medicine and Science in Sports and Exercise* 31 (Suppl.): S663–7.

Colditz, G.A., Willett, W.C., Rotnitzky, A. & Manson, J.E. (1995). Weight gain as a risk factor for clinical diabetes mellitus in women. *Annals of Internal Medicine* 122: 481–6.

Cole, T.J. (2003). The secular trend in human physical growth: a biological view. *Economics and Human Biology* 1: 161–8.

Cole, T.J., Bellizzi, M.C., Flegal, K.M. & Dietz, W.H. (2000). Establishing a standard definition for child overweight and obesity worldwide: international survey. *British Medical Journal* 320: 1240–5.

Colls, R. (2007). Materialising bodily matter: intra-action and the embodiment of fat. *Geoforum* 38: 353–65.

Colls, R. & Evans, B. (2008). Embodying responsibility: children's health and supermarket initiatives. *Environment and Planning A* 40: 615–31.

Colon-Gonzalez, F., Kim, G.W., Lin, J.E., Valentino, M.A. & Waldman, S.A. (2013). Obesity pharmacotherapy: what is next? *Molecular Aspects of Medicine* 34: 71–83.

Commonwealth of Australia (2013). Income inequality in Australia. Economic Roundup Issue 2, 2013. www.treasury.gov.au/PublicationsAndMedia/Publications/2013/Economic-Roundup-Issue-2/Economic-Roundup/Income-inequality-in-Australia (accessed 11 January 2017).

Comuzzie, A.G. (2002). The emerging pattern of the genetic contribution to human obesity. *Best Practice and Research Clinical Endocrinology & Metabolism* 16: 611–21.

Cordain, L., Eaton, S.B., Miller, J.B. & Hill, K. (2002). The paradoxical nature of hunter-gatherer diets: meat-based, yet non-atherogenic. *European Journal of Clinical Nutrition* 56: S42–52.

Cordero, P., Campion, J., Milagro, F.I. et al. (2011). Leptin and TNF-α promoter methylation levels measured by MSP could predict the response to a low-calorie diet. *Journal of Physiological Biochemistry* 67: 463–70.

Cornier, M.-A., von Kaenel, S.S., Bessesen, D.H. & Tregellas, J.R. (2007). Effects of overfeeding on the neuronal response to visual food cues. *American Journal of Clinical Nutrition* 86: 965–71.

Cosgel, M.M. (1992). Rhetoric in the economy: consumption and audience. *Journal of Socio-Economics* 21: 363–77.

Costanza, R., Kubiszewski, I., Giovannini, E. et al. (2014). Development: time to leave GDP behind. *Nature* 505: 283–5.

Costa-Font, J., Mas, N. & Navarro, P. (2013). *Globesity: Is Globalization a Pathway to Obesity?* LSE Health Working Paper No. 31. London: London School of Economics.

Coveney, J.D. (2000). *Food, Morals and Meaning. The Pleasure and Anxiety of Eating.* Abingdon, Oxfordshire: Routledge.

Craig, R. & Mindell, J. (eds.) (2014). *Health Survey for England 2013.* London: The Health and Social Care Information Centre.

Credit Suisse (2014). *Global Wealth Report.* Zurich: Credit Suisse.

Cristea, A.L. & Zaharia, C.N. (1988). Methodology for the development of expert systems of viral epidemiology. *Virologie* 39: 7–13.

Critser, G. (2003). *Fat Land. How Americans Became the Fattest People in the World.* Boston, MA: Houghton Mifflin Company.

Cross, G.S. (2000). *An All-Consuming Century: Why Commercialism Won in Modern America.* New York, NY: Columbia University Press.

Cross-Government Obesity Unit, Department of Health and Department of Children, Schools and Families (2008). *Healthy Weight, Healthy Lives: A Cross-government Strategy for England.* London: Her Majesty's Government.

Crossley, N. (2004). Fat is a sociological issue: obesity rates in late modern, 'body-conscious' societies. *Social Theory and Health* 2: 222–53.

Crow, J.F. (1958). Index of total selection intensity. Some possibilities for measuring selection intensities in man. *Human Biology* 30: 1–3.

Culyer, A.J. & Newhouse, J.P. (2000). *Handbook of Health Economics, Vols. 1A and B*. New York, NY: Elsevier.

Cummins, S. & Macintyre, S. (2006). Food environments and obesity – neighbourhood or nation? *International Journal of Epidemiology* 35: 100–4.

Curry, A., Hodgson, T., Kelnar, R. & Wilson, A. (2006). *Intelligent Infrastructure Futures. The Scenarios – Towards 2055*. London: Office of Science and Technology, Her Majesty's Government.

Cutler, D.M., Glaeser, E.L. & Shapiro, J.M. (2003). Why have Americans become more obese? *Journal of Economic Perspectives* 17: 93–118.

Daar, A.S., Singer, P.A., Persad, D.L. et al. (2007). Grand challenges in chronic non-communicable diseases. *Nature* 450: 494–6.

D'Addio, A.C. (2007). *Intergenerational Transmission of Disadvantage. Mobility or Immobility Across Generations?* OECD Social, Employment and Migration Working Paper Number 52. Paris: Organization for Economic Cooperation and Development.

Dallman, M.F. (2010). Stress-induced obesity and the emotional nervous system. *Trends in Endocrinology and Metabolism* 21: 159–65.

Dallman, M.F., Pecoraro, N., Akana, S.F. et al. (2003). Chronic stress and obesity: a new view of "comfort food." *Proceedings of the National Academy of Sciences USA* 100: 11696–701.

Dallman, M.F., Pecoraro, NC. & la Fleur, S.E. (2005). Chronic stress and comfort foods: self-medication and abdominal obesity. *Brain, Behavior, and Immunity* 19: 275–80.

Darmon, N. & Drewnowski, A. (2008). Does social class predict diet quality? *American Journal of Clinical Nutrition* 87: 1107–17.

Davies, M.J. (2006). Evidence for effects of weight on reproduction in women. *Reproductive BioMedicine Online* 12: 532–41.

Davila-Cervantes, C.A. & Pardo, A.M. (2014). Diabetes mellitus: contribution to changes in the life expectancy in Mexico 1990, 2000, and 2010. *Revista de Salud Publica* 16: 910–23.

Davis, C., Patte, K., Curtis, C. & Reid, C. (2010). Immediate pleasures and future consequences. A neuropsychological study of binge eating and obesity. *Appetite* 54: 208–13.

Davy, B. (1997). *Essential Injustice. When Legal Institutions Cannot Resolve Environmental and Land Use Disputes*. New York, NY: Springer.

Davy, B. (2008). Plan it without a condom! *Planning Theory* 7: 301–17.

Davy, B. (2013). Planning cultures in Europe. Decoding cultural phenomena in urban and regional planning. *Planning Theory* 12: 219–22.

de Castro, J.M. (1994). Family and friends produce greater social facilitation of food intake than other companions. *Physiology and Behavior* 56: 445–55.

de Castro, J.M. (1999). Heritability of hunger relationships with food intake in free-living humans. *Physiology and Behavior* 67: 249–58.

de Garine, I. & Harrison, G.A. (eds.) (1988). *Coping with Uncertainty in Food Supply*. Oxford: Oxford University Press.

de Garine, I. & Koppert, G.J.A. (1991). Guru-fattening session among the Massa. *Ecology of Food and Nutrition* 25: 1–28.

de Vogli, R., Kouvonen, A. & Gimeno, D. (2011). 'Globesization': ecological evidence on the relationship between fast food outlets and obesity among 26 advanced economies. *Critical Public Health* 21: 395–402.

de Vogli, R., Kouvonen, A., Elovainioe, M. & Marmot, M. (2014). Economic globalization, inequality and body mass index: a cross-national analysis of 127 countries. *Critical Public Health* 24: 7–21.

de Vries, J. (2007). The obesity epidemic: medical and ethical considerations. *Science and Engineering Ethics* 13: 55–67.

Dear, M. & Flusty, S. (1998). Postmodern urbanism. *Annals of the Association of American Geographers* 88: 50–72.

Deeks, S.G., Lewin, S.R. & Havlir, D.V. (2013). The end of AIDS: HIV infection as a chronic disease. *Lancet* 382: 2–8.

Dejong, W. (1980). The stigma of obesity: the consequences of naïve assumptions concerning the causes of physical deviance. *Journal of Health and Social Behavior* 21: 75–87.

Deloitte Touche Tohmatsu Ltd (2017). *Global Powers of Retailing*. London: Deloitte.

Department of Health (1992). *The Health of the Nation: A Strategy for Health in England*. London: Her Majesty's Stationery Office.

Department of Health (1999). *Saving Lives: Our Healthier Nation*. London: Her Majesty's Government.

Department of Health (2000). *National Service Framework: Coronary Heart Disease*. London: Her Majesty's Government.

Department of Health (2008). *Healthy Weight, Healthy Lives: A Cross-Government Strategy for England*. London: Her Majesty's Government.

Department of Health (2009). *Change4Life Marketing Strategy. In Support of Healthy Weight, Healthy Lives*. London: Her Majesty's Government.

Department of Health (2010). *White Paper: Healthy Lives, Healthy People: Our Strategy for Public Health in England*. London: Her Majesty's Government.

Department of Health (2011). *Healthy Lives, Healthy People: a Call to Action on Obesity in England*. London: Her Majesty's Government.

Department of Health, Prime Minister's Office, Her Majesty's Treasury and Cabinet Office (2016). *Childhood Obesity: a Plan for Action*. London: Her Majesty's Government.

Department of Trade and Industry (2005). Scoping the Foresight Project on Tackling Obesities: Future Choices. http://webarchive.nationalarchives.gov.uk/20121212135622/http://www.bis.gov.uk/foresight/our-work/projects/current-projects/tackling-obesities/reports-and-publications/results-of-scoping (accessed 11 May 2017).

Design Council (2017). The power of branding. www.designcouncil.org.uk/news-opinion/power-branding (accessed 27 January 2017).

Desmarais, A.A. (2012). La Vía Campesina. In G. Ritzer, ed., *The Wiley-Blackwell Encyclopedia of Globalization*. Oxford: Wiley Blackwell.

Despres, J.-P., Moorjani, S., Lupien, P.J. et al. (1990). Regional distribution of body fat, plasma lipoproteins, and cardiovascular disease. *Arteriosclerosis, Thrombosis, and Vascular Biology* 10: 497–511.

Dethlefsen, A., McFall-Ngai, M. & Relman, D.A. (2007). An ecological and evolutionary perspective on human–microbe mutualism and disease. *Nature* 449: 811–8.

Deurenberg, P., Deurenberg-Yap, M. & Guricci, S. (2002). Asians are different from Caucasians and from each other in their body mass index/body fat per cent relationship. *Obesity Reviews* 3: 141–6.

Diamond, J. (2003). The double puzzle of diabetes. *Nature* 423: 599–602.

Dietz, W.H., Benken, D.E. & Hunter, A.S. (2009). Public health law and the prevention and control of obesity. *Millbank Quarterly* 87: 215–27.

Dinsa, G.D., Goryakin, Y., Fumagalli, E. & Suhrcke, M. (2012). Obesity and socioeconomic status in developing countries: a systematic review. *Obesity Reviews* 13: 1067–79.

Dixon, J. (2002). *The Changing Chicken: Chooks, Cooks and Culinary Culture*. Sydney, NSW: University of New South Wales Press.

Dixon, J. (2009). From the imperial to the empty calorie: how nutrition relations underpin food regime transitions. *Agriculture and Human Values* 26: 321–33.

Dodson, J., Li, X., Ming, K. et al. (2009). Early bronze in two Holocene archaeological sites in Gansu, NW China. *Quaternary Research* 72: 309–14.

Dodson, J.R., Li, X., Zhou, X. et al. (2013). Origin and spread of wheat in China. *Quaternary Science Reviews* 72: 108–11.

Dolan, P., Peasgood, T. & White, M. (2008). Do we really know what makes us happy? A review of the economic literature on the factors associated with subjective well-being. *Journal of Economic Psychology* 29: 94–122.

Doll, H.A., Peterson, S.E.K. & Stewart-Brown, S.L. (2000). Obesity and physical and emotional well-being: associations between body mass index, chronic illness, and the physical and mental components of the SF-36 questionnaire. *Obesity Research* 8: 160–70.

Donovan, M.R., Glue, P., Kolluri, S. & Emir, B. (2010). Comparative efficacy of antidepressants in preventing relapse in anxiety disorders – a meta-analysis. *Journal of Affective Disorders* 123: 9–16.

Douglas, M. (1978). *Cultural Bias.* Occasional Paper No. 35. London: Royal Anthropological Institute.

Douglas, M. (1986). *How Institutions Think.* Syracuse, NY: Syracuse University Press.

Douglas, M. (1996). *Thought Styles: Critical Essays on Good Taste.* Thousand Oaks, CA: Sage Publications.

Drayna, D. (2005). Human taste genetics. *Annual Review of Genomics and Human Genetics* 6: 217–35.

Dreher, A, Gaston, N. & Martens, P. (eds.) (2008). *Measuring Globalisation. Gauging Its Consequences.* New York, NY: Springer Science.

Drewnowski, A. (1998). Energy density, palatability, and satiety: implications for weight control. *Nutrition Reviews* 56: 347–53.

Drewnowski, A. (2012). Statial analyses of obesity and poverty. In A. Offer, R. Pechey & S.J. Ulijaszek, eds., *Insecurity, Inequality and Obesity.* Oxford: Oxford University Press, pp. 83–104.

Drewnowski, A. & Darmon, N. (2005). The economics of obesity: dietary energy density and energy cost. *American Journal of Clinical Nutrition* 82: 265S–73S.

Drewnowski, A. & Greenwood, M.R.C. (1983). Cream and sugar: human preferences for high-fat foods. *Physiology and Behavior* 30: 629–33.

Drewnowski, A. & Popkin, B.M. (1997). The nutrition transition: new trends in the global diet. *Nutrition Reviews* 55: 31–43.

Du, S., Lu, B., Zhai, F. & Popkin, B.M. (2002). A new stage of the nutrition transition in China. *Public Health Nutrition* 5: 169–74.

Due, P., Damsgaard, M.T., Rasmussen, M. et al. (2009). Socioeconomic position, macroeconomic environment and overweight among adolescents in 35 countries. *International Journal of Obesity* 33: 1084–93.

Dulloo, A.G. (2006). Regulation of fat storage via suppressed thermogenesis: a thrifty phenotype that predisposes individuals with catch-up growth to insulin resistance and obesity. *Hormone Research.* 65 (Suppl. 3): 90–7.

Dulloo, A.G. (2013). Translational issues in targeting brown adipose tissue thermogenesis for human obesity management. *Annals of the New York Academy of Sciences USA* 1302: 1–10.

Dunbar, R.I.M. (1998). The social brain hypothesis. *Evolutionary Anthropology* 6: 178–90.

Easterlin, R.A. (2001). Income and happiness: towards a unified theory. *Royal Economic Society* 111: 465–84.

Ebbeling, C., Pawlak, D. & Ludwig, D. (2002). Childhood obesity: public-health crisis, common sense cure. *Lancet* 360: 473–82.

Ebrahim, G.J. (1980). Cross-cultural aspects of pregnancy and breast feeding. *Proceedings of the Nutrition Society* 39: 13–15.

Edwards, F.M., Wise, P.H., Thomas, D.W., Murchland, J.B. & Craig, R.J. (1976). Blood pressure and electrocardiographic findings in the South Australian Aborigines. *Australian and New Zealand Journal of Medicine* 6: 197–205.

Eisenstadt, S.N. (1969). *The Political Systems of Empires.* London: Transaction Publishers.

Eli, K. & Ulijaszek, S.J. (eds.) (2014). *Obesity, Eating Disorders and the Media*. Farnham, Surrey: Ashgate Publishing.

Elinder, L.S. & Jansson, M. (2009). Obesogenic environments – aspects on measurement and indicators. *Public Health Nutrition* 12: 307–15.

Elks, C.E., den Hoed, M., Zhao, J.H. et al. (2012). Variability in the heritability of body mass index: a systematic review and meta-regression. *Frontiers in Endocrinology* 3: 29.

Ellis, L. & Haman, D. (2004). Population increases in obesity appear to be partly due to genetics. *Journal of Biosocial Science* 36: 547–59.

Ellison, P.T. (2001). *On Fertile Ground: a Natural History of Reproduction*. Cambridge, MA: Harvard University Press.

Emmett, P.M. & Heaton, K.W. (1995). Is extrinsic sugar a vehicle for dietary fat? *Lancet* 345: 1537–40.

Engerman, S. (1976). The height of U.S. slaves. *Local Population Studies* 16: 45–9.

Erlichman, J., Kerbey, A.L. & James, W.P.T. (2002). Physical activity and its impact on health outcomes. Paper 2: Prevention of unhealthy weight gain and obesity by physical activity: an analysis of the evidence. *Obesity Reviews* 3: 273–87.

Esping-Andersen, G. (1990). *The Three Worlds of Welfare Capitalism*. Cambridge: Polity Press.

Esping-Andersen, G. (ed.) (2002). *Why We Need a New Welfare State*. Oxford: Oxford University Press.

Evans, B. (2006). 'Gluttony or sloth': critical geographies of bodies and morality in (anti)obesity policy. *Area* 38: 259–67.

Evans, B. & Colls, R. (2009). Measuring fatness, governing bodies: the spatialities of the body mass index (BMI) in anti-obesity politics. *Antipode* 41: 1051–83.

Evans, B. & Colls, R. (2011). Doing more good than harm? The absent presence of children's bodies in (anti-)obesity policy. In E. Rich, L.F. Monaghan & L. Aphramor, eds., *Debating Obesity. Critical Perspectives*. Basingstoke, Hampshire: Palgrave Macmillan, pp. 115–38.

Evans, B., Colls, R. & Horschelmann, K. (2011). 'Change4Life for your kids': embodied collectives and public health pedagogy. *Sport, Education and Society* 16: 323–41.

Exworthy, M. & Hunter, D.J. (2011). The challenge of joined up government in tackling health inequalities. *International Journal of Public Administration* 34: 201–12.

Faith, M.S., Berkowitz, R.I., Stallings, V.A. et al. (2004). Parental feeding attitudes and styles and child body mass index: prospective analysis of a gene–environment interaction. *Pediatrics* 114: e429–36.

Fantom, N.J. & Serajuddin, U. (2016).*The World Bank's Classification of Countries by Income*. World Bank Policy Research Paper 7528. Washington, DC: World Bank.

Farhani, S., Mrizak, S., Chaibi, A. & Rault, C. (2014). The environmental Kuznets curve and sustainability: a panel data analysis. *Energy Policy* 71: 189–98.

Farooqi, I.S., Keogh, K.M., Kamath, S. et al. (2001). Partial leptin deficiency and human adiposity. *Nature* 414: 34–5.

Feigenbaum, E.A. (2003). Some challenges and grand challenges for computational intelligence. *Journal of the ACM* 50: 32–40.

Felt, U., Felder, K., Ohler, T. & Penckler, M. (2014). Timescapes of obesity: coming to terms with a complex socio-medical phenomenon. *Health* 18: 646–64.

Filozof, C., Pinilla, M.C.F. & Fernandez-Cruz, A. (2004). Smoking cessation and weight gain. *Obesity Reviews* 5: 95–103.

Filter, M., Appel, B. & Buschulte, A. (2016). Expert systems for food safety. *Current Opinion in Food Science* 6: 61–5.

Finegood, D.T. (2011). The complex systems science of obesity. In J. Cawley, ed., *Oxford Handbook of the Social Science of Obesity*. Oxford: Oxford University Press.

Finegood, D.T., Merth, D.T.N. & Rutter, H. (2010). Implications of the Foresight Obesity System Map for solutions to childhood obesity. *Obesity* 18: S13–16.

Finkelstein, E.A., Ruhm, C.J. & Kosa, K.M. (2005). Economic causes of and consequences of obesity. *Annual Review of Public Health* 26: 239–57.

Finkelstein, E.A., Trogdon, J.G., Cohen, J.W. & Dietz, W. (2009). Annual medical spending attributable to obesity: payer- and service-specific estimates. *Health Affairs* 28: w822–31.

Finucane, M.L., Alhakami, A., Slovic, P. & Johnson, S.M. (2000). The affect heuristic in judgments of risks and benefits. *Journal of Behavioral Decision Making* 13: 1–17.

Finucane, M.M., Stevens, G.A., Cowan, M.J. et al. (2011). National, regional, and global trends in body-mass index since 1980: systematic analysis of health examination surveys and epidemiological studies with 960 country-years and 9.1 million participants. *Lancet* 377: 557–67.

Fischhoff, B., Slovic, P., Lichtenstein, S., Reid, S. & Combs, B. (1978). How safe is safe enough? A psychometric study of attitudes towards technological risks and benefits. *Policy Sciences* 9: 127–52.

Fisher, R.A. (1930). *The Genetical Theory of Natural Selection*. Oxford: Clarendon Press.

Fjellstrom, C. (2004). Mealtime and meal patterns from a cultural perspective. *Scandinavian Journal of Nutrition* 48: 161–4.

Flegal, K.M., Carroll, M.D., Kuczmarski, R.J. & Johnson, C.L. (1998). Overweight and obesity in the United States: prevalence and trends, 1960–1994. *International Journal of Obesity and Related Metabolic Disorders* 22: 39–47.

Flegal, K.M., Ogden, C.L., Carroll, M.D. et al. (2002). Prevalence and trends in obesity among US adults, 1999–2000. *Journal of the American Medical Association* 288: 1723–7.

Flegal, K.M., Graubard, B.I., Williamson, D.F. & Gail, M.H. (2007). Cause-specific excess deaths associated with underweight, overweight, and obesity. *Journal of the American Medical Association* 298: 2028–37.

Flegal, K.M., Kit, B.K., Orpana, H. & Graubard, B.I. (2013). Association of all-cause mortality with overweight and obesity using standard body mass index categories. A systematic review and meta-analysis. *Journal of the American Medical Association* 309: 71–82.

Flint, S.W., Hudson, J. & Lavallee, D. (2015). UK adults' implicit and explicit attitudes towards obesity. *BMC Obesity* 2: 31.

Flood, R.L. (2010). The relationship of 'systems thinking' to action research. *Systems Practice and Action Research* 23: 269–84.

Florey, C.d.V. (1970). The use and interpretation of ponderal index and other weight-height ratios in epidemiological studies. *Journal of Chronic Diseases* 23: 93–103.

Foley, D.K. (1998). Introduction. In P.S. Albin, ed., *Barriers and Bounds to Rationality: Essays on Economic Complexity and Dynamics in Interactive Systems*. Princeton, NJ: Princeton University Press, pp. 3–72.

Foley, R.A. (1993). The influence of seasonality on hominid evolution. In S.J. Ulijaszek & S.S. Strickland, eds., *Seasonality and Human Ecology*. Cambridge: Cambridge University Press, pp. 17–37.

Food and Agriculture Organization (2002). World agriculture: towards 2015/2030. Summary report. www.fao.org/3/a-y3557e.pdf (accessed 28 March 2017).

Food and Agriculture Organization (2017a). Food supply – Crops Primary Equivalent. www.fao.org/faostat/en/#data/CC (accessed 19 May 2017).

Food and Agriculture Organization (2017b). Food Supply – Livestock and Fish Primary Equivalent. www.fao.org/faostat/en/#data/CL (accessed 19 May 2017).

Foote, R. (2007). Mathematics and complex systems. *Science* 318: 410–2.

Foresight (2007a). *Tackling Obesities: Future Choices. Modelling Future Trends in Obesity and their Impact on Health*. London: Office of Science and Technology, Her Majesty's Government.

Foresight (2007b). *Tackling Obesities: Future Choices – Obesity System Atlas*. London: Government Office for Science.

Foresight (2010). *Tackling Obesities: Future Choices. Mid-Term Review. November 2008–September 2010*. London: Government Office for Science.

Foresight (2017). Foresight projects. www.bis.gov.uk/foresight/our-work/projects (accessed 14 June 2017).

Foresight International Dimensions of Climate Change (2011). *Final Project Report*. London: Her Majesty's Government.

Forth, C.E. & Leitch, A. (eds.) (2014). *Fat: Culture and Materiality*. London: Bloomsbury.

Fox, N.J. (2011). Boundary objects, social meanings and the success of new technologies. *Sociology* 45: 70–85.

Fox, N.J., Ward, K.J. & O'Rourke, A.J. (2005). The 'expert patient': empowerment or medical dominance? The case of weight loss, pharmaceutical drugs and the internet. *Social Science and Medicine* 60: 1299–309.

Franck, C., Grandi, S.M. & Eisenberg, M.J. (2013). Agricultural subsidies and the American obesity epidemic. *American Journal of Preventive Medicine* 45: 327–333.

Frank, L.D., Andresen, M.A. & Schmid, T.L. (2004). Obesity relationships with community design, physical activity, and time spent in cars. *American Journal of Preventive Medicine* 27: 87–96.

Franz, M.J., van Wormer, J.J., Crain, A.L. et al. (2007). Weight-loss outcomes: a systematic review and meta-analysis of weight-loss clinical trials with a minimum 1-year follow-up. *Journal of the American Dietetic Association* 107: 1755–67.

Fraser Institute (2013). *Economic Freedom of the World Annual Report 2013*. Vancouver, BC: Fraser Institute.

Frayling, T.M., Timpson, N.J., Weedon, M.N. et al. (2007). A common variant in the *FTO* gene is associated with body mass index and predisposes to childhood and adult obesity. *Science* 316: 889–94.

Frederick, C.B., Snellman, K. & Putnam, R.D. (2014). Increasing socioeconomic disparities in adolescent obesity. *Proceedings of the National Academy of Sciences USA* 111: 1338–42.

Freedman, D.S. & Sherry, B. (2009). The validity of BMI as an indicator of body fatness and risk among children. *Pediatrics* 124 (Suppl. 1): 1338–42.

Friedman, G.C. (1982). The heights of slaves in Trinidad. *Social Science History* 6: 482–515.

Friedman, M. (2002). Kant, Kuhn, and the rationality of science. *Philosophy of Science* 69: 171–90.

Friedmann, H. (1993). The political economy of food: a global crisis. *New Left Review* 197: 29–57.

Friel, S., Chopra, M. & Satcher, D. (2007). Unequal weight: equity oriented policy responses to the global obesity epidemic. *British Medical Journal* 335: 1241–3.

Frood, S., Johnson, L.M., Matteson, C.L. & Finegood, D.T. (2013). Obesity, complexity, and the role of the health system. *Current Obesity Reports* 2: 320–6.

Fry, J. & Finley, W. (2005). The prevalence and costs of obesity in the EU. *Proceedings of the Nutrition Society* 64: 359–62.

Fryar, C.D. & Ervin, R.B. (2013). *Caloric Intake from Fast Food Among Adults: United States, 2007–2010*. NCHS Data Brief, No. 114. Hyattsville, MD: National Center for Health Statistics.

Furrow, R.E., Christiansen, F.B. & Feldman, M.W. (2011). Environment-sensitive epigenetics and the heritability of complex diseases. *Genetics* 189: 1377–87.

Gallagher, D., Visser, M., Sepulveda, D. et al. (1996). How useful is body mass index for comparison of body fatness across age, sex, and ethnic groups? *American Journal of Epidemiology* 143: 228–39.

Ganley, R.M. (1989). Emotion and eating in obesity: a review of the literature. *International Journal of Eating Disorders* 8: 343–61.

Garaulet, M.P., Pérez-Llamas, F., Fuente, T., Zamora, S. & Tebar, F.J. (2000). Anthropometric, computer tomography and fat cell data in an obese population: relationship with insulin, leptin, tumor necrosis factor-α, sex hormone-binding globulin and sex hormones. *European Journal of Endocrinology* 143: 657–66.

Gard, M. (2011a) Between alarmists and sceptics: on the cultural politics of obesity scholarship and public policy. In K. Bell, D. McNaughton & A. Salmon, eds., *Alcohol, Tobacco and Obesity: Morality, Medicine and the New Public Health*. London: Routledge, pp. 59–72.

Gard, M. (2011b). *The End of the Obesity Epidemic*. Abingdon, Oxfordshire: Routledge.

Gard, M. and Wright, J. (2005). *The Obesity Epidemic. Science, Morality and Ideology*. Abingdon, Oxfordshire: Routledge.

Garrow, J.S. (1978). *Energy Balance and Obesity in Man*, 2nd edn. Amsterdam: Elsevier.

Garrow, J.S. (1985). Quetelet's index (W/H^2) as a measure of fatness. *International Journal of Obesity* 9: 147–53.

Gecas, V. (1979). The influence of social class on socialization. In W.R. Burr, R. Hill, F.I. Nye & I.L. Reiss, eds., *Contemporary Theories about the Family*. New York, NY: Free Press, pp. 365–404.

Gelbach, J.B., Klick, J. & Stratmann, T. (2009). Cheap donuts and expensive broccoli: the effect of relative prices on obesity. Research Paper No. 261. Tallahassee, FL: Florida State University College of Law. http://dx.doi.org/10.2139/ssrn.976484

George, S. (1977). *How the Other Half Dies*. Montclair, NJ: Allanheld, Osmun and Company.

Gerace, T.A. & George, V.A. (1996). Predictors of weight increases over 7 years in fire fighters and paramedics. *Preventive Medicine* 25: 593–600.

German, J.B., Hammock, B.D. & Watkins, S.M. (2005). Metabolomics: building on a century of biochemistry to guide human health. *Metabolomics* 1: 3–9.

Gerstein, D.E., Woodward-Lopez, G., Evans, A.E. et al. (2004). Clarifying concepts about macronutrients' effects on satiation and satiety. *Journal of the American Dietetic Association* 104: 1151–3.

Gewertz, D. & Errington, F. (2010). *Cheap Meat: Flap Food Nations in the Pacific Islands*. Berkeley, CA: University of California Press.

Geyer, S., Hemstrom, O., Peter, R. & Vagero, D. (2006). Education, income, and occupational class cannot be used interchangeably in social epidemiology. Empirical evidence against a common practice. *Journal of Epidemiology and Community Health* 60: 804–10.

Gibson, L.Y., Byrne, S.M., Davis, E.A. et al. (2007). The role of family and maternal factors in childhood obesity. *Medical Journal of Australia* 186: 591–5.

Giddens, A. (1990). *The Consequences of Modernity*. Cambridge: Polity Press.

Giddens, A. (1998). *Conversations with Anthony Giddens: Making Sense of Modernity*. Stanford, CA: Stanford University Press.

Gigerenzer, G. (2010). Moral satisficing: rethinking moral behavior as bounded rationality. *Topics in Cognitive Science* 2: 528–54.

Gillies, V. (2005). Raising the 'meritocracy': parenting and the individualization of social class. *Sociology* 39: 835–53.

Gilman, S.L. (2010). *Obesity: the Biography*. Oxford: Oxford University Press.

Gluckman, P. & Hanson, M. (2004). *The Fetal Matrix: Evolution, Development and Disease*. Cambridge: Cambridge University Press.

Gluckman, P.D., Hanson, M.A. & Low, F.M. (2011). The role of developmental plasticity and epigenetics in human health. *Birth Defects Research Part C: Embryo Today: Reviews* 93: 12–18.

Golden, M.H.N. (1994). Is complete catch-up possible for stunted malnourished children? *European Journal of Clinical Nutrition* 48 (Suppl. 1): S58–71.

Goldman, D., Lakdawalla, D. & Zheng, Y. (2011). Food prices and the dynamics of body weight. In M. Grossman & N. Mocan, eds., *Economic Aspects of Obesity*. National Bureau of Economic Research Conference Report. Chicago, IL: University of Chicago Press, pp. 65–83.

Goodman, A.H. & Leatherman, T.L. (eds.) (1998). *Building a New Biocultural Synthesis. Political-Economic Perspectives on Human Biology*. Ann Arbor, MI: University of Michigan Press.

Goodman, E. & Whitaker, R.C. (2002). A prospective study of the role of depression in the development and persistence of adolescent obesity. *Pediatrics* 110: 497–504.

Goran, M.I., Ulijaszek, S.J. & Ventura, E.E. (2012). High fructose corn syrup and diabetes prevalence: a global perspective. *Global Public Health* 8: 55–64.

Gornall, J. (2015). Sugar: spinning a web of influence. *British Medical Journal* 350: h231.

Gortmaker, S.L., Swinburn, B.A., Levy, D. et al. (2011). Changing the future of obesity: science, policy, and action. *Lancet* 378: 838–47.

Gosby, A.K., Conigrave, A.D., Lau, N.S. et al. (2011). Testing protein leverage in lean humans: a randomised controlled experimental study. *PLoS One* 6: e25929.

Gottlob, G. & Nejdl, W. (1990). *Expert Systems in Engineering, Principles and Applications, International Workshop, Vienna, Austria, September 24–26, 1990, Proceedings*. Lecture Notes in Computer Science 462. New York, NY: Springer.

Government of Western Australia Department for Planning and Infrastructure (2009). *Perth 2009. Public Spaces and Public Life*. Perth, WA: Government of Western Australia Department for Planning and Infrastructure.

Graham, H. (2007). *Unequal Lives: Health and Socioeconomic Inequalities*. Maidenhead, Berkshire: Open University Press.

Green, D.P. & Shapiro, I. (1994). *Pathologies of Rational Choice Theory: a Critique of Applications in Political Science*. New Haven, CT: Yale University Press.

Greener, J., Douglas, F. & van Teijlingen, E. (2010). More of the same? Conflicting perspectives of obesity causation and intervention amongst overweight people, health professionals and policy makers. *Social Science and Medicine* 70: 1042–9.

Greenleaf, C., Chambliss, H., Martin, S.B. & Morrow, J.R. (2006). Weight stereotypes and behavioral intentions toward thin and fat peers among White and Hispanic adolescents. *Journal of Adolescent Health* 39: 546–52.

Grendstad, G., Selle, P. & Thompson, M. (2003). *Cultural Theory as Political Science*. London: Routledge.

Grimley Evans, J. & Prior, I.A.M. (1969). Indices of obesity derived from height and weight in two Polynesian populations. *British Journal of Preventive Social Medicine* 23: 56–9.

Groesz, L.M., McCoy, S., Carl, J. et al. (2012). What is eating you? Stress and the drive to eat. *Appetite* 58: 717–21.

Gross, J.L. & Rayner, S. (1985). *Measuring Culture: a Paradigm for the Analysis of Social Organization*. New York, NY: Columbia University Press.

Grossman, J. & MacKenzie, F.J. (2005). The randomized controlled trial: gold standard, or merely standard? *Perspectives in Biology and Medicine* 48: 516–34.

Grossman, M. & Mocan, N. (2011). *Economic Aspects of Obesity. National Bureau of Economic Research*. Chicago, IL: University of Chicago Press.

Grossmann, I. & Varnum, M.E.W. (2015). Social structure, infectious diseases, disasters, secularism, and cultural change in America. *Psychological Science* 26: 311–24.

Gruber, J. & Frakes, M. (2006). Does falling smoking lead to rising obesity? *Journal of Health Economics* 25: 183–97.

Grundy, S.M. (1998). Multifactorial causation of obesity: implications for prevention. *American Journal of Clinical Nutrition* 67 (Suppl.): 563S–72S.

Guthman, J. (2011). *Weighing In: Obesity, Food Justice, and the Limits of Capitalism*. Berkeley, CA: University of California Press.

Guthman, J. (2013). Fatuous measures: the artifactual construction of the obesity epidemic. *Critical Public Health* 23: 263–73.

Guthman, J. & du Puis, M. (2006). Embodying neoliberalism: economy, culture, and the politics of fat. *Environment and Planning D* 24: 427–48.

Guyenet, S.J. & Schwartz, M.W. (2012). Regulation of food intake, energy balance, and body fat mass: implications for the pathogenesis and treatment of obesity. *Journal of Clinical Endocrinology and Metabolism* 97: 745–55.

Haase, A., Steptoe, A., Sallis, J.F. & Wardle, J. (2004). Leisure-time physical activity in university students from 23 countries: associations with health beliefs, risk awareness, and national economic development. *Preventive Medicine* 39: 182–90.

Hacker, J.S., Rehm, P. & Schlesinger, M. (2013). The insecure American: economic experiences, financial worries, and policy attitudes. *Perspectives on Politics* 11: 23–49.

Hacking, I. (1983). *Representing and Intervening. Introductory Topics in the Philosophy of Natural Science*. Cambridge: Cambridge University Press.

Hall, K.D. & Heymsfield, S.B. (2009). Models use leptin and calculus to count calories. *Cell Metabolism* 9: 3–4.

Hall, K.D., Heymsfield, S.B., Kemnitz, J.W. et al. (2012). Energy balance and its components: implications for body weight regulation. *American Journal of Clinical Nutrition* 95: 989–94.

Hall, P.A. & Soskice, D. (2001). *Varieties of Capitalism*. Oxford: Oxford University Press.

Hall, S.K., Cousins, J.H. & Power, T.G. (1991). Self-concept and perceptions of attractiveness and body size among Mexican-American mothers and daughters. *International Journal of Obesity* 15: 567–75.

Hamid, T.K.A. (2009). *Thinking in Circles about Obesity: Applying Systems Thinking to Weight Management*. New York, NY: Springer.

Hammond, R.A. (2009). Complex systems modeling for obesity research. *Preventing Chronic Disease* 6: A97.

Hancock, A.M., Clark, V.J., Qian, Y. & Di Rienzo, A. (2011). Population genetic analysis of the uncoupling proteins supports a role for UCP3 in human cold resistance. *Molecular Biology and Evolution* 28: 601–14.

Hannerz, H., Albertsen, K., Nielsen, M.L., Tuchsen, F. & Burr, H. (2004). Occupational factors and 5-year weight change among men in a Danish national cohort. *Health Psychology* 23: 283–8.

Hansen, F. & Christensen, S.R. (2007). *Emotions, Advertising and Consumer Choice*. Frederiksberg, Copenhagen: Copenhagen Business School Press.

Hansson, L.M., Karnehed, N., Tynelius, P. & Rasmussen, F. (2009). Prejudice against obesity among 10-year-olds: a nationwide population-based study. *Acta Paediatrica* 98: 1176–82.

Harlow, H.F. & Yudin, H.C. (1933). Social behavior of primates. I. Social facilitation of feeding in the monkey and its relation to attitudes of ascendance and submission. *Journal of Comparative Psychology* 16: 171–85.

Harrington, D.W. & Elliott, S.J. (2009). Weighing the importance of neighbourhood: a multilevel exploration of the determinants of overweight and obesity. *Social Science and Medicine* 68: 593–600.

Hartmann, T. (2009). Clumsy floodplains and the law: towards a responsive land policy for extreme floods. *Built Environment* 35: 531–44.

Hartmann, T. (2010). Reframing polyrational floodplains: land policy for large areas for temporary emergency retention. *Nature and Culture* 5: 15–30.

Hartmann, T. (2012). Wicked problems and clumsy solutions: planning as expectation management. *Planning Theory* 11: 242–56.

Hartmann, T. & Spit, T.J.M. (2012). Managing riverside property: Spatial water management in Germany from a Dutch perspective. In T. Hartmann & B. Needham, eds., *Planning by Law and Property Rights Reconsidered*. Farnham, Surrey: Ashgate Publishing, pp. 97–116.

Hartmann, T. & Spit, T.J.M. (2015). Dilemmas of involvement in land management – comparing an active (Dutch) and a passive (German) approach. *Land Use Policy* 42: 729–37.

Hasnain, M., Victor, W., Vieweg, R. & Hollet, T.B. (2012). Weight gain and glucose dysregulation with second-generation antipsychotics and antidepressants: a review for primary care physicians. *Postgraduate Medicine* 124: 154–67.

Haug, M.R. (1977). Measurement in social stratification. *Annual Review of Sociology* 3: 51–77.

Hawkes, C. (2005). The role of foreign direct investment in the nutrition transition. *Public Health Nutrition* 8: 357–65.

Hawkes, C. (2006). Uneven dietary development: linking the policies and processes of globalization with the nutrition transition, obesity and diet-related chronic diseases. *Globalization and Health* 2: 4.

Hayes-Roth, F., Waterman, D. & Lenat, D. (1983). *Building Expert Systems*. Reading, MA: Addison-Wesley.

Haymes, S., Vidal de Haymes, M. & Miller, R. (eds.) (2015). *The Routledge Handbook of Poverty in the United States*. London: Routledge.

Haynes, A.S., Derrick, G.E., Chapman, S. et al. (2011). From "our world" to the "real world": exploring the views and behaviour of policy-influential Australian public health researchers. *Social Science and Medicine* 72: 1–11.

Head, B.W. (2008). Three lenses of evidence-based policy. *Australian Journal of Public Administration* 67: 1–11.

Healthy Together Geelong (2014). *Greater Geelong Community Health Needs Assessment 2014*. Geelong, VIC: Healthy Together Governance Group.

Healthy Together Geelong (2016). Geelong bucks the trend in obesity. www.geelongaustralia.com.au/healthygeelong/news/item/8d3e6e2d4c46919.aspx (accessed 26 November 2016).

Heijmans, B., Tobi, E., Stein, E. et al. (2008). Persistent epigenetic differences associated with prenatal exposure to famine in humans. *Proceedings of the National Academy of Sciences USA* 105: 17046–9.

Helleiner, E. (1994). *States and the Reemergence of Global Finance*. Ithaca, NY: Cornell University Press.

Hemmingsson, E. (2014). A new model of the role of psychological and emotional distress in promoting obesity: conceptual review with implications for treatment and prevention. *Obesity Reviews* 15: 769–79.

Hendrie, G.A., Coveney, J. & Cox, D.N. (2012). Defining the complexity of childhood obesity and related behaviours within the family environment using structural equation modelling. *Public Health Nutrition* 15: 48–57.

Her Majesty's Government (1999). *Saving Lives: Our Healthier Nation*. London: Her Majesty's Government.

Herrera, B.M., Keildson, S. & Lindgren, C.M. (2011). Genetics and epigenetics of obesity. *Maturitas* 69: 41–9.

Herrick, C. (2009). Shifting blame/selling health: corporate social responsibility in the age of obesity. *Sociology of Health and Illness* 31: 51–65.

Hess, R.D. (1970). Social class and ethnic influences on socialization. In P.H. Mussen, ed., *Carmichael's Manual of Child Psychology*, 3rd edn., Vol. 2. New York, NY: Wiley, pp. 457–557.

Hetherington, M.M., Anderson, A.S., Norton, G.N.M. & Newson, L. (2006). Situational effects on meal intake: a comparison of eating alone and eating with others. *Physiology and Behavior* 88: 498–505.

Hill, J.O., Peters, J.C. & Wyatt, H.R. (2007). The role of public policy in treating the epidemic of global obesity. *Clinical Pharmacology and Therapeutics* 81: 772–5.

Hill, J.O., Wyatt, H.R. & Peters, J.C. (2012). Energy balance and obesity. *Circulation* 126: 126–32.

Hines, P., Holweg, M. & Rich, N. (2004). Learning to evolve: a review of contemporary lean thinking. *International Journal of Operations and Production Management* 24: 994–1011.

Hladik, C.M.(1988). Seasonal variations in food supply for wild primates. In I. de Garine and G.A. Harrison, eds., *Coping with Uncertainty in Food Supply*. Oxford: Clarendon Press, pp. 1–25.

Hoek, H.W. & van Hoeken, D. (1996). Risk factors for eating disorders: differences in incidence rates in relation to urbanization and culture. *European Psychiatry* 11 (Suppl. 4): 220.

Hoelscher, D.M., Kirk, S., Ritchie, L. & Cunningham-Sabo, L. (2013). Position of the Academy of Nutrition and Dietetics: interventions for the prevention and treatment of pediatric overweight and obesity. *Journal of the Academy of Nutrition and Dietetics* 113: 1375–94.

Hoff, E., Laursen, B. & Tardif, T. (2002). Socioeconomic status and parenting. In M.H. Bornstein, ed., *Handbook of Parenting. Vol. 2. Biology and Ecology of Parenting*. London: Lawrence Erlbaum Associates, Publishers, pp. 231–52.

Holm, L. & Fruhbeck, G. (2013). *Executive Summary. Workshop on Social Sciences and Humanities' Contribution to Tackle the Obesity Epidemic*. Copenhagen: University of Copenhagen.

Holt, D.B. (1998). Does cultural capital structure American consumption? *Journal of Consumer Research* 25: 1–25.

Hood, L., Heath, J.R., Phelps, M.E. & Lin, B. (2004). Systems biology and new technologies enable predictive and preventative medicine. *Science* 306: 640–3.

House of Commons Health Committee (2004). *Obesity. Third Report of Session 2003–04. Vol. I. Report, Together with Formal Minutes.* London: The Stationery Office.

Howe, L.D., Tilling, K., Galobardes, B. et al. (2010). Socioeconomic disparities in trajectories of adiposity across childhood. *International Journal of Pediatriatric Obesity* 6: e144–53.

Hruschka, D.J. (2012). Do economic constraints on food choice make people fat? A critical review of two hypotheses for the poverty–obesity paradox. *American Journal of Human Biology* 24: 277–85.

Hu, F.B. (2008). Obesity and mortality. In F. Hu, ed., *Obesity Epidemiology.* Oxford: Oxford University Press, pp. 216–33.

Huang, T., Drewnowski, A., Kumanyika, S. & Glass, T. (2009). A systems-oriented multilevel framework for addressing obesity in the 21st century. *Preventing Chronic Disease* 6: A82.

Hudson, J.I., Hiripi, E., Pope, H.G. Jr. & Kessler, R.C. (2007). The prevalence and correlates of eating disorders in the national comorbidity survey replication. *Biological Psychiatry* 61: 348–58.

Huneault, L., Mathieu, M.-E. & Tremblay, A. (2011). Globalization and modernization: an obesogenic combination. *Obesity Reviews* 12: e64–72.

Hurrelmann, K., Rathmann, K. & Richter, M. (2011). Health inequalities and welfare state regimes. A research note. *Journal of Public Health* 19: 3–13.

Huss-Ashmore, R., Schall, J. & Hediger, M. (1992). *Health and Lifestyle Change.* MASCA Research Papers in Science and Archaeology, Vol. 9. Philadelphia, PA: University of Pennsylvania.

Huxley, R., Mendis, S., Zheleznyakov, E., Reddy, S. & Chan, J. (2010). Body mass index, waist circumference and waist:hip ratio as predictors of cardiovascular risk – a review of the literature. *European Journal of Clinical Nutrition* 64: 16–22.

Ideker, T., Galitski, T. & Hood, L. (2001). A new approach to decoding life: systems biology. *Annual Review of Genomics and Human Genetics* 2: 343–72.

Ifland, J.R., Preuss, H.G., Marcus, M.T. et al. (2009). Refined food addiction: a classic substance use disorder. *Medical Hypotheses* 72: 518–26.

Innes, J.E. & Booher, D.E. (2010). *Planning with Complexity: An Introduction to Collaborative Rationality for Public Policy.* London: Routledge.

International Labour Organization (2016). ILOSTAT: the world's leading source on labour statistics. www.ilo.org/ilostat/faces/wcnav_defaultSelection;ILOSTATCOOKIE=4-CSXYOxBfIp1KyThm LEUlKC98el70yWfHSBKrQlWag2aiSf8m–!1554508336?_afrLoop=73679078641796&t_afrWin dowMode=0&t_afrWindowId=null#!%40%40%3F_afrWindowId%3Dnull%26_afrLoop% 3D73679078641796%26_afrWindowMode%3D0%26_adf.ctrl-state%3Ds3u82ujj5_4 (accessed 6 January 2017).

Ioannidis, J.P.A. (2005). Why most published research findings are false. *PLoS Medicine* 2: e124.

Ismail, M.N., Chee, S., Nawawi, H. et al. (2002). Obesity in Malaysia. *Obesity Reviews* 3: 203–8.

Jabs, J. & Devine, C.M. (2006). Time scarcity and food choices: an overview. *Appetite* 47: 196–204.

Jack, A. (2007). Obesity plan lacks foresight. *Lancet* 370: 1528–9.

Jacobs, D. & Myers, L. (2014). Union strength, neoliberalism, and inequality. Contingent political analyses of U.S. income differences since 1950. *American Sociological Review* 79: 752–74.

Jahns, L., Siega-Riz, A.M. & Popkin, B.M. (2001). The increasing prevalence of snacking among US children from 1977 to 1996. *Journal of Pediatrics* 138: 493–8.

James, W.P.T. (2004). Obesity: the worldwide epidemic. *Clinics in Dermatology* 22: 276–80.

Jang, H. & Serra, C. (2014). Nutrition, epigenetics, and diseases. *Clinical Nutrition Research* 3: 1–8.

Janssen, I., Katzmarzyk, P.T. & Ross, R. (2004). Waist circumference and not body mass index explains obesity-related health risk. *American Journal of Clinical Nutrition* 79: 379–84.

Janz, K.F., Levy, S.M., Burns, T.L. et al. (2002). Fatness, physical activity, and television viewing in children during the adiposity rebound period: the Iowa bone development study. *Preventive Medicine* 35: 563–71.

Jarosz, D. & Pasztor, M. (2007). An attempt at a history of meat in people's Poland. *Acta Poloniae Historica* 95: 139–87.

Jebb, S.A., Aveyard, P.N. & Hawkes, C. (2013). The evolution of policy and actions to tackle obesity in England. *Obesity Reviews* 14 (Suppl. 2): 42–59.

Jelliffe, D.B. (1966). The assessment of the nutritional status of the community (with special reference to field surveys in developing regions of the world). *Monograph Series of the World Health Organization* 53: 3–271.

Jevons, W.S. (1866). A brief account of a general mathematical theory of political economy. *Journal of the Royal Statistical Society* 29: 282–87.

Jevons, WS. (1871). *The Theory of Political Economy*. London: Macmillan.

Joffe, B. & Zimmet, P. (1998). The thrifty genotype in type 2 diabetes: an unfinished symphony moving to its finale? *Endocrine* 9: 139–41.

Johnson, R. (2007). Post-hegemony? I don't think so. *Theory, Culture and Society* 24: 95–110.

Johnston, F.E. (1998). The ecology of post-natal growth. In S.J. Ulijaszek, F.E. Johnston & M.A. Preece, eds., *Cambridge Encyclopedia of Human Growth and Development*. Cambridge: Cambridge University Press, pp. 315–9.

Johnston, J. (2005). Rawls's Kantian educational theory. *Educational Theory* 55: 201–18.

Johnston, J. & Baumann, S. (2007). Democracy versus distinction: a study of omnivorousness in gourmet food writing. *American Journal of Sociology* 113: 165–204.

Jones, A., Bentham, G., Foster, C., Hillsdon, M. & Panter, J. (2007). *Foresight. Tackling Obesities: Future Choices – Obesogenic Environments – Evidence Review*. London: Government Office for Science.

Jones, G. & Ledger, J. (1986). Expert systems in decision support: opportunities for the retailer. *Retail and Distribution Management* 14: 18–9.

Jones, G. & Morgan, N.J. (eds.) (1994). *Adding Value: Brands and Marketing in Food and Drink*. London: Routledge.

Jou, C. (2014). The biology and genetics of obesity – a century of inquiries. *New England Journal of Medicine* 370: 1874–7.

Jou, J. & Techakehakij, W. (2012). International application of sugar-sweetened beverage (SSB) taxation in obesity reduction: factors that may influence policy effectiveness in country-specific contexts. *Health Policy* 107: 83–90.

Jutel, A. (2005). Weighing health: the moral burden of obesity. *Social Semiotics* 15: 113–25.

Kahan, S. & Zvenyach, T. (2016). Obesity as a disease: current policies and implications for the future. *Current Obesity Reports* 5: 291–97.

Kahn, H.S. & Williamson, D.F. (1994). Abdominal obesity and mortality risk among men in nineteenth-century North America. *International Journal of Obesity* 18: 686–91.

Kahneman, D. (2003). Maps of bounded rationality: psychology for behavioral economics. *American Economic Review* 93: 1449–75.

Kahneman, D. & Tversky, A. (1972). Subjective probability: a judgment of representativeness. *Cognitive Psychology* 3: 430–54.

Kalberg, S. (1980). Max Weber's types of rationality: cornerstones for the analysis of rationalization processes in history. *American Journal of Sociology* 85: 1145–79.

Kamadjeu, R.M., Edwards, R., Atanga, J.S. et al. (2006). Anthropometry measures and prevalence of obesity in the urban adult population of Cameroon: an update from the Cameroon Burden of Diabetes Baseline Survey. *BMC Public Health* 6: 228.

Kanarek, R.B. & Hirsch, E. (1977). Dietary-induced overeating in experimental animals. *Federation Proceedings* 36: 154–58.

Kant, I. (1785). *Grounding for the Metaphysics of Morals*. Translated by J. Ellington, 1993. Indianapolis, IN: Hackett Publishing Company.

Kant, I. (1891). *Principles of Politics*. Translated by W. Hastie. Edinburgh: T. and T. Clark.

Kant, I. (1997). *Practical Philosophy*. Translated and edited by M.J. McGregor. Cambridge: Cambridge University Press.

Kantar Worldpanel (2013). Coca Cola leads global ranking of the most chosen brands. www.kantarworldpanel.com/global/News/Coca-Cola-leads-Kantar-Worldpanel-global-ranking-of-the-most-chosen-FMCG-brands- (accessed 15 January 2017).

Kanter, R. & Caballero, B. (2012). Global gender disparities in obesity: a review. *Advances in Nutrition* 3: 491–8.

Kaplan, H., Hill, K., Lancaster, J. & Hurtado, A.M. (2000). A theory of human life history evolution: diet, intelligence, and longevity. *Evolutionary Anthropology* 9: 156–85.

Kapoor, A.K. & Kaur, J. (2012). Natural selection in a population group of Andaman and Nicobar Islands. *Journal of Natural Science, Biology and Medicine* 3: 71–7.

Kapoor, A.K., Kshatriya, G.K. & Kapoor, S. (2003). Fertility and mortality differentials among the population groups of the Himalayas. *Human Biology* 75: 729–47.

Kassel, J.D. & Unrod, M. (2000). Smoking, anxiety, and attention: support for the role of nicotine in attentionally mediated anxiolysis. *Journal of Abnormal Psychology* 109: 161–6.

Keith, S.W., Redden, D.T., Katzmarzyk, P.T. et al. (2006). Putative contributors to the secular increase in obesity: exploring the roads less travelled. *International Journal of Obesity* 30: 1585–94.

Keles, A., Yavuz, U. & Keles, A. (2011). Expert system based on neuro-fuzzy rules for diagnosis breast cancer. *Expert Systems with Applications* 38: 5719–26.

Kelly, P. (2003). Growing up as risky business? Risks, surveillance and the institutionalised mistrust of youth. *Journal of Youth Studies* 6: 165–80.

Kelly, Y.J. & Watt, R.G. (2005). Breast-feeding initiation and exclusive duration at 6 months by social class – results from the Millennium Cohort Study. *Public Health Nutrition* 8: 417–21.

Kennedy, M. & Garcia, E. (1994). Assessing linkages between body mass index and morbidity in adults: evidence from four developing countries. *European Journal of Clinical Nutrition* 48 (Suppl. 3): S90–6.

Keys, A., Fidanza, F., Karvonen, M.J., Kimura, N. & Taylor, H.L. (1972). Indices of relative weight and obesity. *Journal of Chronic Diseases* 25: 329–43.

Khosla, T. & Lowe, C.R. (1967). Indices of obesity derived from body weight and height. *British Journal of Preventive and Social Medicine* 21: 122–28.

Kim, G.W., Lin, J.E., Valentino, M.A., Colon-Gonzalez, F. & Waldmann, S.A. (2011). Regulation of appetite to treat obesity. *Expert Review of Clinical Pharmacology* 4: 243–59.

Kim, J.K., Samaranayake, M. & Pradhan, S. (2009). Epigenetic mechanisms in mammals. *Cellular and Molecular Life Sciences* 66: 596–612.

Kim, T.J., Wiggins, L.L. & Wright, J.R. (eds.) (1990). *Expert Systems: Applications to Urban Planning*. New York, NY: Springer.

King, T., Kavanagh, A.M., Jolley, D., Turrell, G. & Crawford, D. (2006). Weight and place: a multilevel cross-sectional survey of area-level social disadvantage and overweight/obesity in Australia. *International Journal of Obesity* 30: 281–7.

Kingdon, J.W. (1984). *Agendas, Alternatives, and Public Policies*. Boston, MA: Little, Brown and Company.

Kirk, S.F.L., Penney, T.L. & McHugh, T.-L.F. (2009). Characterizing the obesogenic environment: the state of the evidence with directions for future research. *Obesity Reviews* 11: 109–17.

Kitano, H. (2002). Systems biology: a brief overview. *Science* 295: 1662–4.

Klassen, M.L., Jasper, C.R. & Harris, R.J. (1993). The role of physical appearance in managerial decisions. *Journal of Business and Psychology* 8: 181–98.

Klein, M. & Dwyer, J. 2008). Role of probiotics stakeholders in future research and policy on probiotics use in the United States. *Clinical Infectious Diseases* 46: S144–51.

Klesges, R.C & Shumaker, S.A. (1992). Understanding the relations between smoking and body weight and their importance to smoking cessation and relapse. *Health Psychology* 11 (Suppl.): 1–3.

Komlos, J. & Lauderdale, B. (2007). Underperformance in affluence: the remarkable relative decline in U.S. heights in the second half of the 20th century. *Social Science Quarterly* 88: 283–305.

Kootte, R.S., Vrieze, A., Holleman, F. et al. (2012). The therapeutic potential of manipulating gut microbiota in obesity and type 2 diabetes mellitus. *Diabetes, Obesity and Metabolism* 14: 112–20.

Korsgaard, C.M. (1997). The normativity of instrumental reason. In G. Cullity & B. Gaut, eds., *Ethics and Practical Reason*. Oxford: Clarendon Press, pp. 215–54.

Koziel, S., Ulijaszek, S.J., Szklarska, A. & Bielicki, T. (2007). The effects of fatness and fat distribution on respiratory function. *Annals of Human Biology* 34: 123–31.

Krieger, N., Williams, D.R. & Moss, N.E. (1997). Measuring social class in US public health research: concepts, methodologies, and guidelines. *Annual Review of Public Health* 18: 341–78.

Kringelbach, M.L. (2015). The pleasure of food: underlying brain mechanisms of eating and other pleasures. *Flavour* 4: 20.

Kubiszewski, I., Costanza, R., Franco, C. et al. (2013). Beyond GDP: measuring and achieving global genuine progress. *Ecological Economics* 93: 57–68.

Kumanyika, S., Jeffery, R.W., Morabia, A., Ritenbaugh, C. & Antipatis, V.J. (2002). Obesity prevention: the case for action. Public health approaches to the prevention of obesity. *International Journal of Obesity* 26: 425–36.

Kumar, V.R., Chung, C.Y.C. & Lindley, C.A. (1994). Toward building an expert system for weather forecasting operations. *Expert Systems with Applications* 7: 373–81.

Kuo, L.E., Czarnecka, M., Kitlinska, J.B. et al. (2008). Chronic stress, combined with a high-fat/high-sugar diet, shifts sympathetic signaling toward neuropeptide Y and leads to obesity and the metabolic syndrome. *Stress, Neurotransmitters, and Hormones: Neuroendocrine and Genetic Mechanisms* 1148: 232–7.

Kuserow, A. (2004). *American Individualism: Child Rearing and Social Class in Three Neighborhoods*. New York, NY: Palgrave Macmillan.

Kuzawa, C.W. (1998). Adipose tissue in human infancy and childhood: an evolutionary perspective. *Yearbook of Physical Anthropology* 41: 177–209.

Kwa, C. (2002). Romantic and baroque conceptions of complex wholes in the sciences. In J. Law & A. Mol, eds., *Complexities. Social Studies of Knowledge Practices*. Durham, NC: Duke University Press, pp. 23–52.

Ladyman, J., Lambert, J. & Wiesner, K. (2013). What is a complex system? *European Journal for Philosophy of Science* 3: 33–67.

Lakdawalla, D. & Philipson, T. (2002). *The Growth of Obesity and Technological Change: a Theoretical and Empirical Examination*. NBER Working Paper No. 8946. Cambridge, MA: National Bureau of Economic Research.

Lakdawalla, D., Philipson, T. & Bhattacharya, J. (2005). Welfare-enhancing technological change and the growth of obesity. *American Economic Review* 95: 253–7.

Lake, J.K., Power, C. & Cole, T.J. (1997). Child to adult body mass index in the 1958 British birth cohort: associations with parental obesity. *Archives of Disease in Childhood* 77: 376–80.

Lambert, P.M. (2009). Health versus fitness: competing themes in the origins and spread of agriculture? *Current Anthropology* 50: 603–8.

Lancet Editorial (2011). Malaria: control vs elimination vs eradication. *Lancet* 378: 1117.

Lancy, D. (2008). *The Anthropology of Childhood: Cherubs, Chattel, Changelings*. Cambridge: Cambridge University Press.

Landecker, H. (2011). Food as exposure: nutritional epigenetics and the new metabolism. *BioSocieties* 6: 167–94.

Landon, J. & Graff, H. (2012). What is the role of health-related food duties? National Heart Forum. tinyurl.com/ctvm2uf (accessed 15 May 2017).

Lane, P.R. & Milesi-Ferretti, G.M. (2007). The external wealth of nations mark II: revised and extended estimates of foreign assets and liabilities, 1970–2004. *Journal of International Economics* 73: 223–50.

Lang, T. & Heasman, M. (2015). *Food Wars. The Global Battle for Mouths, Minds and Markets*. London: Earthscan Books.

Lang, T. & Rayner, G. (2005). Obesity: a growing issue for European policy? *Journal of European Social Policy* 15: 301–27.

Lang, T. & Rayner, G. (2007). Overcoming policy cacophony on obesity: an ecological public health framework for policymakers. *Obesity Reviews* 8 (Suppl. 1): 165–81.

Lang, T. & Rayner, G. (2014). Ecological public health: the 21st century's big idea? An essay by Tim Lang and Geof Rayner. *British Medical Journal* 345: e5466.

Larnkjaer, A., Schroder, S.A., Schmidt, I.M. et al. (2006). Secular change in adult stature has come to a halt in northern Europe and Italy. *Acta Paediatrica* 93: 754–55.

Lascoumes, P. & le Gales, P. (2007). Introduction: understanding public policy through its instruments – from the nature of instruments to the sociology of public policy instrumentation. *Governance* 20: 1–21.

Latour, B. (2004). Why has critique run out of steam? *Critical Inquiry* 30: 225–48.

Latour, B. & Woolgar, S. (1986). *Laboratory Life: The Construction of Scientific Facts*. Princeton, NJ: Princeton University Press.

Lau, C., Ambalavanan, N., Chakraborty, H., Wingate, M.S. & Carlo, W.A. (2013). Extremely low birth weight and infant mortality rates in the United States. *Pediatrics* 131: 855–60.

Laurier, D., Guiget, M., Chau, N.P. et al. (1992). Prevalence of obesity: a comparative survey in France, the United Kingdom and the United States. *International Journal of Obesity* 16: 565–72.

Law, J. (2004a). And if the global were small and noncoherent? Method, complexity, and the baroque. *Environment and Planning D: Society and Space* 22: 13–26.

Law, J. (2004b). *After Method: Mess in Social Science Research*. London: Routledge.

Lawn, P.A. (2003). A theoretical foundation to support the Index of Sustainable Economic Welfare (ISEW), Genuine Progress Indicator (GPI), and other related indexes. *Ecological Economics* 44: 105–18.

Lawrence, R.G. (2004). Framing obesity: the evolution of news discourse on a public health issue. *Politics* 9: 56–75.

Lawton, C.L., Burley, V.L., Wales, J.K. & Blundell, J.E. (1993). Dietary fat and appetite control in obese subjects: weak effects on satiation and satiety. *International Journal of Obesity* 17: 409–16.

Lee, C.M.Y., Huxley, R.R., Wildman, R.P. & Woodward, M. (2008). Indices of abdominal obesity are better discriminators of cardiovascular risk factors than BMI: a meta-analysis. *Journal of Clinical Epidemiology* 61: 646–53.

Lee, G.A., Crawford, G.W., Liu, L. & Xingcan, C. (2007). Plants and people from the early Neolithic to Shang periods in North China. *Proceedings of the National Academy of Sciences USA* 104: 1087–92.

Leibel, R.L. (2008). Molecular physiology of weight regulation in mice and humans. *International Journal of Obesity* 32: S98–108.

Lenski, G. & Nolan, P.D. (1984). Trajectories of development: a test of ecological evolutionary theory. *Social Forces* 63: 1–23.

Leonard, W.R. & Ulijaszek, S.J. (2002). Energetics and evolution: an emerging research domain. *American Journal of Human Biology* 14: 547–50.

Lerner, J.S., Gonzalez, R.M., Small, D.A. & Fischhoff, B. (2003). Effects of fear and anger on perceived risks of terrorism: a national field experiment. *Psychological Science* 14: 144–50.

Lev-Ran, A. (2001). Human obesity: an evolutionary approach to understanding our bulging waistline. *Diabetes/Metabolism Research and Reviews* 17: 347–62.

Levin, K., Cashore, B., Bernstein, S. & Auld, G. (2012). Overcoming the tragedy of super wicked problems: constraining our future selves to ameliorate global climate change. *Policy Sciences* 45: 123–52.

Levy, D.T., Mabry, P.L., Wang, Y.C. et al. (2011). Simulation models of obesity: a review of the literature and implications for research and policy. *Obesity Reviews* 12: 378–94.

Lexchin, J., Djulbegovic, B. & Clark, O. (2003). Pharmaceutical industry sponsorship and research outcome and quality: systematic review. *British Medical Journal* 326: 1167–70.

Ley, R.E., Bäckhed, F., Turnbaugh, P. et al. (2005). Obesity alters gut microbial ecology. *Proceedings of the National Academy of Sciences USA* 102: 11070–5.

Li, G., Chen, X., Jang, Y. et al. (2002). Obesity, coronary heart disease risk factors and diabetes in Chinese: an approach to the criteria of obesity in the Chinese population. *Obesity Reviews* 3: 167–72.

Li, L., Law, C., Conte, R.L. et al. (2009). Intergenerational influences on childhood body mass index: the effect of parental body mass index trajectories. *American Journal of Clinical Nutrition* 89: 551–7.

Lindberg, L., Ek, A., Nyman, J. et al. (2015). Low grandparental social support combined with low parental socioeconomic status is closely associated with obesity in preschool-aged children: a pilot study. *Pediatric Obesity* 11: 313–6.

Lindgren, C.M., Heid, I.M., Randall, J.C. et al. (2009). Genome-wide association scan meta-analysis identifies three loci influencing adiposity and fat distribution. *PLoS Genetics* 5: e1000508.

Lissner, L., Visscher, T.L., Rissanen, A. & Heitmann, B.L. (2013). Prevention and Public Health Task Force of European Association for the Study of Obesity. Monitoring the obesity epidemic into the 21st century – weighing the evidence. *Obesity Facts* 6: 561–5.

Liu, Y., Tong, G., Tong, W., Lu, L. & Qin, X. (2011). Can body mass index, waist circumference, waist-hip ratio and waist-height ratio predict the presence of multiple metabolic risk factors in Chinese subjects? *BMC Public Health* 11: 35.

Llewellyn, C., van Jaarsveld, C., Boniface, D., Carnell, S. & Wardle, J. (2008). Eating rate is a heritable phenotype related to weight in children. *American Journal of Clinical Nutrition* 88: 1560–6.

Lloyd, L.J., Langley-Evans, S.C. & McMullen, S. (2010). Childhood obesity and adult cardiovascular disease risk: a systematic review. *International Journal of Obesity* 34: 18–28.

Lloyd, L.J., Langley-Evans, S.C. & McMullen, S. (2012). Childhood obesity and risk of the adult metabolic syndrome: a systematic review. *International Journal of Obesity* 36: 1–11.

Lobstein, T., Baur, L. & Uauy, R. (2004). Obesity in children and young people: a crisis in public health. *Obesity Reviews* 5 (Suppl. 1): 4–85.

Lodge, M. & Wegrich, K. (2014). *Rational Tools of Government in a World of Bounded Rationality.* Discussion Paper No. 75. London: London School of Economics.

Lodge, M. & Wegrich, K. (2016). The rationality paradox of nudge: rational tools of government in a world of bounded rationality. *Law and Policy* 38: 250–67.

Lopez, R.P. (2007). Neighborhood risk factors for obesity. *Obesity* 15: 2111–9.

Loughlin, J. (2000). Regional autonomy and state paradigm shifts in Western Europe. *Regional and Federal Studies* 10: 10–34.

Lovejoy, J.C., Sainsbury, A. & Stock Conference 2008 Working Group (2009). Sex differences in obesity and the regulation of energy homeostasis. *Obesity Reviews* 10: 154–67.

Lowe, M.R. & Butryn, M.L. (2007). Hedonic hunger: a new dimension of appetite? *Physiology and Behavior* 91: 432–9.

Lowe, M.R., Miller-Kovach, K. & Phelan, S. (2001). Weight-loss maintenance in overweight individuals one to five years following successful completion of a commercial weight loss program. *International Journal of Obesity and Related Metabolic Disorders* 25: 325–31.

Lubchenco, L.O., Searls, D.T. & Brazie, J.V. (1972). Neonatal mortality rate: relationship to birth weight and gestational age. *Journal of Pediatrics* 81: 814–22.

Ludwig, D.S., Peterson, K.E. & Gortmaker, S.L. (2001). Relation between consumption of sugar-sweetened drinks and childhood obesity: a prospective, observational analysis. *Lancet* 357: 505–8.

Luger, G. & Stubblefield, W. (2004). *Artificial Intelligence: Structures and Strategies for Complex Problem Solving*, 5th edn. Reading, MA: Benjamin/Cummings Publishing Company.

Lukka, A. & Lukka, M. (1988). Expert systems: a role in transportation planning. *International Journal of Physical Distribution and Materials Management* 18: 3–8.

Lumey, L., Terry, M., Delgado-Cruzata, L. et al. (2012). Adult global DNA methylation in relation to pre-natal nutrition. *International Journal of Epidemiology* 41: 116–23.

Lundborg, P., Bolin, K., Hojgard, S. & Lindgren, B. (2006). Obesity and occupational attainment among the 50+ of Europe. In K. Bolin & J. Cawley, eds., *The Economics of Obesity.* Advances in Health Economics and Health Services Research, Vol. 17. Bingley, West Yorkshire: Emerald Group Publishing Limited, pp. 219–51.

Lundborg, P., Nystedt, P. & Rooth, D.A. (2014). Body size, skills, and income: evidence from 150,000 teenage siblings. *Demography* 51: 1573–96.

Lupton, D. (1996). *Food, the Body and the Self.* London: Sage Publications.

Macadam, S. & Dettwyler, K. (eds.) (1995). *Breastfeeding: Biocultural Perspectives.* Chicago, IL: Aldine Transaction.

MacDiarmid, J.I., Vail, A., Cade, J.E. & Blundell, J.E. (1998). The sugar–fat relationship revisited: differences in consumption between men and women of varying BMI. *International Journal of Obesity* 22: 1053–61.

Macht, M. (2008). How emotions affect eating: a five-way model. *Appetite* 50: 1–11.

Mackett, R. & Edwards, M. (1996). An expert system to advise on urban public transport technologies. *Computers, Environment and Urban Systems* 20: 261–73.

Maher, J.M., Fraser, S. & Lindsay, J. (2010). Between provisioning and consuming? Children, mothers and childhood obesity. *Health Sociology Review* 19: 304–16.

Maio, G.R., Haddock, G.G. & Jarman, H.L. (2007). Social psychological factors in tackling obesity. *Obesity Reviews* 8 (Suppl. 1): 123–5.

Malik, M. & Bakir, A. (2007). Prevalence of overweight and obesity among children in the United Arab Emirates. *Obesity Reviews* 8: 15–20.

Malik, V.S., Schulze, M.B. & Hu, F.B. (2006). Intake of sugar-sweetened beverages and weight gain: a systematic review. *American Journal of Clinical Nutrition* 84: 274–88.

Malik, V.S., Willett, W.C. & Hu, F.B. (2013). Global obesity: trends, risk factors and policy implications. *Nature Reviews Endocrinology* 9: 13–27.

Mamadouh, V. (1999). Grid-group cultural theory: an introduction. *GeoJournal* 47: 395–409.

Manktelow, K.I. & Over, D.E. (eds.) (1993). *Rationality: Psychological and Philosophical Perspectives.* Florence, KY: Taylor & Francis/Routledge.

Marmot, M.G. (2004). *Status Syndrome: How Your Social Standing Directly Affects Your Health and Life Expectancy.* London: Bloomsbury.

Marmot, M.G., Allen, J., Goldblatt, P. et al. (2010). *Fair Society, Healthy Lives. Strategic Review of Health Inequalities in England Post-2010. The Marmot Review.* London: Strategic Review of Health Inequalities in England Post-2010.

Marshall, G., Rose, D., Newby, H. & Vogle, C. (1988). *Social Class in Modern Britain.* London: Routledge.

Martens, E.A., Lemmens, S.G. & Westerterp-Plantenga, M.S. (2013). Protein leverage affects energy intake of high-protein diets in humans. *American Journal of Clinical Nutrition* 97: 86–93.

Martínez-Cordero, C., Kuzawa, C.W., Sloboda, D.M. et al. (2012). Testing the protein leverage hypothesis in a free-living human population. *Appetite* 59: 312–5.

Matan, A. & Newman, P. (2016). *People Cities: The Life and Legacy of Jan Gehl.* Washington, DC: Island Press.

Mathers, C.D. & Loncar, D. (2006). Projections of global mortality and burden of disease from 2002 to 2030. *PLoS Medicine* 3: e442.

Maybury-Lewis, D. (1960). The analysis of dual organization: a methodological critique. *Journal of the Humanities and Social Sciences of Southeast Asia* 116: 17–44.

Mayer, J. (1955). Regulation of energy intake and the body weight: the glucostatic theory and the lipostatic hypothesis. *Annals of the New York Academy of Sciences* 63: 15–43.

Mazzocchi, M., Traill, W.B. & Shogren, J.F. (2009). *Fat Economics: Nutrition, Health, and Economic Policy*. Oxford: Oxford University Press.

McCarthy, H.D., Ellis, S.M. & Cole, T.J. (2003). Central overweight and obesity in British youth aged 11–16 years: cross sectional surveys of waist circumference. *British Medical Journal* 326: 624.

McCrady, S.K. & Levine, J.A. (2009). Sedentariness at work: how much do we really sit? *Obesity* 17: 2103–5.

McCullough, M.B. & Hardin, J.A. (eds.) (2013). *Reconstructing Obesity: The Meaning of Measures and the Measure of Meanings*. Oxford: Berghahn Books.

McGartland, M.R. & Hendrickson, C.T. (1985). Expert systems for construction project monitoring. *Journal of Construction Engineering and Management* 111: 293–307.

McGarvey, S.T. (1991). Obesity in Samoans and a perspective on its etiology in Polynesians. *American Journal of Clinical Nutrition* 53: 1586S.

McGarvey, S.T. & Baker, P. (1979). The effects of modernization on Samoan blood pressure. *Human Biology* 51: 461–79.

McGee, D.L. (2005). Body mass index and mortality: a meta-analysis based on person-level data from twenty-six observational studies. *Annals of Epidemiology* 15: 87–97.

McGuire, M.T., Wing, R.R., Klem, M.L., Lang, W. & Hill, J.O. (1999). What predicts weight regain in a group of successful weight losers? *Journal of Consulting and Clinical Psychology* 67: 177–85.

McKinion, J.M. & Lemmon, H.E. (1985). *Symbolic Computers and AI Tools for a Cotton Expert System*. ASAE Tech Paper 85-5520. St Joseph, MI: American Society for Agricultural Engineers.

McLaren, L. (2007). Socioeconomic status and obesity. *Epidemiologic Reviews* 29: 29–48.

McLennan, A. & Ulijaszek, S.J. (2015). An anthropological insight into the Pacific island diabetes crisis and its clinical implications. *Diabetes Management* 5: 143–5.

McLennan, A. Ulijaszek, S.J. & Eli, K. (2014). Social aspects of dietary sugars. In M. Goran, L. Tappy & K.-A. Le, eds., *Dietary Sugars and Health*. Boca Raton, FL: CRC Press, pp. 1–11.

McMillen, M., MacLaughlin, S.M., Muhlhausler, B.S. et al. (2008). Developmental origins of adult health and disease: the role of periconceptional and foetal nutrition. *Basic and Clinical Pharmacology and Toxicology* 102: 82–9.

McPherson, K., Marsh, T. & Brown, M. (2007). *Foresight. Tackling Obesities: Future Choices – Modelling Future Trends in Obesity and the Impact on Health*. London: Government Office for Science.

Mechanick, J.I., Garber, A.J., Handelsman, Y. & Garvey, W.T. (2012). American Association of Clinical Endocrinologists' position statement on obesity and obesity medicine. *Endocrine Practice* 18: 642–8.

Mele, R. & Rawling, P. (2004). Introduction. Aspects of rationality. In A.R. Mele & P. Rawling, eds., *The Oxford Handbook of Rationality*. Oxford: Oxford University Press, pp. 3–13.

Meloni, M. (2013). Biology without biologism: social theory in a postgenomic age. *Sociology* 48: 731–46.

Meloni, M. (2014). How biology became social and what it means for social theory. *Sociological Review* 62: 593–614.

Meyer, W. (1990). *Expert Systems in Factory Management*. Upper Saddle River, NJ: Prentice Hall.

Milanovic, B. (2016). *Global Inequality: A New Approach for the Age of Globalization*. Cambridge, MA: Harvard University Press.

Milio, N. (1981). Promoting health through structural change: analysis of the origins and implementation of Norway's farm-food-nutrition policy. *Social Science and Medicine* 15A: 721–34.

Mintz, S. (1985). *Sweetness and Power: The Place of Sugar in Modern History*. New York, NY: Viking.

Mitchell, S.D. (2009). *Unsimple Truths: Science, Complexity and Policy*. Chicago, IL: University of Chicago Press.

Mizuno, T.M., Makimura, H. & Mobbs, C.V. (2003). The physiological function of the agouti-related peptide gene: the control of weight and metabolic rate. *Annals of Medicine* 35: 425–33.

Mohebati, L., Lobstein, T., Millstone, E. & Jacobs, M. (2007). Policy options for responding to the growing challenge from obesity in the United Kingdom. *European Journal of Public Health* 8: 109–15.

Mokdad, A.H., Ford, E.S., Bowman, B.A. et al. (2003). Prevalence of obesity, diabetes, and obesity-related health risk factors, 2001. *Journal of the American Medical Association* 289: 76–9.

Mol, A. (2009). Good taste: the embodied normativity of the consumer-citizen. *Journal of Cultural Economics* 2: 269–83.

Molarius, A. (2003). The contribution of lifestyle factors to socioeconomic differences in obesity in men and women – a population-based study in Sweden. *European Journal of Epidemiology* 18: 227–34.

Molarius, A., Seidell, J.C., Sans, S., Tuomilehto, J. & Kuulasmaa, K. (2000). Educational level, relative body weight, and changes in their association over 10 years: an international perspective from the WHO MONICA Project. *American Journal of Public Health* 90: 1260–8.

Monaghan, L. (2005). Discussion piece: a critical take on the obesity debate. *Social Theory and Health* 3: 302–14.

Monbiot, G. (2015). Slim chance. http://www.monbiot.com/2015/08/11/slim-chance/ (accessed 25 August 2016).

Moncrieff, J. (2006). Psychiatric drug promotion and the politics of neoliberalism. *British Journal of Psychiatry* 188: 301–2.

Monteiro, C.A., Mondini, L., Medeiros de Souza, A.L. & Popkin, B.M. (1995). The nutrition transition in Brazil. *European Journal of Clinical Nutrition* 49: 105–13.

Monteiro, C.A., Cannon, G., Moubarac, J.C. et al. (2015). Dietary guidelines to nourish humanity and the planet in the twenty-first century. A blueprint from Brazil. *Public Health Nutrition* 18: 2311–22.

Monteiro, P.O.A., Victora, C.G., Barros, F.C. & Monteiro, L.M.A. (2003). Birth size, early childhood growth, and adolescent obesity in a Brazilian birth cohort. *International Journal of Obesity* 27: 1274–82.

Morowitz, H.J. (1991). *The Thermodynamics of Pizza: Essays on Science in Everyday Life*. Newark, NJ: Rutgers University Press.

Morris, S.D. (1999). Reforming the nation: Mexican nationalism in context. *Journal of Latin American Studies* 31: 363–97.

Moschis, G.P. & Churchill, G.A. (1979). An analysis of the adolescent consumer. *Journal of Marketing* 43: 40–8.

Muhlhausler, B.S., Gugusheff, J.R., Ong, Z.Y. & Vithayathil, M. (2013). Nutritional approaches to breaking the intergenerational cycle of obesity. *Canadian Journal of Physiology and Pharmacology* 91: 421–8.

Mulgan, G. (1997). *Connexity: How to Live in a Connected World*. London: Chatto and Windus.

Muller, M.J., Bosy-Westphal, A. & Heymsfield, S.B. (2010). Is there evidence for a set point that regulates human body weight? *F1000 Medicine Reports* 2: 59.

Munster, E., Ruger, H., Ochsmann, E., Letzel, S. & Toschke, A.M. (2009). Over-indebtedness as a marker of socioeconomic status and its association with obesity: a cross-sectional study. *BMC Public Health* 9: 286.

Murgatroyd, C. & Spengler, D. (2011). Epigenetics of early child development. *Frontiers in Psychiatry* 2: 16.

Murtagh, L. & Ludwig, D.S. (2011). State intervention in life-threatening childhood obesity. *Journal of the American Medical Association* 306: 206–7.

Must, A., Spadano, J., Coakley, M.S. et al. (1999). The disease burden associated with overweight and obesity. *Journal of the American Medical Association* 282: 1523–9.

Nagel, T. (1997). *The Last Word*. New York, NY: Oxford University Press.

Nathan, S.A., Develin, E., Grove, N. & Zwi, A.B. (2005). An Australian childhood obesity summit: the role of data and evidence in 'public' policy making. *Australia and New Zealand Health Policy* 2: 17.

National Audit Office (2001). *Tackling Obesity in England.* London: The Stationery Office.

National Obesity Observatory (2012). Fast food outlets by local authority. Relationship between density of fast food outlets and deprivation in England. http://webarchive.nationalarchives .gov.uk/20160805121933/http://www.noo.org.uk/visualisation (accessed 11 May 2017).

Navarrete, A., van Schaik, C.P. & Isler, K. (2011). Energetics and the evolution of human brain size. *Nature* 480: 91–3.

Navarro, V. (2007). *Neoliberalism, Globalization, and Inequalities: Consequences for Health and Quality of Life.* Amityville, NY: Baywood Publishing.

Nedergaard, J., Bengtsson, T. & Cannon, B. (2007). Unexpected evidence for active brown adipose tissue in adult humans. *American Journal of Physiology – Endocrinology and Metabolism* 293: E444–52.

Neel, J. (1962). Diabetes mellitus: a "thrifty" genotype rendered detrimental by "progress"? *American Journal of Human Genetics* 14: 353–62.

Neel, J.V., Weder, A.B. & Julius, S. (1998). Type II diabetes, essential hypertension, and obesity as "syndromes of impaired genetic homeostasis": the "thrifty genotype" hypothesis enters the 21st century. *Perspectives in Biology and Medicine* 42: 44–74.

Nestle, M. (2002). *Food Politics: How the Food Industry Influences Nutrition and Health.* Berkley, CA: University of California Press.

Nestle, M. & Jacobsen, M.F. (2000). Halting the obesity epidemic: a public health policy approach. *Public Health Reports* 115: 12–24.

Ng, M., Fleming, T., Robinson, M. et al. (2014). Global, regional, and national prevalence of overweight and obesity in children and adults during 1980–2013: a systematic analysis for the Global Burden of Disease Study 2013. *Lancet* 384: 766–81.

Nicholls, D.G. & Locke, R.M. (1984). Thermogenic mechanisms in brown fat. *Physiological Reviews* 64: 65–102.

Nichols, M.S., de Silva-Sanigorski, A.M., Cleary, J.E. et al. (2011). Decreasing trends in overweight and obesity among an Australian population of preschool children. *International Journal of Obesity* 35: 916–24.

Nicholson, J.K. & Lindon, J.C. (2008). Systems biology: metabonomics. *Nature* 455: 1054–56.

Norgan, N.G. (1994). Population differences in body composition in relation to the body mass index. *European Journal of Clinical Nutrition* 48 (Suppl. 3): S10–27.

Norton, G.N., Anderson, A.S. & Hetherington, M.M. (2006). Volume and variety: relative effects on food intake. *Physiology and Behavior* 87: 714–22.

Novak, N.L. & Brownell, K.D. (2011). Taxation as prevention and as a treatment for obesity: the case of sugar-sweetened beverages. *Current Pharmaceutical Design* 17: 1218–22.

Novak, N.L. & Brownell, K.D. (2012). Role of policy and government in the obesity epidemic. *Circulation* 126: 2345–52.

Nuffield Council on Bioethics (2007). *Public Health: Ethical Issues.* London: Nuffield Council on Bioethics.

Oakes, J.M. & Rossi, P.H. (2003). The measurement of SES in health research: current practice and steps toward a new approach. *Social Science and Medicine* 56: 769–84.

Ochs, E. & Izquierdo, C. (2009). Responsibility in childhood: three developmental trajectories. *Ethos* 37: 391–413.

Offer, A. (2016). Obesity and welfare regimes. In J. Komlos & I.R. Kelly, eds., *The Oxford Handbook of Economics and Human Biology.* Oxford: Oxford University Press.

Offer, A., Pechey, R. & Ulijaszek, S.J. (2010). Obesity under affluence varies by welfare regimes: the effect of fast food, insecurity, and inequality. *Economics and Human Biology* 8: 297–308.

Offer, A., Pechey, R. & Ulijaszek, S.J. (eds.) (2012). *Insecurity, Inequality and Obesity.* Oxford: Clarendon Press.

Ogden, C.L. & Carroll, M.D. (2010). Prevalence of overweight, obesity, and extreme obesity among adults: United States, trends 1960–1962 through 2007–2008. Centers of Disease Control: NCHS

Health and Stats. https://www.cdc.gov/nchs/data/hestat/obesity_adult_07_08/obesity_adult_07_08.pdf (accessed 11 May 2017).

Ogden, C.L., Carroll, M.D., Curtin, L.R. et al. (2006). Prevalence of overweight and obesity in the United States, 1999–2004. *Journal of the American Medical Association* 295: 1549–55.

Ogden, C.L., Carroll, M.D., Fryar, C.D. & Flegal, K.M. (2015). *Prevalence of Obesity Among Adults and Youth: United States, 2011–2014*. NCHS Data Brief No. 219. Hyattsville, MD: National Center for Health Statistics.

Oken, E. & Gillman, M.W. (2003). Fetal origins of obesity. *Obesity Research* 11: 496–506.

Olds, T., Maher, C., Zumin, S., Peneau, S. et al. (2011). Evidence that the prevalence of overweight is plateauing: data from nine countries. *International Journal of Pediatric Obesity* 6: 342–60.

Oliver, A. (2011). Is nudge an effective public health strategy to tackle obesity? Yes. *British Medical Journal* 342: d2168.

Olshansky, S.J., Passaro, D.J., Hershow, R.C., et al. (2005). A potential decline in life expectancy in the United States in the 21st century. *New England Journal of Medicine* 352: 1138–45.

O'Rourke, K. & Williamson, J.G. (1999). *Globalization and History: The Evolution of a Nineteenth-Century Atlantic Economy*. Cambridge, MA: MIT Press.

Oswald, A.J. & Powdthavee, N. (2007). Obesity, unhappiness, and the challenge of affluence: Theory and evidence. *Economic Journal* 117: F441–54.

Ouellet, V., Labbe, S.M., Blondin, D.P. et al. (2012). Brown adipose tissue oxidative metabolism contributes to energy expenditure during acute cold exposure in humans. *Journal of Clinical Investigation* 122: 545–52.

Ozbilgin, M. & Tatli, A. (2011). Mapping out the field of equality and diversity: rise of individualism and voluntarism. *Human Relations* 64: 1229–53.

Padez, C., Mourao, I., Moreira, P. & Rosado, V. (2005). Prevalence and risk factors for overweight and obesity in Portuguese children. *Acta Paediatrica* 94: 1550–7.

Paeratakul, S., Ferdinand, M.N., Champagne, C.M., Ryan, D.H. & Bray, G.A. (2003). Fast-food consumption among US adults and children: dietary and nutrient intake profile. *Journal of the American Dietetic Association* 103: 1332–8.

Pagan, J.A. & Davila, A. (1997). Obesity, occupational attainment, and earnings. *Social Science Quarterly* 78: 756–70.

Palsson, B.O. (2015). *Systems Biology: Constraint-based Reconstruction and Analysis*. Cambridge: Cambridge University Press.

Pandza, H. & Masic, I. (1999). Expert systems in medicine. *Medical Archives* 53 (Suppl. 3): 25–7.

Panjwani, C. & Caraher, M. (2014). The public health responsibility deal: brokering a deal for public health, but on whose terms? *Health Policy* 114: 163–73.

Papp, K. & Alcorn, J. (2013). Right scale, resilient watersheds: managing complexity through nodal networks. *Minding Nature* 6: 35–47.

Paquette, M.-C. & Raine, K. (2004). Sociocultural context of women's body image. *Social Science and Medicine* 59: 1047–58.

Parkin, D. and Ulijaszek, S.J. (eds.) (2007). *Holistic Anthropology: Convergence and Emergence*. Oxford: Berghahn Books.

Parsons, T.J., Power, C., Logan, S. & Summerbell, C.D. (1999). Childhood predictors of adult obesity: a systematic review. *International Journal of Obesity* 23 (Suppl. 8): S1–107.

Parsons, W. (2002). From muddling through to muddling up – evidence based policy making and the modernization of British government. *Public Policy and Administration* 17: 43–60.

Pasco, J.A., Nicholson, G.C., Brennan, S.L. & Kotowicz, M.A. (2012). Prevalence of obesity and the relationship between the body mass index and body fat: cross-sectional, population-based data. *PLoS One* 7: e29580.

Pechlaner, G. & Otero, G. (2010). The neoliberal food regime: neoregulation and the new division of labor in North America. *Rural Sociology* 75: 179–208.

Pennington, A.W. (1953). A reorientation on obesity. *New England Journal of Medicine* 248: 959–64.

Philipson, T.J. & Posner, R.A. (1999). *The Long-run Growth in Obesity as a Function of Technological Change*. National Bureau of Economic Research Working Paper 7423. Cambridge, MA: National Bureau of Economic Research.

Philipson, T.J. & Posner, R.A. (2008). *Is the Obesity Epidemic a Public Health Problem?* National Bureau of Economic Research Working Paper 14010. Cambridge, MA: National Bureau of Economic Research.

Pickett, K., Kelly, S., Brunner, E., Lobstein, T. & Wilkinson, R.G. (2005). Wider income gaps, wider waistbands? An ecological study of obesity and income inequality. *Journal of Epidemiology and Community Health* 59: 670–4.

Pidd, M. (2004). *Systems Modelling: Theory and Practice*. Chichester, West Sussex: John Wiley & Sons.

Pinkhasov, R.M., Wong, J., Kashanian, J. et al. (2010). Are men shortchanged on health? Perspective on health care utilization and health risk behavior in men and women in the United States. *International Journal of Clinical Practice* 64: 475–87.

Piperno, D.R. & Flannery, K.V. (2001). The earliest archaeological maize (*Zea mays* L.) from highland Mexico: new accelerator mass spectrometry dates and their implications. *Proceedings of the National Academy of Sciences USA* 98: 2101–3.

Platte, P., Herbert, C., Pauli, P. & Breslin, P.A.S. (2013). Oral perceptions of fat and taste stimuli are modulated by affect and mood induction. *PLoS One* 8: e65006

Pollock, N. (1995). Social fattening patterns in the Pacific: the positive side of obesity: a Nauru case study. In I. de Garine & N. Pollock, eds., *Social Aspects of Obesity and Fatness*. New York, NY: Gordon and Breach, pp. 87–110.

Popkin, B.M. (1999). Urbanization, lifestyle changes and the nutrition transition. *World Development* 27: 1905–16.

Popkin, B.M. (2001). The nutrition transition and obesity in the developing world. *Journal of Nutrition* 131: 871S–3S.

Popkin, B.M. (2002). Part II. What is unique about the experience in lower- and middle income less-industrialised countries compared with the very-high income industrialised countries? The shift in stages of the nutrition transition in the developing world differs from past experiences! *Public Health Nutrition* 5: 205–14.

Popkin, B.M. (2004). The nutrition transition: an overview of world patterns of change. *Nutrition Reviews* 62: S140–3.

Popkin, B.M. (2009). *The World is Fat: The Fads, Trends, Policies, and Products that are Fattening the Human Race*. New York, NY: Avery.

Popkin, B.M. & Doak, C.M. (1998). The obesity epidemic is a worldwide phenomenon. *Nutrition Reviews* 56: 106–14.

Popkin, B.M. & Hawkes, C. (2016). Sweetening of the global diet, particularly beverages: patterns, trends, and policy responses. *Lancet Diabetes and Endocrinology* 4: 174–86.

Popkin, B.M., Richards, M.K. & Monteiro, C.A. (1996). Stunting is associated with overweight in children of four nations that are undergoing the nutrition transition. *Journal of Nutrition* 126: 3009–16.

Popovich, P.M., Everton, W.J., Campbell, K.L. et al. (1997). Criteria used to judge obese persons in the workplace. *Perceptual and Motor Skills* 85: 859–66.

Prader, A., Tanner, J.M. & von Harnack, G.A. (1963). Catch-up growth following illness or starvation: an example of developmental canalization in man. *Journal of Pediatrics* 62: 646–59.

Prakash, D.S.R.S. & Sudhakar, G. (2011). Natural selection intensity in Settibalija, a Mendelian human population from South India. *Journal of Anthropology* 7: 111–5.

Prasad, E., Rogoff, K., Wei, S.-J. & Kose, M.A. (2005). Effects of financial globalisation on developing countries: some empirical evidence. In W. Tseng & D. Cowen, eds., *India's and China's Recent Experience with Reform and Growth*. Washington, DC: International Monetary Fund, pp. 201–28.

Prentice, A.M. & Jebb, S.A. (1995). Obesity in Britain: gluttony or sloth? *British Medical Journal* 311: 437–9.

Prentice, A.M. & Jebb, S.A. (2003). Fast foods, energy density and obesity: a possible mechanistic link. *Obesity Reviews* 4: 187–94.

Prentice, A.M., Hennig, B.J. & Fulford, A.J. (2008). Evolutionary origins of the obesity epidemic: natural selection of thrifty genes or genetic drift following predation release? *International Journal of Obesity* 32, 1607–10.

Prior, I. & Tasman-Jones, C. (1981). New Zealand Maori and Pacific Polynesians. In H.C. Trowell & D.P. Burkitt, eds., *Western Diseases: Their Emergence and Prevention*. London: Edward Arnold, pp. 227–67.

Prospective Studies Collaboration (2009). Body mass index and cause-specific mortality in 900 000 adults: collaborative analyses of 57 prospective studies. *Lancet* 373: 1083–96.

Public Health England (2015a). *Changes in Children's Body Mass Index between 2006/07 and 2013/14: National Child Measurement Programme*. London: Public Health England.

Public Health England (2015b). *Sugar Reduction: The Evidence for Action*. London: Public Health England.

Public Health England (2016). PHE Obesity. http://webarchive.nationalarchives.gov.uk/20170210161227/http://www.noo.org.uk/index.php (accessed 11 May 2017).

Puhl, R. & Brownell, K.D. (2001). Bias, discrimination, and obesity. *Obesity Research* 9: 788–805.

Puhl, R.M. & Brownell, K.D. (2003). Psychosocial origins of obesity stigma: toward changing a powerful and pervasive bias. *Obesity Reviews* 4: 213–27.

Puhl, R.M. & Heuer, C.A. (2009). The stigma of obesity: a review and update. *Obesity* 17: 941–64.

Puhl, R.M. & Latner, J.D. (2007). Stigma, obesity, and the health of the nation's children. *Psychological Bulletin* 133: 557–80.

Quinn, D., Schindler, M. & Toyoda, A.M. (2011). Assessing measures of financial openness and integration. *IMF Economic Review* 59: 488–522.

Raberg, M., Kumar, B., Holmboe-Ottesen, G. & Wandel, M. (2010). Overweight and weight dissatisfaction related to socio-economic position, integration and dietary indicators among South Asian immigrants in Oslo. *Public Health Nutrition* 13: 695–703.

Rabin, B.A., Boehmer, T.K. & Brownson, R.C. (2007). Cross-national comparison of environmental and policy correlates of obesity in Europe. *European Journal of Public Health* 17: 53–61.

Rada, P., Avena, N.M. & Hoebel, B.G. (2005). Daily bingeing on sugar repeatedly releases dopamine in the accumbens shell. *Neuroscience* 134: 737–44.

Rail, G., Holmes, D. & Murray, S. (2010). The politics of evidence on 'domestic terrorists': obesity discourses and their effects. *Social Theory and Health* 8: 259–79.

Rao, M.P. & Miller, D.M. (2004). Expert systems applications for productivity analysis. *Industrial Management and Data Systems* 104: 776–85.

Rashad, I. & Grossman, M. (2004). The economics of obesity. *Public Interest* 156: 104–12.

Rasmussen, N. (2008). America's first amphetamine epidemic 1929–1971. *American Journal of Public Health* 98: 974–85.

Rasmussen, N. (2015). Stigma and the addiction paradigm for obesity: lessons from 1950s America. *Addiction* 110: 217–25.

Ravelli, G.P. & Belmont, L. (1979). Obesity in nineteen-year-old men: family size and birth order associations. *American Journal of Epidemiology* 109: 66–70.

Ravelli, G.P., Stein, Z.A. & Susser, M.W. (1976). Obesity in young men after famine exposure in utero and early infancy. *New England Journal of Medicine* 295: 349–53.

Raymond, C.A. (1986). Biology, culture, dietary changes conspire to increase incidence of obesity. *Journal of the American Medical Association* 256: 2157–8.

Rayner, G. & Lang, T. (2011). Is nudge an effective public health strategy to tackle obesity? No. *British Medical Journal* 342: d2177.

Rayner, S. (2014). Wicked problems. *Environmental Scientist* 23: 4–6.

Razer, M., Friedmann, V.J. & Warshofsky, B. (2013). Schools as agents of social exclusion and inclusion. *International Journal of Inclusive Education* 17: 1152–70.

Reardon, T. & Berdegué, J. (2002). The rapid rise of supermarkets in Latin America: challenges and opportunities for development. *Development Policy Review* 20: 371–88.

Reidpath, D., Burns, C., Garrard, J., Mahoney, M. & Townsend, M. (2002). An ecological study of the relationship between social and environmental determinants of obesity. *Health and Place* 8: 141–5.

Reilly, J.J. & Kelly, J. (2011). Long-term impact of overweight and obesity in childhood and adolescence on morbidity and premature mortality in adulthood: systematic review. *International Journal of Obesity* 35: 891–8.

Reilly, J.J., Armstrong, J., Dorosty, A.R. et al. (2005). Early life risk factors for obesity in childhood: cohort study. *British Medical Journal* 330: 1357.

Reis, J.P., Macera, C.A., Araneta, M.R. et al. (2009). Comparison of overall obesity and body fat distribution in predicting risk of mortality. *Obesity* 17: 1232–9.

Reynolds, R.M., Jacobsen, G.H. & Drake, A.J. (2013). What is the evidence in humans that DNA methylation changes link events in utero and later life disease? *Clinical Endocrinology* 78: 814–22.

Rich, E. (2011). 'I see her being obesed!': public pedagogy, reality media and the obesity crisis. *Health* 15: 3–21.

Rich, E., Monaghan, L. & Aphramor, L. (eds.) (2011). *Debating Obesity: Critical Perspectives.* Basingstoke, Hampshire: Palgrave Macmillan.

Ritchey, T. (2012). Outline for a morphology of modelling methods contribution to a general theory of modelling. *Acta Morphologica Generalis* 1: 1–20.

Rittel, H.W.J. & Webber, M.M. (1973). Dilemmas in a general theory of planning. *Policy Sciences* 4: 155–69.

Rivera, J.A., Barquera, S., Campirano, F. et al. (2002). Epidemiological and nutritional transition in Mexico: rapid increase of non-communicable chronic diseases and obesity. *Public Health Nutrition* 5: 1–11.

Rivera, J.A., Barquera, S., González-Cossío, T., Olaiz, G. & Sepúlveda, J. (2004). Nutrition transition in Mexico and in other Latin American countries. *Nutrition Reviews* 62: S149–57.

Roberto, C.A., Swinburn, B., Hawkes, C. et al. (2015). Patchy progress on obesity prevention: emerging examples, entrenched barriers, and new thinking. *Lancet* 385: 13–9.

Rodionov, S.N. & Martin, J.H. (1999). An expert system-based approach to prediction of year-to-year climatic variations in the North Atlantic region. *International Journal of Climatology* 19: 951–74.

Roehling, M.V., Roehling, P.V. & Pichler, S. (2007). The relationship between body weight and perceived weight-related employment discrimination: the role of sex and race. *Journal of Vocational Behavior* 71: 300–18.

Rokholm, B., Baker, J.L. & Sorensen, T.I.A. (2010). The levelling off of the obesity epidemic since the year 1999 – a review of evidence and perspectives. *Obesity Reviews* 11: 835–46.

Rokholm, B., Andersen, C.S. & Sorensen, T. (2011). Developmental origins of obesity – genetic and epigenetic determinants. *Open Obesity Journal* 3: 27–33.

Rolland-Cachera, M.F., Deheeger, M., Bellisle, F. et al. (1984). Adiposity rebound in children: a simple indicator for predicting obesity. *American Journal of Clinical Nutrition* 39: 129–35.

Rolland-Cachera, M.F., Deheeger, M., Maillot, M. & Bellisle, F. (2006). Early adiposity rebound: causes and consequences for obesity in children and adults. *International Journal of Obesity* 30: S11–17.

Room, G. (2015). Complexity, power and policy. In R. Geyer & P. Cairney, eds., *Handbook on Complexity and Public Policy.* Abingdon, Oxfordshire: Edward Elgar Publishing, pp. 19–31.

Rönn, T., Volkov, P., Davegårdh, C. et al. (2013). A six months exercise intervention influences the genome-wide DNA methylation pattern in human adipose tissue. *PLoS Genetics* 9: e1003572.

Rooney, B.L., Mathiason, M.A. & Schauberger, C.W. (2011). Predictors of obesity in childhood, adolescence, and adulthood in a birth cohort. *Maternal and Child Health Journal* 15: 1166–75.

Rose, N. (1999). *The Power of Freedom: Reframing Political Thought.* Cambridge: Cambridge University Press.

Rose, N. (2013). The human sciences in a biological age. *Theory, Culture and Society* 30: 3–34.

Rosenbaum, M. & Leibel, R.L. (1998). The physiology of body weight regulation: relevance to the etiology of obesity in children. *Pediatrics* 101: 525–39.

Roskam, A.-J.R., Kunst, A.E., van Oyen, H. et al. (2010). Comparative appraisal of educational inequalities in overweight and obesity among adults in 19 European countries. *International Journal of Epidemiology* 39: 392–404.

Rosser, J., Rosser, M V. & Ahmed, E. (2000). Income inequality and the informal economy in transition economies. *Journal of Comparative Economics* 28: 156–71.

Rothwell, N.J. & Stock, M.J. (1981). Regulation of energy balance. *Annual Review of Nutrition* 1: 235–56.

Royal College of Physicians (1983). Obesity: Report of the Royal College of Physicians. *Journal of the Royal College of Physicians* 17: 1–58.

Ruhm, C.J. (2010). *Understanding Overeating and Obesity.* National Bureau of Economic Research Working Paper 16149. Cambridge, MA: National Bureau of Economic Research.

Rull, J.A., Aguilar-Salinas, C.A., Rojas, R. et al. (2005). Epidemiology of type 2 diabetes in Mexico. *Archives of Medical Research* 36: 188–96.

Rundle, A., Diez-Roux, A.V., Freeman, L.M. et al. (2007). The urban built environment and obesity in New York City: a multilevel analysis. *American Journal of Health Promotion* 21 (Suppl.): 326–34.

Sabanayagam, C., Shankar, A., Wong, T.Y., Saw, S.M. & Foster, P.J. (2007). Socioeconomic status and overweight/obesity in an adult Chinese population in Singapore. *Journal of Epidemiology,* 17, 161–8.

Sacks, G., Swinburn, B.A. & Lawrence, M.A. (2008). A systematic policy approach to changing the food system and physical activity environments to prevent obesity. *Australia and New Zealand Health Policy* 5: 13.

Saguy, A.C. (2006). French women don't get fat? French news reporting on obesity. *Health at Every Size* 19: 219–34.

Saguy, A.C. & Almeling, R. (2014). Making the 'obesity epidemic': the role of science and the news media. In K. Eli & S. Ulijaszek, eds., *Obesity, Eating Disorders and the Media.* Farnham, Surrey: Ashgate Publishing, pp. 107–23.

Saito, M., Okamatsu-Ogura, Y., Watanabe, K. et al. (2009). High incidence of metabolically active brown adipose tissue in healthy adult humans. *Diabetes* 58: 1526–31.

Saltonstall, R. (1993). Healthy bodies, social bodies. Men's and women's concepts and practices of health in everyday life. *Social Science and Medicine* 36: 7–14.

Samuels, R. & Stich, S. (2004). Rationality and psychology. In A.R. Mele & P. Rawling, eds., *The Oxford Handbook of Rationality.* Oxford: Oxford University Press, pp. 279–300.

Sanabria, E. & Yates-Doerr, E. (2015). Alimentary uncertainties: from contested evidence to policy. *BioSocieties* 10: 117–24.

Sargent, J.D. & Blanchflower, D.G. (1994). Obesity and stature in adolescence and earnings in young adulthood: analysis of a British birth cohort. *Archives of Pediatrics and Adolescent Medicine* 148: 681–7.

Sassatelli, R. & Scott, A. (2001). Novel food, new markets and trust regimes: responses to the erosion of consumers' confidence in Austria, Italy and the UK. *European Societies* 3: 213–44.

Savage, M. (2000). *Class Analysis and Social Transformation.* Buckingham, Buckinghamshire: Open University Press.

Schmidhuber, J. & Shetty, P. (2005). The nutrition transition to 2030. Why developing countries are likely to bear the major burden. *Acta Agriculturae Scandinavica, Section C – Food Economics* 2: 150–66.

Schmidt, I.M., Jorgensen, M.H. & Michaelsen, K.F. (1995). Heights of conscripts in Europe: is postneonatal mortality a predictor? *Annals of Human Biology* 22: 57–67.

Schmidt Morgen, C., Rokholm, B., Brixval, C.S. et al. (2013). Trends in prevalence of overweight and obesity in Danish, children and adolescents – are we still on a plateau? *PLoS One* 8: e69860.

Schneider, H.J., Friedrich, N., Klotsche, J. et al. (2010). The predictive value of different measures of obesity for incident cardiovascular events and mortality. *Journal of Clinical Endocrinology and Metabolism* 95: 1777–85.

Schoeller D (1990). How accurate is self-reported dietary energy intake? *Nutrition Reviews* 48: 373–9.

Schrecker, T. & Bambra, C. (2015). *How Politics Makes Us Sick*. Basingstoke, Hampshire: Palgrave Macmillan.

Schrecker, T., Labonte, R. & de Vogli, R. (2008). Globalization and health: the need for a global vision. *Lancet* 372: 1670–6.

Schultz, K.F., Altman, D.G., Moher, D. and the CONSORT Group (2010). CONSORT 2010 Statement: updated guidelines for reporting parallel group randomised trials. *BMC Medicine* 8: 18.

Schutz, Y. (1995). Macronutrients and energy balance in obesity. *Metabolism* 44: 7–11.

Schwarz, M. & Thompson, M. (1990). *Divided We Stand: Re-Defining Politics, Technology and Social Choice*. Philadelphia, PA: University of Pennsylvania Press.

Schwartz, M.B. & Puhl, R. (2003). Childhood obesity: a societal problem to solve. *Obesity Reviews* 4: 57–71.

Sclafani, A. (1984). Animal models of obesity: classification and characterization. *International Journal of Obesity* 8: 491–508.

Seale, P., Kajimura, S., Yang, W. et al. (2007). Transcriptional control of brown fat determination by PRDM16. *Cell Metabolism* 6: 38–54.

Sellayah, D., Cagampang, F.R. & Cox, R.D. (2014). On the evolutionary origins of obesity: a new hypothesis. *Endocrinology* 155: 1573–88.

Serdula, M.K., Mokdad, A.H., Williamson, D.F. et al. (1999). Prevalence of attempting weight loss and strategies for controlling weight. *Journal of the American Medical Association* 282: 1353–8.

Serretti, A. & Mandelli, L. (2010). Antidepressants and body weight: a comprehensive review and meta-analysis. *Journal of Clinical Psychiatry* 71: 1259–72.

Shafir, E. & LeBoeuf, R.A. (2002). Rationality. *Annual Review of Psychology* 53: 491–517.

Shah, N.P. (2007). Functional cultures and health benefits. *International Dairy Journal* 17: 1262–77.

Share, M. & Strain, M. (2008). Making schools and young people responsible: a critical analysis of Ireland's obesity strategy. *Health and Social Care in the Community* 16: 234–43.

Sharma, L.L., Teret, S.P. & Brownell, K.D. (2010). The food industry and self-regulation: standards to promote success and to avoid public health failures. *American Journal of Public Health* 100: 240–6.

Shen, T., Habicht, J.P. & Chang, Y. (1996). Effect of economic reforms on child growth in urban and rural areas of China. *New England Journal of Medicine* 335: 400–6.

Shetty, P.S. & James, W.P.T. (1994). *Body Mass Index. A Measure of Chronic Energy Deficiency in Adults*. FAO Food and Nutrition Paper 56. Rome: Food and Agriculture Organization.

Shill, J., Mavoa, H., Allender, S. et al. (2012). Government regulation to promote healthy food environments – a view from inside state governments. *Obesity Reviews* 13: 162–173.

Shove, E. (2010). Beyond the ABC: climate change policy and theories of social change. *Environment and Planning A* 42: 1273–85.

Shrewsbury, V. & Wardle, J. (2008). Socioeconomic status and adiposity in childhood: a systematic review of cross-sectional studies 1990–2005. *Obesity* 16: 275–84.

Shugart, H.A. (2014). Heavy viewing: emergent frames in contemporary news coverage of obesity. In K. Eli & S. Ulijaszek, eds., *Obesity, Eating Disorders and the Media*. Farnham, Surrey: Ashgate Publishing, pp. 141–68.

Shugart, H. (2016). *Heavy: The Obesity Crisis in Cultural Context.* New York, NY: Oxford University Press.

Simon, H.A. (1955). A behavioral model of rational choice. *Quarterly Journal of Economics* 69: 99–118.

Simon, H.A. (1956). Rational choice and the structure of the environment. *Psychological Review* 60: 129–38.

Simon, H.A. (1962). The architecture of complexity. *Proceedings of the American Philosophical Society* 106: 467–82.

Simpson, S.J. & Raubenheimer, D. (2005). Obesity: the protein leverage hypothesis. *Obesity Reviews* 6: 133–42.

Simpson, S.J., Raubenheimer, D., Charleston, M.A. & Clissold, F.J. (2010). Modelling nutritional interactions: from individuals to communities. *Trends in Ecology and Evolution* 25: 53–60.

Singh, G.K., Siahpush, M. & Kogan, M.D. (2010). Rising social inequalities in US childhood obesity, 2003-2007. *Annals of Epidemiology* 20: 40–52.

Sinha, R. & Jastreboff, A.M. (2013). Stress as a common risk factor for obesity and addiction. *Biological Psychiatry* 73: 827–35.

Skogen, J.C. & Overland, S. (2012). The fetal origins of adult disease: a narrative review of the epidemiological literature. *Journal of the Royal Society of Medicine* 3: 59.

Sleddens, E.F.C., Gerards, S.M.P.L., Thijs, C. et al. (2011). General parenting, childhood overweight and obesity-inducing behaviors: a review. *International Journal of Pediatric Obesity* 6: e12–27.

Sloboda, D.M., Beedle, A.S., Cupido, C.L., Gluckman, P.D. & Vickers, M.H. (2009). Impaired perinatal growth and longevity: a life history perspective. *Current Gerontology and Geriatrics Research* 2009: 608740.

Smil, V. (2008). *Energy in Nature and Society: General Energetics of Complex Systems.* Cambridge, MA: MIT Press.

Smith, B.D. (1997). The initial domestication of *Cucurbita pepo* in the Americas 10,000 years ago. *Science* 276: 932–4.

Smith, C. (1998). *The Science of Energy – a Cultural History of Energy Physics in Victorian Britain.* Chicago, IL: University of Chicago Press.

Smith, M.E. (1984). The Aztlan migrations of the Nahuatl chronicles: myth or history? *Ethnohistory* 31: 153–86.

Snodgrass, J.J., Leonard, W.R., Sorensen, M.V. et al. (2006). The emergence of obesity among indigenous Siberians. *Journal of Physiological Anthropology* 25: 75–84.

Sobal, J. (1991). Obesity and socioeconomic status: a framework for examining relationships between physical and social variables. *Medical Anthropology* 13: 231–47.

Sobal, J. & Stunkard, A.J. (1989). Socioeconomic status and obesity: a review of the literature. *Psychological Bulletin* 105: 260–75.

Sorensen, T.I.A., Rokholm, B. & Ajslev, T.A. (2012). The history of the obesity epidemic in Denmark. In. A. Offer, R. Pechey & S.J. Ulijaszek, eds., *Insecurity, Inequality and Obesity.* Oxford: Oxford University Press, pp. 161–78.

Spahlholz, J., Baer, N., König, H.-H., Riedel-Heller, S.G. & Luck-Sikorski, C. (2016). Obesity and discrimination – a systematic review and meta-analysis of observational studies. *Obesity Reviews* 17: 43–55.

Speakman, J.R. (2006). The genetics of obesity: five fundamental problems with the famine hypothesis. In G. Fantuzzi & T. Mazzone, eds., *Adipose Tissue and Adipokines in Health and Disease.* New York, NY: Humana Press, pp. 221–36.

Speakman, J.R. (2007). A nonadaptive scenario explaining the genetic predisposition to obesity: the "predation release" hypothesis. *Cell Metabolism* 6: 5–12.

Speakman, J.R. (2008). Thrifty genes for obesity, an attractive but flawed idea, and an alternative perspective: the 'drifty gene' hypothesis. *International Journal of Obesity* 32: 1611–7.

Speakman, J.R. (2013). Evolutionary perspectives on the obesity epidemic: adaptive, maladaptive, and neutral viewpoints. *Annual Review of Nutrition* 33: 289–317.

Speakman, J., Hambly, C., Mitchell, S. & Król, E. (2007). Animal models of obesity. *Obesity Reviews* 8 (Suppl. 1): 55–61.

Stamatakis, E., Wardle, J. & Cole, T.J. (2010). Childhood obesity and overweight prevalence in England: evidence for growing socio-economic disparities. *International Journal of Obesity* 34: 41–7.

Steckel, R.H. (1995). Stature and the standard of living. *Journal of Economic Literature* 33: 1903–40.

Steckel, R.H. (1998). Stature and the standard of living. In J. Komlos & T. Cuff, eds., *Classics in Anthropometric History*. St Katharinen, Neuwied: Scripta Mercaturae Verlag, pp. 63–114.

Stephenson, G. & Hepburn, J.A. (1955). *Plan for the Metropolitan Region, Perth and Fremantle, Western Australia: A Report Prepared for the Government of Western Australia*. Perth, WA: Government Printing Office.

Stern, D., Piernas, C., Barquera, S., Rivera, J.A. & Popkin, B.M. (2014). Caloric beverages were major sources of energy among children and adults in Mexico, 1999–2012. *Journal of Nutrition* 144: 949–56.

Stevens, A. (2011). Telling policy stories: an ethnographic study of the use of evidence in policy-making in the UK. *Journal of Social Policy* 40: 237–55.

Stevens, G.A., Singh, G.M., Lu, Y. et al. (2012). National, regional, and global trends in adult overweight and obesity prevalences. *Population Health Metrics* 10: 22.

Story, M., Kaphingst, K.M., Robinson-O'Brien, R. & Glanz, K. (2008). Creating healthy food and eating environments: policy and environmental approaches. *Annual Review of Public Health* 29: 253–72.

Strickland, S.S. & Ulijaszek, S.J. (1994). Body mass index and illness in Sarawak. *European Journal of Clinical Nutrition* 48 (Suppl. 3): S98–108.

Striegel-Moore, R.H. & Franko, D.L. (2004). Body image issues among girls and women. In T.F. Cash & T. Pruzinsky, eds., *Body Image: A Handbook of Theory, Research, and Clinical Practice*. New York, NY: Guilford Press, pp. 183–91.

Strine, T.W., Mokdad, A.H., Balluz, L.S. et al. (2008). Depression and anxiety in the United States: findings from the 2006 Behavioral Risk Factor Surveillance System. *Psychiatric Services* 59: 1383–90.

Stubbs, R.J. & Whybrow, S. (2004). Energy density, diet composition and palatability: influences on overall food energy intake in humans. *Physiology and Behavior* 81: 755–64.

Stubbs, R.J., Ferres, S. & Horgan, G. (2000). Energy density of foods: effects on energy intake. *Critical Reviews in Food Science and Nutrition* 40: 481–515.

Stunkard, A.J. (1959). Eating patterns and obesity. *Psychological Bulletin* 33: 284–94.

Sugarman, J. (2015). Neoliberalism and psychological ethics. *Journal of Theoretical and Philosophical Psychology* 35: 103–16.

Sui, D.Z. (2003). Musings on the fat city: are obesity and urban forms linked? *Urban Geography* 24: 75–84.

Sunder, M. & Woitek, U. (2005). Boom, bust, and the human body: further evidence on the relationship between height and business cycles. *Economics and Human Biology* 3: 450–66.

Swan, G. & Carmelli, D. (1995). Characteristics associated with excessive weight gain after smoking cessation in men. *American Journal of Public Health* 85: 73–7.

Swank, D. (2004). *The Spread of Neoliberalism: U.S. Economic Power and the Diffusion of Market-oriented Tax Policy*. Harvard University Center for European Studies Working Paper No. 120. Cambridge, MA: Harvard University Center for European Studies.

Swinburn, B., Sacks, G. & Ravussin, E. (2009). Increased food energy supply is more than sufficient to explain the US epidemic of obesity. *American Journal of Clinical Nutrition* 90: 1453–6.

Swinburn, B., Kraak, V., Rutter, H. et al. (2015). Strengthening of accountability systems to create healthy food environments and reduce global obesity. *Lancet* 385: 2534–45.

Swinburn, B.A., Egger, G. & Raza, F. (1999a). Dissecting obesogenic environments: the development and application of a framework for identifying and prioritizing environmental interventions for obesity. *Preventive Medicine* 29: 563–70.

Swinburn, B.A., Ley, S.J., Carmichael, M.H.E. & Plank, L.D. (1999b). Body size and composition of Polynesians. *International Journal of Obesity and Related Metabolic Disorders* 23: 1178–83.

Swinburn, B.A., Gill, T. & Kumanyika, S. (2005). Obesity prevention: a proposed framework for translating evidence into action. *Obesity Reviews* 6: 23–33.

Swinburn, B.A., Sacks, G., Hall, K.D. et al. (2011). The global obesity pandemic: shaped by global drivers and local environments. *Lancet* 378, 804–14.

Szyf, M. (2015). Nongenetic inheritance and transgenerational epigenetics. *Trends in Molecular Medicine* 21: 134–44.

Tandler, P.J., Butcher, J.A., Tao, H. & Harrington, P.d.B. (1995). Analysis of plastic recycling products by expert systems. *Analytica Chimica Acta* 312: 231–44.

Tanner, J.M. (1981). *A History of the Study of Human Growth*. Cambridge: Cambridge University Press.

Tanner, J.M. (1987). Growth as a mirror of the condition of society: secular trends and class distinctions. *Acta Paediatrica Japonica* 29: 96–103.

Tartaglia, L.A., Dembski, M., Weng, X. et al. (1995). Identification and expression cloning of a leptin receptor, OB-R. *Cell* 83: 1263–71.

Tausch, A. (2012). A globalization-oriented perspective on health, inequality and socio-economic development. *International Journal of Health Planning and Management* 27: 2–33.

Taylor, J. (2003). *Foresight Cognitive Systems Project*. London: Office of Science and Technology, Her Majesty's Government.

Taylor, P.J. (2012). Extraordinary cities: early 'city-ness' and the origins of agriculture and states. *International Journal of Urban and Regional Research* 36: 415–47.

Teegarden, S.L. & Bale, T.L. (2007). Decreases in dietary preference produce increased emotionality and risk for dietary relapse. *Biological Psychiatry* 61: 1021–9.

Telch, C.F. & Agras, W.S. (1994). Obesity, binge eating and psychopathology: are they related? *International Journal of Eating Disorders* 15: 53–61.

Tencati, A. & Zsolnai, L. (2009). The collaborative enterprise. *Journal of Business Ethics* 85: 367–76.

Thaler, R.H. (2015). *Misbehaving. The Making of Behavioral Economics*. New York, NY: W.W. Norton and Company.

Thaler, R.H. & Sunstein, C.R. (2008). *Nudge. Improving Decisions about Health, Wealth, and Happiness*. New Haven, CT: Yale University Press.

Thomas, D.M., Bouchard, C., Church, T. et al. (2012). Why do individuals not lose more weight from an exercise intervention at a defined dose? An energy balance analysis. *Obesity Reviews* 13: 835–47.

Thomas, R.B. (1997). Wandering toward the edge of adaptability: adjustments of Andean people to change. In S.J. Ulijaszek & R.A. Huss-Ashmore, eds., *Human Adaptability: Past, Present and Future*. Oxford: Oxford University Press, pp. 183–232.

Thompson, A.L. (2012). Developmental origins of obesity: early feeding environments, infant growth, and the intestinal microbiome. *American Journal of Human Biology* 24: 350–60.

Thompson, M., Ellis, R.J. & Wildavsky, A.B. (1990). *Cultural Theory*. Boulder, CO: Westview Press.

Thow, A. & Hawkes, C. (2009). The implications of trade liberalization for diet and health: a case study from Central America. *Globalization and Health* 5: 5.

Thow, A.-M., Jan, S., Leeder, S. & Swinburn, B. (2010). The effect of fiscal policy on diet, obesity and chronic disease: a systematic review. *Bulletin of the World Health Organization* 88: 609–14.

Throsby, K. (2007). "How could you let yourself get like that?": stories of the origins of obesity in accounts of weight loss surgery. *Social Science and Medicine* 65: 1561–71.

Throsby, K. (2012). 'I'd kill anyone who tried to take my band away': obesity surgery, critical fat politics and the 'problem' of patient demand. *Somatechnics* 2: 107–26.

Tolman, C.W. (1964). Social facilitation of feeding behaviour in the domestic chick. *Animal Behavior* 12: 245–51.

Toussaint, O. & Schneider, E.D. (1998). The thermodynamics and evolution of complexity in biological systems. *Comparative Biochemistry and Physiology Part A: Molecular & Integrative Physiology* 120: 3–9.

Trentmann, F. (2007). Citizenship and consumption. *Journal of Consumer Culture* 7: 147–58.

Triandis, H.C. (1995). *Individualism and Collectivism (New Directions in Social Psychology)*. Boulder, CO: Westview Press.

Triandis, H.C. (2001). Individualism-collectivism and personality. *Journal of Personality* 69: 907–924.

Trowbridge, F.L., Marks, J.S., Deromana, G.L. et al. (1987). Body composition of Peruvian children with short stature and high weight-for-height. 2. Implications for the interpretation of weight-for-height as an indicator of nutritional status. *American Journal of Clinical Nutrition* 46: 411–8.

Trowell, H. (1975). Obesity in the Western world. *Plant Foods for Man* 1: 157–65.

Tsai, F. & Coyle, W.J. (2009). The microbiome and obesity: is obesity linked to our gut flora? *Current Gastroenterology Reports* 11: 307–13.

Tseng, Y.-H., Cypess, A.M. & Kahn, C.R. (2010). Cellular bioenergetics as a target for obesity therapy. *Nature Reviews Drug Discovery* 9: 465–82.

Turnbaugh, P.J., Hamady, M., Yatsunenko, T. et al. (2009). A core gut microbiome in obese and lean twins. *Nature* 457: 480–84.

Turok, I. (2009). The distinctive city: pitfalls in the pursuit of differential advantage. *Environment and Planning A* 41: 13–30.

Twenge, J.M. (2000). The age of anxiety? Birth cohort change in anxiety and neuroticism, 1952–1993. *Journal of Personality and Social Psychology* 79: 1007–21.

Ulijaszek, S.J. (1990). Nutritional status and susceptibility to infectious disease. In G.A. Harrison & J.C. Waterlow, eds., *Diet and Disease*. Cambridge: Cambridge University Press, pp. 137–54.

Ulijaszek, S.J. (1991). Human dietary change. *Philosophical Transactions of the Royal Society of London, Series B* 334: 271–9.

Ulijaszek, S.J. (1992). Energetics methods in biological anthropology. *Yearbook of Physical Anthropology* 35: 215–42.

Ulijaszek, S.J. (1993). Evidence for a secular trend in heights and weights of adults in Papua New Guinea. *Annals of Human Biology* 20: 349–55.

Ulijaszek, S.J. (1995). *Human Energetics in Biological Anthropology*. Cambridge: Cambridge University Press.

Ulijaszek, S.J. (1996a). Energetics, adaptation, and adaptability. *American Journal of Human Biology* 8: 169–82.

Ulijaszek, S.J. (1996b). Relationships between undernutrition, infection, and growth and development. *Human Evolution* 11: 233–48.

Ulijaszek, S.J. (1999). Physical activity, lifestyle and health of urban populations. In L.M. Schell & S.J. Ulijaszek, eds., *Urbanism, Health and Human Biology in Industrialised Countries*. Cambridge: Cambridge University Press, pp. 250–79.

Ulijaszek, S.J. (2000). Nutrition, infection, and child growth in Papua New Guinea. *Collegium Antropologicum* 24: 423–9.

Ulijaszek, S.J. (2001a). Increasing body size and obesity among Cook Islanders between 1966 and 1996. *Annals of Human Biology* 28: 363–73.

Ulijaszek, S.J. (2001b). Body mass index and physical activity levels of adults on Rarotonga, the Cook Islands. *International Journal of Food Science and Nutrition* 52: 453–61.

Ulijaszek, S.J. (2001c). Socioeconomic status, body size and physical activity of adults on Rarotonga, the Cook Islands. *Annals of Human Biology* 28: 554–63.

Ulijaszek, S.J. (2001d). Ethnic differences in patterns of human growth in stature. In R. Martorell & F. Haschke, eds., *Nutrition and Growth*. Philadelphia, PA: Lippincott Williams & Wilkins, pp. 1–20.

Ulijaszek, S.J. (2001e). Secular trends in growth and the narrowing of ethnic differences in stature. *Nutrition Bulletin*, 26, 43–51.

Ulijaszek, S.J. (2002a). Human eating behaviour in an evolutionary ecological context. *Proceedings of the Nutrition Society* 61: 517–26.

Ulijaszek, S.J. (2002b). Modernization and the diet of adults on Rarotonga, the Cook Islands. *Ecology of Food and Nutrition* 41: 203–28.

Ulijaszek, S.J. (2003). Trends in body size, diet and food availability in the Cook Islands in the second half of the twentieth century. *Economics and Human Biology* 1: 123–37.

Ulijaszek, S.J. (2006). The International Growth Reference for Children and Adolescents project: environmental influences on preadolescent and adolescent growth in weight and height. *Food and Nutrition Bulletin* 27 (Suppl.): S279–94.

Ulijaszek, S.J. (2007a). Frameworks of population obesity and the use of cultural consensus modeling in the study of environments contributing to obesity. *Economics and Human Biology* 5: 443–57.

Ulijaszek, S.J. (2007b). Obesity: a disorder of convenience. *Obesity Reviews* 8 (Suppl. 1): 183–7.

Ulijaszek, S.J. (2008). Seven models of population obesity. *Angiology* 59 (Suppl.): 34S–8S.

Ulijaszek, S.J. (2010). Variation in human growth patterns due to environmental factors. In M.P. Muehlenbein, ed., *Human Evolutionary Biology*. Cambridge: Cambridge University Press, pp. 396–404.

Ulijaszek, S.J. (2012). Socio-economic status, forms of capital and obesity. *Journal of Gastrointestinal Cancer* 43: 3–7.

Ulijaszek, S.J. (2014). Obesity, government and the media. In K. Eli & S. Ulijaszek, eds., *Obesity, Eating Disorders and the Media*. Farnham, Surrey: Ashgate Publishing, pp. 125–40.

Ulijaszek, S.J. (2015). With the benefit of Foresight: obesity, complexity and joined-up government. *BioSocieties* 10: 213–28.

Ulijaszek, S.J. & Bryant, E.J. (2016). Binge eating, disinhibition and obesity. In A. Alvergne, C. Jenkinson & C. Faurie, eds., *Evolutionary Thinking in Medicine: From Research to Policy and Practice*. New York, NY: Springer, pp. 105–17.

Ulijaszek, S.J. & Koziel, S. (2007). Nutrition transition and dietary energy availability in Eastern Europe after the collapse of communism. *Economics and Human Biology* 5: 359–69.

Ulijaszek, S.J. & Lofink, H. (2006). Obesity in biocultural perspective. *Annual Review of Anthropology* 35: 337–60.

Ulijaszek, S.J. & McLennan, A.K. (2016). Framing obesity in UK policy from the Blair years, 1997–2015: persistent individualistic approaches despite overwhelming evidence of societal and economic factors, and the need for collective responsibility. *Obesity Reviews* 17: 397–411.

Ulijaszek, S.J. & Strickland, S.S. (1993). *Nutritional Anthropology: Prospects and Perspectives in Human Nutrition*. London: Smith-Gordon and Company.

Ulijaszek, S.J., Hyndman, D.C., Lourie, J.A. & Pumuye, A. (1987). Mining, modernisation and dietary change among the Wopkaimin of Papua New Guinea. *Ecology of Food and Nutrition* 20: 148–56.

Ulijaszek, S.J., Mann, N. & Elton, S. (2012). *Evolving Human Nutrition. Implications for Public Health*. Cambridge: Cambridge University Press.

Ulijaszek, S.J., Graff, H. & McLennan, A.K. (2016a). Conceptualizing ecobiosocial interactions: lessons from obesity. In M. Singer, ed., *A Companion to the Anthropology of Environmental Health*. New York, NY: John Wiley & Sons, pp. 85–100.

Ulijaszek, S.J., Pentecost, M., Marcus, C. et al. (2016b). Inequality and childhood overweight and obesity: a commentary. *Pediatric Obesity* 12: 195–202.

Uller, T. (2008). Developmental plasticity and the evolution of parental effects. *Trends in Molecular Medicine* 23: 432–8.

UNAIDS (2013). *Global Report. UNAIDS report on the global AIDS epidemic 2013*. Geneva: UNAIDS.

UNAIDS (2016). UNAIDS/WHO Policy on HIV testing. http://data.unaids.org/una-docs/hivtesting policy_en.pdf (accessed 5 July 2016).

Unerman, J. & O'Dwyer, B. (2007). The business case for regulation of corporate social responsibility and accountability. *Accounting Forum* 31: 332–53.

United Nations Development Program (2016). Human Development Index (HDI). http://hdr.undp .org/en/content/human-development-index-hdi (accessed 14 July 2016).

United Nations Development Programme (2006). *Beyond Scarcity: Power, Poverty and the Global Water Crisis*. Basingstoke, Hampshire: Palgrave Macmillan.

United Nations Statistical Office (1980). *Towards More Effective Measurement of Levels of Living, and Review of Work of the United Nations Statistical Office (UNSO) Related to Statistics of Levels of Living*. LSMS Working Paper No. 4. Washington, DC: World Bank.

United States Anxiety Disorder Industry (2016). *2016 Market Research Report*. Puyallup, WA: QY Research Groups.

US Department of Health and Human Services (2000). *Healthy People 2000. Final Review*. Hyattsville, MD: National Center for Health Statistics.

US Department of Health and Human Services (2001). *The Surgeon General's Call to Action to Prevent and Decrease Overweight and Obesity*. Rockville, MD: US Department of Health and Human Services, Office of the Surgeon General.

US Department of Health and Human Services (2010). *The Surgeon General's Vision for a Healthy and Fit Nation 2010*. Rockville, MD: US Department of Health and Human Services, Office of the Surgeon General.

Valavanis, I. & Kosmopoulos, D. (2010). Multiclass defect detection and classification in weld radiographic images using geometric and texture features. *Expert Systems with Applications* 37: 7606–14.

Vallgarda, S., Nielsen, M.E.J., Harlev, M. & Sandoe, P. (2015). Backward-and forward-looking responsibility for obesity: policies from WHO, the EU and England. *European Journal of Public Health* 25: 845–8.

van Boom, W., Garde, A. & Akseli, O. (eds.) (2014). *The European Unfair Commercial Practices Directive – Impact, Enforcement Strategies and National Legal Systems*. Farnham, Surrey: Ashgate Publishing.

van der Lans, A.A.J.J., Hoeks, J., Brans, B. et al. (2013). Cold acclimation recruits human brown fat and increases nonshivering thermogenesis. *Journal of Clinical Investigation* 123: 3395–3403.

van Dijk, S.J., Molloy, P.L., Varinli, H. et al. (2015). Epigenetics and human obesity. *International Journal of Obesity* 39: 85–97.

Vandegrift, D. & Yoked, T. (2004). Obesity rates, income, and suburban sprawl: an analysis of US states. *Health and Place* 10: 221–9.

Vandenbroeck, P., Goossens, J. & Clemens, M. (2007a). *Tackling Obesities: Future Choices – Building the Obesity System Map*. London: Government Office for Science.

Vandenbroeck, P., Goossens, J. & Clemens, M. (2007b). *Tackling Obesities: Future Choices – Obesity System Atlas*. London: Government Office for Science.

Vazquez, G., Duval, S., Jacobs, D.R. & Silventoinen, K. (2007). Comparison of body mass index, waist circumference, and waist/hip ratio in predicting incident diabetes: a meta-analysis. *Epidemiologic Reviews* 29: 115–128.

Veblen, T. (1994). *The Theory of the Leisure Class: An Economic Study of Institutions*. Mineola, NY: Dover Publications.

Veenendaal, M.V., Painter, R.C., de Rooij, S.R. et al. (2013). Transgenerational effects of prenatal exposure to the 1944–45 Dutch famine. *British Journal of Obstetrics and Gynaecology* 120: 548–53.

Venator, J. & Reeves, R.V. (2015). Weight and social mobility: taking the long view on childhood obesity. Brookings Institute Social Mobility Paper. www.brookings.edu/research/weight-and-social-mobility-taking-the-long-view-on-childhood-obesity (accessed 26 April 2016).

Verloigne, M., van Lippevelde, W., Maes, L., Brug, J. & de Bourdeaudhuij, I. (2012). Family- and school-based correlates of energy balance-related behaviours in 10–12-year-old children:

a systematic review within the ENERGY (EuropeaN Energy balance Research to prevent excessive weight Gain among Youth) project. *Public Health Nutrition* 15: 1380–95.

Vickers, M.H. (2014). Early life nutrition, epigenetics and programming of later life disease. *Nutrients* 6: 2165–78.

Vickers, M.H., Cupido, C.L. & Gluckman, P.D. (2007). Developmental programming of obesity and type 2 diabetes. *Fetal and Maternal Medicine Review* 18: 1–23.

Vignerova, J., Humenıkova, L., Brabec, M. et al. (2007). Long-term changes in body weight, BMI, and adiposity rebound among children and adolescents in the Czech Republic. *Economics and Human Biology* 5: 409–25.

Vikhlyaev, A.A. (2005). Science on the tap, not on the top. *International Journal of Technology and Globalisation* 1: 145–61.

Viner, R.M., Roche, E., Maguire, S.A. & Nicholls, D.E. (2010). Childhood protection and obesity: framework for practice. *British Medical Journal* 341: c3074.

Visscher, T.L. & Seidell, J.C. (2001). The public health impact of obesity. *Annual Review of Public Health* 22: 355–75.

Visscher, T.L., Seidell, J.C., Molarius, A. et al. (2001). A comparison of body mass index, waist–hip ratio and waist circumference as predictors of all-cause mortality among the elderly: the Rotterdam study. *International Journal of Obesity and Related Metabolic Disorders* 25: 1730–5.

Visscher, T.L., Heitmann, B.L., Rissanen, A., Lahti-Koski, M. & Lissner, L. (2015). A break in the obesity epidemic? Explained by biases or misinterpretation of the data? *International Journal of Obesity* 39: 189–98.

Wabitsch, M., Moss, A. & Kromeyer-Hauschild, K. (2014). Unexpected plateauing of childhood obesity rates in developed countries. *BMC Medicine* 12: 17.

Wacquant, L. (2009). *Punishing the Poor. The Neoliberal Government of Social Insecurity*. Durham, NC: Duke University Press.

Wade, T.J. & Cooper, M. (1999). Sex differences in the links between attractiveness, self-esteem and the body. *Personality and Individual Differences* 27: 1047–56.

Walker, A. (1981). South African black, Indian and coloured populations. In H.C. Trowell & D.P. Burkitt, eds., *Western Diseases: Their Emergence and Prevention*. London: Edward Arnold, pp. 285–318.

Wallace, D.C. (2010). Bioenergetics, the origins of complexity, and the ascent of man. *Proceedings of the National Academy of Sciences USA* 107 (Suppl. 2): 8947–53.

Walley, A.J., Asher, J.E. & Froguel, P. (2009). The genetic contribution to non-syndromic human obesity. *Nature Reviews Genetics* 10: 431–42.

Wang, D., Liu, X., Zhou, Y. et al. (2012). Individual variation and longitudinal pattern of genome-wide DNA methylation from birth to the first two years of life. *Epigenetics* 7: 594–605.

Wang, G. & Dietz, W.H. (2002). Economic burden of obesity in youths aged 6 to 17 years: 1979–1999. *Pediatrics* 109: E81.

Wang, Y.C., McPherson, K., Marsh, T., Gortmaker, S.L. & Brown, M. (2011). Health and economic burden of the projected obesity trends in the USA and the UK. *Lancet* 378: 815–25.

Wansink, B., Cheney, M.M. & Chan, N. (2003). Exploring comfort food preferences across age and gender. *Physiology and Behavior* 79: 739–47.

Wardle, J. & Griffith, J. (2001). Socio-economic status and weight control practices in British adults. *Journal of Epidemiology and Community Health* 55: 185–90.

Wardle, J., Waller, J. & Jarvis, M.J. (2002). Sex differences in the association of socioeconomic status with obesity. *American Journal of Public Health* 92: 1299–1304.

Wardle, J., Haase, A.M., Steptoe, A., et al. (2004). Gender differences in food choice: the contribution of health beliefs and dieting. *Annals of Behavioral Medicine* 27: 107–16.

Warin, M., Zivkovic, T., Moore, V. & Davies, M. (2012). Mothers as smoking guns: fetal overnutrition and the reproduction of obesity. *Feminism and Psychology* 22: 360–75.

Warin, M., Moore, V., Davies, M. & Ulijaszek, S.J. (2015). Epigenetics and obesity: the reproduction of habitus through intracellular and social environments. *Body and Society* 22: 53–78.

Warren, E. & Tyagi, A.W. (2003). *The Two-income Trap: Why Families Went Broke When Mothers Went to Work.* New York, NY: Basic Books.

Waterlow, J.C. (1988). Observations on the natural history of stunting. In J.C. Waterlow, ed., *Linear Growth Retardation in Less Developed Countries.* New York, NY: Raven Press, pp. 1–12.

Waters, T. & Waters, D. (2015). *Weber's Rationalism and Modern Society: New Translations on Politics, Bureaucracy, and Social Stratification.* New York, NY: Palgrave Macmillan

Watson, J.D. & Crick, F.H.C. (1953). The structure of DNA. *Cold Spring Harbor Symposia on Quantitative Biology* 18: 123–31.

Webber, J. (2003). Energy balance in obesity. *Proceedings of the Nutrition Society* 62: 539–43.

Weber, M. (1946). Politics as a vocation. In H.H. Gerth & C.W. Mills, eds., *Max Weber: Essays in Sociology.* New York, NY: Oxford University Press, pp. 77–128.

Weber, M. (1978). *Economy and Society.* Berkeley, CA: University of California Press.

Webster, E., Lambert, R. & Bezuidenhout, A. (2008). *Grounding Globalization. Labour in the Age of Insecurity.* Oxford: Blackwell Publishing.

Wedel, J.R., Shore, C., Feldman, G. & Lathrop, S. (2005). Toward an anthropology of public policy. *Annals of the American Academy of Political and Social Science* 600: 30–51.

Weigly, E.S. (1984). Average? Ideal? Desirable? A brief overview of weight tables in the United States. *Journal of the American Dietetic Association* 84: 417–23.

Weirich, P. (2004). Economic rationality. In A.R. Mele & P. Rawling, eds., *The Oxford Handbook of Rationality.* Oxford: Oxford University Press, pp. 380–98.

Wells, J.C.K. (2010). *The Evolutionary Biology of Human Body Fatness.* Cambridge: Cambridge University Press.

Wells, J.C.K., Marphatia, A.A., Cole, T.J. & McCoy, D. (2012). Associations of economic and gender inequality with global obesity prevalence: understanding the female excess. *Social Science and Medicine* 75: 482–90.

Wen, C.P., Cheng, T.Y.D., Tsai, S.P. et al. (2009). Are Asians at greater mortality risks for being overweight than Caucasians? Redefining obesity for Asians. *Public Health Nutrition*: 12: 497–506.

Wen, W. (2010). An intelligent traffic management expert system with RFID technology. *Expert Systems with Applications* 37: 3024–35.

Whitaker, R.C. (2004). Predicting preschooler obesity at birth: the role of maternal obesity in early pregnancy. *Pediatrics* 114: e29–36.

White, T.D., Asfaw, B., Beyene, Y. et al. (2009). *Ardipithecus ramidus* and the paleobiology of early hominids. *Science* 326: 64–86.

Widmaier, E.P. (1999). *Why Geese Don't Get Obese (and We Do): How Evolution's Strategies for Survival Affect Our Everyday Lives.* New York, NY: Henry Holt and Company.

Winter, J.E., MacInnis, R.J., Wattanapenpaiboon, N. & Nowson, C.A. (2014). BMI and all-cause mortality in older adults: a meta-analysis. *American Journal of Clinical Nutrition* 99: 875–90.

Weissner, P. & Schiefenhovel, W. (eds.)(1996). *Food and the Status Quest.* Oxford: Berghahn Books.

Wilcoxon, A.J. & Russell, I.T. (1983). Birthweight and perinatal mortality: II. On weight-specific mortality. *International Journal of Epidemiology* 12: 319–25.

Wildavsky, A.B., Ellis, R.J. & Thompson, M. (1997). *Culture Matters: Essays in Honor of Aaron Wildavsky.* Boulder, CO: Westview Press.

Wilkinson, R.G. & Pickett, K. (2009). *The Spirit Level: Why More Equal Societies Almost Always Do Better.* London: Allen Lane.

Wimsatt, W.C. (1994). The ontology of complex systems: levels of organization, perspectives, and causal thickets. *Canadian Journal of Philosophy* 20: 207–74.

Wing, R.R. & Phelan, S. (2005). Long-term weight loss maintenance. *American Journal of Clinical Nutrition* 82: 222S–5S.

Winterhalder, B. & Kennett, D.J. (2009). Four neglected concepts with a role to play in explaining the origins of agriculture. *Current Anthropology* 50: 645–8.

Wisman, J.D. & Capehart, H.W. (2012). Creative destruction, economic and security, stress, and epidemic obesity. In A. Offer, R. Pechey & S.J. Ulijaszek, eds., *Insecurity, Inequality and Obesity*. Oxford: Oxford University Press, pp. 5–53.

Witt, A.A. & Lowe, M.R. (2014). Hedonic hunger and binge eating among women with eating disorders. *International Journal of Eating Disorders* 47: 273–80.

Wolf, A.M. & Colditz, G.A. (1998). Current estimates of the economic cost of obesity in the United States. *Obesity Research* 6: 97–106.

Woolgar, S. & Neyland, D. (2013). *Mundane Governance: Ontology and Accountability*. Oxford: Oxford University Press.

World Bank (2016a). GDP per capita, PPP (current international $). World Bank, International Comparison Program database. http://data.worldbank.org/indicator/NY.GDP.PCAP.PP.CD (accessed 9 November 2016).

World Bank (2016b). Cause of death, by communicable diseases and maternal, prenatal and nutrition conditions (% of total). http://data.worldbank.org/indicator/SH.DTH.COMM.ZS/coun tries (acccessed 15 January 2016).

World Bank (2016c). Fertility rates, total (births per woman). http://data.worldbank.org/indicator/ SP.DYN.TFRT.IN (accessed 15 September 2016).

World Health Organization (2000). *Obesity: Preventing and Managing the Global Epidemic. Report of a WHO Consultation*. Geneva: World Health Organization.

World Health Organization (2006). *European Charter on Counteracting Obesity*. Geneva: World Health Organization.

World Health Organization (2009a). *Global Health Risks: Mortality and Burden of Disease Attributable to Selected Major Risks*. Geneva: World Health Organization.

World Health Organization (2009b). *2008–2013 Action Plan for the Global Strategy for the Prevention and Control of Noncommunicable Diseases*. Geneva: World Health Organization.

World Health Organization (2011). *Waist Circumference and Waist–Hip Ratio: Report of a WHO Expert Consultation*. Geneva: World Health Organization.

World Health Organization (2014). *Ten Facts About Obesity*. Geneva: World Health Organization.

World Health Organization (2015a). Global database on body mass index. http://apps.who.int/bmi/ index.jsp (accessed 15 December 2015).

World Health Organization (2015b). Global and regional food consumption patterns and trends. http://who.int/nutrition/topics/3_foodconsumption/en/ (accessed 15 December 2015).

World Health Organization (2015c). World Malaria Report 2015. www.who.int/malaria/publica tions/world-malaria-report-2015/en/ (accessed 21 December 2015).

World Health Organization (2016a) Malaria. Diagnostic testing. www.who.int/malaria/areas/diag nosis/en/ (accessed 5 July 2016).

World Health Organization (2016b). *Consideration of the Evidence on Childhood Obesity for the Commission on Ending Childhood Obesity. Report of the Ad hoc Working Group on Science and Evidence for Ending Childhood Obesity*. Geneva: World Health Organization.

World Health Organization Expert Consultation (2004). Appropriate body-mass index for Asian populations and its implications for policy and intervention strategies. *Lancet* 363: 157–63.

World Health Organization/Food and Agriculture Organization/United Nations University (2001). *Human Energy Requirements. Report of a Joint FAO/WHO/UNU Expert Consultation, Rome, Italy, 17–24 October 2001*. Geneva: World Health Organization.

World Obesity Federation (2017). World map of obesity. www.worldobesity.org/data/ (accessed 12 May 2017).

Worrall, J. (1989). Structural realism: the best of both worlds? *Dialectica* 43: 99–124.

Wright, S.M. & Aronne, L.J. (2012). Causes of obesity. *Abdominal Radiology* 37: 730–2.

Wu, T., Gao, X., Chen, M. & van Dam, R.M. (2009). Long-term effectiveness of diet-plus-exercise interventions vs. diet-only interventions for weight loss: a meta-analysis. *Obesity Reviews* 10: 313–23.

Xu, F., Yin, X.M., Zhang, M. et al. (2005). Family average income and body mass index above the healthy weight range among urban and rural residents in regional Mainland China. *Public Health Nutrition* 8: 47–51.

Yajnik, C.S. & Deshmukh, U.S. (2008). Maternal nutrition, intrauterine programming and consequential risks in the offspring. *Reviews in Endocrine and Metabolic Disorders* 9: 203.

Yang, J., Manolio, T.A., Pasquale, L.R. et al. (2011). Genome partitioning of genetic variation for complex traits using common SNPs. *Nature Genetics* 43: 519–25.

Yates-Doerr, E. (2013). The mismeasure of obesity. In M.B. McCullough & J.A. Hardin, eds., *Reconstructing Obesity: The Meaning of Measures and the Measure of Meanings*. Oxford: Berghahn Books, pp. 49–70.

Yeo, G.S.H. & Heisler, L.K. (2012). Unraveling the brain regulation of appetite: lessons from genetics. *Nature Neuroscience* 15: 1343–9.

Yoshizawa, R. (2012). The Barker hypothesis and obesity: connections for transdisciplinarity and social justice. *Social Theory and Health* 10: 348–67.

Yu, Y., Hui, P.C.-L. & Choi, T.-M. (2012). An empirical study of intelligent expert systems on forecasting of fashion color trend. *Expert Systems with Applications* 39: 4383–9.

Zeeck, A., Stelzer, N., Linser, H.W., Joos, A. & Hartmann, A. (2011). Emotion and eating in binge eating disorder and obesity. *European Eating Disorders Review* 19: 426–37.

Zemel, M.B., Kim, J.H., Woychik, R.P. et al. (1995). Agouti regulation of intracellular calcium: role in the insulin resistance of viable yellow mice. *Proceedings of the National Academy of Sciences USA* 92: 4733–7.

Zhang, Y., Proenca, R., Maffei, M. et al. (1994). Positional cloning of the mouse *obese* gene and its human homologue. *Nature* 372: 425–32.

Zhou, B.-F. (2002). Predictive values of body mass index and waist circumference for risk factors of certain related diseases in Chinese adults – study on optimal cut-off points of body mass index and waist circumference in Chinese adults. *Biomedical and Environmental Sciences* 15: 83–95.

Zivkovic, T., Warin, M., Moore, V., Ward, P. & Jones, M. (2015). The sweetness of care: biographies, bodies and place. In E.-J. Abbots, A. Lavis & L. Attala, eds., *Careless Eating: Bodies, Food and Care*. Farnham, Surrey: Ashgate Publishing, pp. 109–126.

Index

abstraction, 31–2
action, 6, 10–11, 22–3, 26
  collective, 164
  consistency of, 10
  ethical, 141
  facilitation of, 148
  governmental, 20
  individual, 141
  personal, 104
  policy, 6, 53, 135
  political, 56, 149
  pragmatic, 24
  public health, 146
  rational, 107
  regulatory, 93
  self-directed, 24
  singular, 170
Action Plan for the Global Strategy
    for the Prevention and Control of
    Noncommunicable Diseases, 146
activism
  food, viii
activity, 51
  anti-obesity, 150
  brown adipose tissue, 39
  corporate, 167
  government, 153
  habitual, 83
  physical, 4, 11, 19, 37, 42, 50, 71,
    78, 83, 104, 120, 128, 141, 154,
    156, 163, 172
  physical patterns, 156
  promoting, 143
adaptation, 42, 52, 106, 170
  behavioural, 37
  cold, 35, 47
  developmental, 125
  evolutionarily based, 106
  feeding, 108
addiction, 135, 152
  food, 147
adipose tissue, 9, 41, 44
  brown, 39
  development, 128
  DNA methylation in, 128

adiposity rebound, 128
adolescence, 58, 66–7, 76, 82, 128
advertising, 85, 93, 105, 144, 158,
    164, 175
Africa, 16, 45–6, 64, 99
  South, 62, 129
  sub-Saharan, 114
agentive organizations, 173
agriculture, 3, 14, 99, 111, 174
  commoditization of, 100
  diversification of, 97
  emergence of, 97
  European systems of, 99
  Mid-Western, 101
  origins of, 19, 47, 96
  transition to, 94
American Medical Association, 5, 9,
    146
amphetamine, 173
animal models
  of obesity, 7, 31
anthropology, 20, 33, 134, 156
  of the body, 168
anthropometry, 15, 56
  political, 56
anti-depressants, 91
anxiety, 86, 88, 107, 109
  disorders, 91
  parental, 93
appearance, 79
appetite, 18, 20, 35, 39, 41–2, 48
  behaviour, 155, 173
  control, 18, 20, 158
  dysregulation, 9
  human, 96
  individual, 106
  neurophysiology of, 169
  physiological, 174
  regulation, 30, 95, 106
  self-control of, 107
attractiveness, 79
Australia, 35, 39, 50–1, 54, 86, 88,
    95, 101, 109, 140
  Melbourne, 84
  Perth, 50

Australians, Indigenous, 45
Austria, 80
authorities, 124, 136
  local, 84

beauty, 78, 120
  ideals, 74, 79
behaviour, 1, 11, 18, 23, 104, 107,
    135, 137, 160, 175
  change, 19, 165
  chaotic, 141
  consumer, 105, 164
  consumption, 109, 166, 175
  eating, 28, 48
  formally rational, 79
  health, 11, 74
  health-seeking, 69, 81
  human, 33
  immoral, 8
  individual, 4, 6, 26, 161, 164
  individualized, 26
  maladaptive, 91, 172
  non-rational, 166
  obesogenic, 1
  organizational, 23
  population, 131
  sinful, 147
  social, 47
  unhealthy, 91
Berio, Luciano, viii
binge-eating, 43, 108, 181
biocultural relations, 171
biology, 170
biosciences, 164
birth, 44, 54, 77, 93, 112, 126–7,
    130
  weight, 73, 91, 112, 126
  weight, low, 113, 125
Blair
  administration, 151, 153, 162
  government, 171
  Labour administration, 92,
    151
  Tony, 153
blame, 93, 146, 154

body, 9, 37, 72
  advisory, 163
  arm's length, 163
  composition, 128, 155
  energy stores, 57
  extreme fatness, 5
  fat, 59
  fat distribution, 71
  fat reduction, 173
  fat stores, 42
  fatness, 8, 10, 12, 18, 34, 41, 44,
    64, 71, 80, 93, 128, 134
  frame, 58
  healthy, 3, 78, 135
  healthy weight, 106
  ideals, 74
  image, 74
  individual, 5
  large size, 82
  legislative, 145
  lower, 44
  mass, 42
  materiality of, 8
  maternal weight, 126
  physiology, 7
  proportions, 58
  shape, 79
  size, 19, 37, 42, 56, 79, 130,
    172
  size phenotypes, 48
  size, healthy, 172
  size, small, 56, 126
  slender female, 79
  slim ideals, 82
  small size, 126
  temperature, 46
  upper, 44
  weight, 29, 74
  weight, constant, 38
body mass index, 2, 10, 58, 60–2,
    64, 66, 68, 123
  average, 161
  cut-offs, 137
  inequality, 73
  population level, 122
boundaries, viii
boundary object, 163
Box, George E.P., 1
brand, 102
  advertised food, 85
  burger, 85

commercial, 165
  foods, 79
  global, 85, 103
  icons, 102
  killer, 167
  specific, 105
  value, 93, 103
branding, 85, 102, 105, 147
Brazil, 16, 112, 129, 138, 176
breastfeeding, 91
Brown, Gordon, 92, 152, 165,
    171
bureaucracies.
  growth of, 25
bureaucracy, 23–5, 111, 178

cacophony, viii
caffeine, 173
Call to Action on Obesity, 165
capital, 18, 77–8, 116
  cognitive, 93
  cultural, 79
  economic, 79
  embodied cultural, 79, 82
  flows, 88, 116
  flows of, 116
  human, 56
  international, 88
  liberalization of, 122
  mental, 152
  objectified cultural, 85
  social, 72, 78
capitalism, 24
  global, 5, 171
carbohydrate, 19, 39, 97
  processed, 113
  refined, 38, 100, 112
care, 140
  health, 6, 18, 55, 80, 145
  health costs, 67
  health provision, 136
  maternal, 11
  medical, 10, 67
  preventative, 69
  private health, 55
  social, 156
cars, 28, 49, 107, 138, 141
causal loops, 158, 162
cause and effect, 29–30, 41
Centers for Disease Control and
    Prevention, 54

cereals, 94, 114
  breakfast, 101
chair, 49, 157
  desk–, 171
change, 154
  body mass index, 58
  climate, 21, 153
  consumer-driven, 175
  demographic, 6
  dietary, 94, 100, 111
  ecological, 28, 111
  economic, 51, 111
  environmental, 70
  epigenetic, 124
  evolutionary, 47
  in energy balance, 37
  in family structure, 123
  in fetal physiology, 125
  in growth and development, 129
  in ideology, 149
  in political ideology, 165
  metabolic, 113
  nutritional, 124
  social, 20, 164, 175
  social policy, 148
  societal, 169
  structural, 52
  technological, 53, 97
Change4Life, 154, 164, 175
childhood obesity, 58, 72
  classification of, 57
  inequalities in, 92
  prevention and treatment, 135
  rates of, 76
  regulation of, 93
Childhood Obesity: a Plan for
    Action, 147
children, 2, 8, 10–12
  cycles of deprivation, 105
  growth rates, 57
  healthy eating among, 143
  in high-income countries, 75, 81,
    93
  in the US, 85
  of high socioeconomic status,
    76
  of low socioeconomic status,
    105
  of obese parents, 71
  preschool, 72
  primary school, 166

children (cont.)
  privately educated, 179
  school, 138
  young, 46, 104
China, 16, 99, 112, 129
choice, 107, 137
  consumer, 33
  drug of, 92
  food, 11, 96, 156, 173
  free, 149
  'good', 18
  guiding, 139
  health, 147
  healthier, 175
  healthy, 2
  incentivizing, 139
  individual, 9, 52, 93, 169
  lifestyle, 164
  past, 11
  rational, 11, 147
  restricting, 139
  rhetoric of, 109, 147
  self-interested, 28
chronic disease, 6, 14, 35, 53, 63, 66,
    94, 111, 125, 170, 181
  burden, 67
  epidemiology, 62
  markers, 150
  predispositions to, 131
  risk, 58, 80
  risk factors, 8
chronic energy deficiency, 60
citizenship, 180
  consumer, 107
  consumption and, 107, 147
  responsibilized, 143
  responsibilized consumer, 106
class, 62, 85, 99, 165
  English upper, 5
  occupational, 72
  social, 73, 105
  working, 21
clumsy solutions, 180
Cold War, 174
Collected Essays in the Sociology of
    Religion, 24
colonial
  domination, 103
  geography, 100
  nations, 99–100
  powers, 99

colonialism, 99
colonizers, 100
  Spanish, 99
comfort eating, 86, 91, 104, 109
commercialism, 104
commodities, 101
  agricultural, 94, 101
  cereal-based, 103
  food, 90, 117
  macronutrient, 95
communications, 171
communism, 25, 120–1, 181
  Soviet-styled, 120
complex adaptive framework, 151
complex systems, 152, 173, 176
complexity, viii, 14, 20, 29, 32, 34,
    50, 53, 131, 142–3, 150–1, 162,
    164, 166
  baroque, 155, 172, 174
  cultural, 97
  discourse of, 164
  internal, 156
  obesity, 167, 181
  of human appetite, 96
  romantic, 155, 172, 174
  science, 168
  systems, 151
computer, 49
  personal, 107
  trading, 152
computer-facilitated work, 171
computing, 5, 166
  interactive, 175
Conservative–Liberal Democrat
    coalition, 163, 165
Consideration of the Evidence on
    Childhood Obesity for the
    Commission on Ending
    Childhood Obesity, 146
consumer, 92, 101, 158
  citizens, 172
  credit, 57
  finances, 105
  good, 103
  goodwill, 93
  individual, 107
  information, 165, 175
  protection, 92
  rational, 165
  society, 147
consumer price index, 57

consumerism, 102, 108, 178
  enlightened, 165
  market, 175
consumption, 2, 42, 94, 101, 147,
    180
  and social status, 103
  behaviour, 166
  food, 29, 37, 39, 44, 103, 105,
    108, 112, 175
  in late modern society, 147
  of addictive substances, 11
  of caloric beverages, 100
  of energy-dense foods, 104
  of fast food, 84–5
  of high-energy-density foods,
    124
  of high-status food, 79
  of highly palatable energy-dense
    foods, 90
  of motor cars, 107
  of sugar, 103
  patterns, 33
  per capita, 113
  rational, 11
  sugar, 5
  theory of, 11
control, 133
  biological, 38
  complex, 97
  corporate, 18
  cultural, 128
  dietary, 43
  ecological, 47
  feedback, 38
  flood, 169
  genetic, 45
  individual, 149
  lack of, 74
  obesity, 20, 28, 41, 66, 106, 139,
    168, 172
  personal, 36
  physiological, 42
  political, 97
  self, 19, 104, 107
  social epigenetic, 128
  state, 174
  system, 38
convenience, 11, 35, 51, 107, 176
  devices, 49
  foods, 101
  of fast food, 83

Cook Islands, 19, 45, 62
cooking
  traditional, 100
Copenhagen, viii
corporate social responsibility, 92,
    165, 167
corporations, 6, 27, 34, 52, 86, 92,
    111, 124, 168, 173, 175, 177–9
  food, 93, 108, 112, 165, 170
  global food, 103
  major, 155
  pharmaceutical, 174
  transnational, 94, 100, 117
cost
  economic, 67, 137
  effectiveness, 144
  environmental, 181
  health, 6
  illness, 67, 69
  medical, 67, 139
  of convenience, 51
  of diabetes, 69
  of food calories, 53
  of obesity, 6, 54–5, 161
  private medical, 88
  psychological health, 88
  social, 123
  to employers, 53
  to nations, 53
country
  Asian, 97, 129
credibility, 171
crops, 99
  cereal, 99
  staple, 97
Cross-Government Obesity Unit,
    154, 164
Crowe's index, 47
culture, 25, 62
  of politics, 131
cut-off
  body mass index, 10, 54, 60, 64
  for ideal weight, 60
  obesity, 58
  overweight and obesity, 58

data
  actuarial, 58
  aggregate, 122
  big, 150
  collection, 54, 137

country, 15
  epidemiological, 30, 53, 170
  health economics, 161
  panel, 122
  stratification, 31
death rates, 54, 65, 69
decision making, 23–4, 26, 29, 108,
    147, 161, 177
decisions, 11, 23, 26, 33, 147, 177
  culturally based, 142
  difficult, 139
  ecological, 28, 130
  economic, 11
  personally bounded, 172
  rational, 11
  time-limited, 11
Denmark, 39, 80, 86
designer-labelled clothes, 79
desirability
  of non-medical treatments, 54
  social, 8
diet, 19, 93
  American, 99
  British, 131
  composition, 39
  cosmopolitan, 99
  energy-dense, 38
  English, 103
  European, 99
  healthier, 3, 74
  healthy, 172
  high-energy-density, 126
  high-fat, 104
  in pregnancy and lactation, 124
  induced thermogenesis, 39
  industrial, 107
  macronutrient composition of, 38
  Mexican, 99
  obesogenic, 18, 106
  plant-based, 113
  quality, 74
  unbalanced, 39
  unhealthy, 136
dietary
  change, 94
  cosmopolitanism, 101
  energy, 39, 96, 113
  energy availability, 120
  energy intake, 39, 86
  guidelines, 138
  habits, 3, 158

intake, 81, 139
  intervention, 4
  preference, 96, 103
  quantity, 128
  recommendations, 176
  regulation, 44, 105
  restriction, 34, 42
  risk factors, 6
  tradition, 96
dinitrophenol, 173
disadvantage, 71, 93, 105
  social, 18, 82
  socioeconomic, 72, 91
discrimination, 10, 80
distress, 88
  childhood, 91
  psychological, 72, 91
DNA methylation, 124, 128
domain
  governmental, 168
  public, 104, 147
  social and societal, 171
  societal, 181
doubly labelled water method, 41
drifty genotype, 45
drivers of obesity, 155, 158,
    170
drugs, 91, 152, 173
  anti-obesity, 43
  approved, 43
  new, 171
  safe, 174

Eastern Europe, 120
eating, 3, 11, 19, 37–8, 74, 107,
    169
  ambivalence, 103
  comfort, 51
  disorder, 147
  disordered, 103
  distracted, 108
  gratifications of, 11
  healthily, 104
  healthy, 165, 172
  out, 83
  patterns, 7, 94, 104
  pleasure, 28
  regulation of, 106
  social and cultural mediators of,
    108
  together, 50

Eckersberg, Christoffer, viii
ecology, 35, 40, 49
  changing, 7
  changing food, 106
  energy, 41
  gut microbiota, 107
  human, 44, 168
  human gut microbiotic, 138
  nutritional, 125
  of obesity, 142, 151
  of obesity, 67
  political, 72, 84, 113, 133, 141
  reproductive, 77
  urban, 84
Economic Freedom of the World
    Index, 88
economics, 14, 23, 25–6, 53, 62, 69,
    99, 134, 147, 153, 170
  behavioural, 26
  free-market, 120, 162
  mainstream, 10
  obesity and, 57
economies
  market, 86
Economy and Society, 24
education, 1, 3, 10, 18, 72–3, 77, 87,
    133, 138, 144, 176
  system, 82
emotion, 23, 28, 72, 91, 104, 178,
    180
employment, 10, 14, 74, 81, 93
  inequalities in, 80
  patterns of, 54
energy, 36, 41, 162
  availability, 113, 120
  balance, 9, 18, 29, 34–5, 39, 141,
    146, 154, 167, 169
  density, 19, 38, 95, 102
  expenditure, 39, 41, 47, 106
  flow, 36, 40
  flux, 36
  homeostasis, 36
  imbalance, 40, 45, 96
  intake, 37, 42, 53, 86, 114, 155
  investment, 131
  metabolism, 43
  nutrition, 41
  partitioning, 125
  stores, 44
energy balance, 35, 37–8, 41–2,
    155, 169

discourses, 36
  homeostatic system, 20
  positive, 14, 19, 36
  research, 7, 43
  rhetoric, 172
  susceptibilities, 7
  systems, 174
  theory, 40
energy balance models, viii, 7, 40,
    42, 44, 141, 168, 179
energy dense, 96
  food, 18, 38, 53, 82, 90, 96, 104,
    106, 109, 171
  palatable foods, 96
energy imbalance, 2, 37, 40–1, 51
engineering, 15
environment, 2, 7, 32
  adverse, 125
  built, 83, 152
  early post-natal, 126
  food, 158
  household, 71
  nutritional, 170
  obesogenic, 7, 35, 49, 93, 111,
    169, 172, 175
  physical, 6
  political, 145
  post-natal, 125
  risk, 105
  seasonal, 44, 46
  social, 131, 161
  threatening, 125
  transitional, 126
  unstable, 18
  urban, 35, 51, 175
epidemiology, 14, 53, 62, 65, 69,
    134, 150, 153, 156, 170
epigenetics, 35, 113, 124–5, 134,
    156, 168, 173, 180
equilibrium, 36
ethics, 20, 135–6, 152, 170
evidence, 11, 20
  clinical, 9
  in obesity policy, 145
  qualitative, 153
  scientific, 135, 143, 147–8, 151
  types of, 144
evolution, 43
  brain size, 96
  hominin, 44
  human, 37

evolutionary
  change, 47
  genetics, 7
  history, 45
  models, 125
  processes, 40
  studies, 79
  success, 28
  time, 18, 44
exercise, 4, 42, 74, 81, 128, 154, 169
expert systems
  interactions of, 21
expert systems software, 14

famine, 19, 41, 47
  Dutch winter, 124
fast food, 84, 105, 117
  chains, 71
  outlets, 51
fat, 19, 39, 80, 95, 114, 117, 131,
    173
  abdominal, 44
  accumulation, 2, 44
  accumulation of, 130
  activism, 33
  babies, 126
  bodies, viii, 10, 65
  body, 9, 105
  brown, 38, 40
  chair, viii
  consumption of, 111
  critical scholars, 33
  critical studies, 8, 33, 134
  dietary preference for, 96
  distribution, 134
  gain, 47
  harmful, 64
  lower body, 44
  mass, 128
  overeating, 39
  overeating on, 96
  passive consumption, 96
  prediction, 59
  reducing intake, 104
  reduction, 173
  stigma, 80
  storage, 35, 125
  taste stimulus, 96
  taxation, 181
  total intake, 3
  visceral, 40

fattening
  ritual, 34
fecundity, 19
feeding constraints, 94
fertility, 9, 44, 126
  average, 47
  differential, 47
  rates, 40
  rates, total, 130
fetal
  development, 66
  epigenome, 126
  growth, 134
  starvation, 124
financial crisis
  global, 90
financial integration
  global, 116
Fisher, R.A., 47
fitness
  expectations, 120
  physiological, 29
  reproductive, 29, 125, 180
fluoxetine (Prozac), 91
food, 14, 20, 85, 96, 138, 145, 156,
    173
  and eating, 28
  and nutrition policy, 133
  availability, 37, 44, 173
  branded fast, 79
  calorific, 2
  cheap energy-dense, 169
  choice, 11, 18, 92, 96, 106
  companies, 140, 158, 175
  complex system, 96, 102
  consumption, 28, 42, 108
  corporations, 109, 147
  cues, 106
  demand, 101
  demand for, 53
  digestion of, 39
  energy-dense, 7, 35, 49, 74, 90,
    108, 158
  energy-dense processed, 78
  Eurasian systems, 99
  European economies, 101
  fast, 84, 101
  globalized, 7
  high-energy-density, 176
  high-fat, 38
  high-fat high-sugar products, 105

high-status, 85
  imports, 111
  industry, 52, 101, 136, 140, 165
  insecurity, 91
  intake, 11, 40, 42, 71, 94
  international, 124
  manufacture, 100
  Mexican system, 100
  Mexico, 124
  minimally processed, 139
  native, 99
  Native American systems, 101
  nutrient-rich, 118
  obesogenic, 93, 139, 146
  packaging, 139
  palatable, 162
  policy, 100
  portion size, 44
  preference, 72
  price, 53, 90, 111
  probiotic, 138
  producers, 141
  production, 14, 96, 139, 174
  production, global, 176
  products, 103
  refined carbohydrate, 49
  regime, global, 96
  retail, 102, 142
  retail companies, global, 94
  safety, 14–15, 133, 174
  scarcity, 108
  security, 38, 40, 100, 106, 114
  shopping, 50
  shortage, 74
  supply, 94, 130
  supply system, 156
  sweet high-fat, 96
  system, 18, 20, 52, 94
  system, Brazilian, 139
  system, expert, 171
  system, global, 14, 94, 96, 106,
    168, 174, 179
  systems, 92, 97, 99
  taxation, 30
  trade global, 101
  traditional, 124
  traditional role of, 82
  transnational corporations, 122
  ultra processed, 117
  uncertainty, 108
  unhealthy, 93

US system, 100
  waste, 96
Food Network Responsibility Deal,
    165
Food and Drug Administration, 9,
    43, 173
Food Network Responsibility Deal,
    109, 175
Foresight, 7, 146, 150
  Obesities, 20, 154, 158, 161
  programme, 153, 163
Foresight Obesity Systems Map, 20,
    157
framework
  analytical, 50
  ANGELO, 50
  bounded rationality, 147
  dimensional, 160
  ecological, 154
  evolutionary, 36
  explanatory, 19
  for hypothesis generation, 40
  human evolutionary, 28
  legal, 146
  neoliberal, 55, 160
  normative institutional, 24
  of insurances, 181
frameworks
  neoliberal, 176
France, 16, 39, 95, 140
  obesity in, 62
Friedrich, Caspar David, viii
future scenarios, 155, 159

Geelong, 50
gender, 56, 71, 88
  and medical expenditure, 67
  difference in economic costs of
    obesity, 69
  disparity, 77
  inequality, 72, 77
generality, 29, 50, 81
genes, 20, 45, 47, 124
  obesity susceptibility, 49, 71
  search for, 49
  system of, 20
  thrifty, 46, 48
genetic
  basis for obesity, 44
  contribution, 'missing', 48
  predispositions, 35, 43, 50

genetic (cont.)
  regulation of energy balance, 45
  systems, 7
  variation, 31, 46
genetics, 32, 134, 151
  human, 7
  modern, 44
  molecular, 49
  obesity, 179
  of energy balance, 45
  of obesity, 31
  of obesity, population, 35
genome-wide association studies,
    48
genotype
  drifty, 45
  thrifty, 1, 45–6, 62
Genuine Progress Indicator, 123
Gini coefficient, 80
global
  food system, 100
Global Database on Body Mass
    Index, 57
global financialization of markets, 7
globalization, viii, 19, 24, 71, 94, 96,
    99, 111, 116, 122, 170, 176
  and food, 99
  of neoliberal values, 109
governance, 56, 100, 153
  food, 174
  global, 140
  mundane, 143
  obesity, 107, 164
  of obesity, 57
government, 27, 29, 52, 92, 108,
    124, 133, 136, 138, 141–2, 147,
    153, 156, 160, 174–5, 178, 182
  Conservative, 166
  departments, 162
  ideology, 160
  joined-up, 154, 156, 164
  Mexican, 100
  national, 165
  neoliberalization of, 88
  policy, 105
  UK, 7, 136, 146, 151, 163, 165
  US, 101
gradient
  social, 73, 109
  social and economic, 73
gross domestic product, 55, 120

gross national product, 56
growth
  and cellular differentiation, 49
  catch-up, 113, 128
  child, 56
  early, 125
  economic, 67, 74, 88, 117, 123,
    135
  fetal, 113, 125
  in global wealth, 73
  market, 165
  of civilizations, 99
  of consumerism, 104
  of fast-food sales, 85
  of institutions, 97
  of neoliberalism, 175
  of obesity, 101
  of transnational corporations,
    122
  physical, 36, 73, 125
  plasticity, 128
  slow, 126

Hamburg, viii
health, 3–4, 87, 140
  burden, 54
  care, 55, 69, 80–1
  global public, 57
  inequalities, 72
  intervention, 66
  interventions, 18, 164
  maternal, 131
  mental, 63, 123
  nutritional, 36, 109, 139, 170
  outcomes, 6, 86
  percieved, 63
  policy, 136–7
  promotion, 11, 143
  public, 1, 7, 10, 27, 92, 94, 134,
    162
  risk, 58, 64, 69, 140
  services, 6
  status, 63
  strategies, 175
Health Survey for England, 161
Healthy Lives, Healthy People, 154
Healthy Weight, Healthy Lives, 164
heart disease, 2, 65, 173
hedonic response, 96
hedonism, 25
heritability, 4, 48, 126

high-fructose corn syrup, 103
high-income countries, 7, 38, 53,
    71, 101, 111, 139–40, 174
history, 131, 134, 156
  chequered, 173
  life, 112, 168
  of humanity, 96
  twentieth century, 120
holistic approaches, 20
homeostasis, 40–1
  genetic, 45
  metabolic, 125
  physiological, 7, 36
hominin, 44
  brain size, 96
Human Development Index, 18,
    73
Hume, David, 24
humoral theory, 36
hypertension, 9, 45, 65, 113
hypometabolism, 44
hypothesis production, 29, 81

ideology
  of democratic cultural
    consumption, 102
  of individualism, 96, 109
  of modernization, 100
  of neoliberalism, 104
  party political, 151
  political, 142, 149
in utero, 73, 113, 125
inactivity, 9
  physical, 8, 35, 107, 136
income
  discretionary, 101
  disposible, 88
  generation, 165
  increased, 120
  increasing, 73
  inequality, 123
  personal, 57
  reliable, 136
  rising, 53
indebtedness, 74
individualism, 24, 27, 103
  hard, 105
  logic of, 95
  soft, 105, 107
industrialization, 25–6, 101, 103,
    111

inequality, 56, 69, 77, 90, 99, 134, 141, 161, 177–8
  and obesity, 167
  between countries, 122
  economic, 33, 51, 72, 85, 97, 120, 146
  income, 121
  obesity, 14, 72–3
  obesity and policy, 92
  social, 86, 92, 105, 179
  stress and, 176
infant feeding, 11, 77, 128, 130
infectious disease, 111, 126, 137, 152
information, 11, 23, 26, 138, 166
  incomplete, 180
  lack of complete, 147
  misleading, 72
  nutritional, 139
  time series, 144
information technology, 5
infrastructure, 96
  distribution, 111
  global, 109
  highway, 50
  intelligent, 153
  material, 175
insecurity, 18, 72, 81, 86, 91, 108, 122, 166
  economic, 85
  household, 93
  individual, 51, 109
  measures, 88
  obesity and, 85
  social, 88
  wealth, 87
  work, 90
institutions, 24, 177, 179, 181
  educational, 79
  governmental, 65
  of late modern society, 8
  political, 24
  research, 178
  social, 18, 104
instrumental principle, 24
insurance, 9, 21, 180
  life, 58
interaction, 1, 32, 48, 52, 100, 142, 158, 171
  complex, 169
  gene–environment, 71, 155, 173

  of people, 160
  social, 44
interactions, 18, 20
interdisciplinarity, 164
International Health and Behaviour Survey, 120
International Monetary Fund, 116
internet, 176
intervention, 8, 14, 42, 144
  biases, 143
  clinical, 31
  economic, 162
  effectiveness of, 135
  ethical, 141
  governmental, 54
  ladder, 138
  ladder, Nuffield, 136, 139, 149
  macro-level, 175
  medical, 136, 154, 174
  minimal political, 109
  obesity, 1, 20, 26, 53, 135, 141–2, 163
  pharmaceutical, 34, 55, 171
  physiological, 154
  policy, 153
  public health, 106, 136
  social, 171
  state, 137, 180
  structural, 92
  surgical, 1
  upstream, 162
  weight-loss, 42, 128
investment, 117, 125
  commercial, 179
  energy, 19
  foreign, 71
  foreign direct, 88
  parental, 131
  social, 93, 131

James, Philip, 157
judgement
  moral, 10

Kant, Immanuel, viii, 24
  ghost of, 26
Kuwait, 62, 75, 82

Labour administration, 105, 135, 147, 161, 165–6
lactation, 36–7, 44, 126

Latin America, 100, 114, 120, 176
Latour, Bruno, viii
leptin, 9, 45
life
  daily, 143, 169, 172
  early, 19, 71, 107, 112, 128–9
  early history, 77
  everyday, 14, 23, 25, 35, 50, 80, 85, 92, 178
life course, 20, 71, 73, 113, 126, 134
  framing, 125
  perspective, 125
  science, 112
lipase inhibitor, 173
Living Standards Measurement Study, 57
Locke
  John, 24
low-income countries, 15, 78, 111
lower middle-income countries, 111

machinery, 176
macronutrient, 38, 96, 196
  intake, 5, 7, 105
maize, 97, 99
malfunction
  pathological, 106
management, 150
  flood plain, 180
  obesity, 166
  of a scientific consensus, 133
  of conflict, 146
  of non-communicable diseases, 146
  of overweight and obesity, 158
  river, 181
  weight, 142, 173
manufacturers, 101, 141
  fast-food, 85
  food, 85, 96
map, 29, 53–4, 155, 158, 163
  shift[n], 157
  zero, 157
mapping, 10, 30, 134, 150
market
  economies, 24, 86
market forces, 29, 109, 179
marketing, 3, 18, 85, 94, 96, 102, 105, 111, 117, 138–9, 143–4, 147, 156

marketing (cont.)
food, 103
social, 1, 164
markets, 100, 176
diverse, 102
financial, 152
free, 129
labour and consumption, 88
open, 120
unregulated, 71
measurement, 40, 54, 73, 179
anthropometric, 56, 64
error, 41
obesity, 15
of heights and weights, 162
of obesity, 61
physical, 56
population, 52
mechanism
cost, 74
endocrine, 169
epigenetic, 126
neural feed-forward, 106
physiological, 124
social, 94
mechanization, 100
media, 81, 108, 120, 143, 164, 172
discourses, 79
representations, 10
medical
aspects of obesity, 154
crisis, 140
establishment, 108
expenses, 87
management, 15
practice, 5
research, 182
scrutiny, 135
treatment, 150
medicalization
of body fatness, 8
of fat, 65
Medicare, 5
medication, 173
obesity, 174
self-, 90
weight-loss, 173
medicine, 10, 27, 143, 156, 164, 174
privatized, 54
Western, 36
metabolic disease, 124, 126

metabolism, 36, 40, 47
metabolomics, 150
metabonomics, 150
Metropolitan Life Insurance
Company, 58
Mexico, 97, 99, 112, 117
microbiome 134
ecology, 107
microbiota
gut, 106, 138
middle-class values, 105
migrant
Asian, 82
model
business process, 155
causal loop, 162–3
econometric, 10, 23, 30, 56, 162
genetics, 71
multilevel, 32
quantified, 30
modelling, 32, 158
econometric, 53, 63
effects of taxation, 139
general theory of, 30
language, 30, 40
macro-level, 170
obesity, 34
of obesity, 111
predictive, 69
scientific, 29
systems, 155
modernity, 34, 109, 169, 179
late, 34, 131
modernization, viii, 45, 71, 94, 111,
126, 170, 179
departmental, 163
monitoring
obesity, 162, 179
population, 63
moral
guidance, 105
guide, 33
judgement, 8
kudos, 165
principles, 24
responsibility, 105, 135
voice, 181
morally responsible agents, 104
Morandi, Georgio, viii
mortality, 4, 10, 29, 61, 120, 125,
146

differential, 47
due to chronic disease, 135
excess, 69
global risk, 8
prediction, 57
premature, 65
rates, 54
rates, global, 166
risk, 33
selection, 47
motivation, 105, 172
motor car, 28, 50, 171

narrative, 31, 134
governmental, 148
nation states, 54, 62, 176, 179
National Audit Office, 6, 141
National Child Measurement
Programme, 138, 162, 179
National Governors Association
'Healthy America' task force, 93
National Institute for Health and
Care Excellence, 145, 164
National Obesity Observatory, 162
National Service Framework for
Coronary Heart Disease, 6
National Statistics status, 162
nature, 171
Nauru, 62
neighbourhood, 50, 72, 79, 160
poorer, 84
neocortical feed-forward
mechanisms, 28
networks, viii, 150
social, 79, 81
neuropathy, 173
New Zealand, 82, 101
non-governmental organizations,
143, 165, 178
Nordic
nations, 86
welfare states, 53
norms, 8, 24, 36, 65, 100, 146, 154,
160
body mass index, 65
body size, 82
group, 28
healthy, 137
individual, 26
political, 148
social, 50, 124

North American Free Trade
    Agreement, 117
nudge, 165
    tactics, 143
    theory, 28
Nuffield Council on Bioethics, 136
nutrition, 44, 94, 126, 130
    child, 19
    grand-maternal, 49
    maternal, 77
    over-, 126
    poor, 128
    research, 133
    scientists, 133
    under-, 61
nutrition transition, 19, 34, 111
    Pattern Four, 110, 112, 125, 129,
        168
    theory, 123
nutritional status, 56, 59

obesity, 40, 182
    alarmists, 33
    as chronic relapsing condition,
        14
    as chronic relapsing neurological
        disease, 7
    changing rates of, 54
    collection, viii
    complexity, 151, 153, 156, 163
    control, 24, 139, 145
    cultural models of, 170
    early-life predispositions to, 131
    emergence, 137
    emergence of, viii, 135, 170
    endogenous, 44
    exogenous, 44
    familial, 71
    genetics, models of, 49
    high rates of, 18
    highest rates of, 114
    individual predispositions to, 69
    lower rates of, 129
    models of, 1, 5, 19, 23, 29, 67,
        141, 167
    monitoring of, 61, 66
    policy cacophony, 142
    policy, childhood, 54
    political ecology of, 71
    population, 6, 15, 24, 39, 51, 113,
        123, 170, 180

    predispositions to, 47–8, 112,
        126, 150, 173
    rates of, 51
    regulation of, 5, 21, 28, 54, 62,
        67, 104, 107, 136, 141, 147,
        171–2, 176–7, 182
    regulation, models of, 104
    reporting, 57
    research, 31, 33, 44, 64, 92, 148,
        150, 162–3, 169, 172
    science and policy, 142
    scientific models of, 149
    sceptics, 33
opportunity, 152
    economic, 56
    for natural selection, 47
order
    social, 18
organizations, 14, 26, 92, 178
    non-governmental, 140, 181
origins
    developmental, 71, 112
    fetal, 20
    secular trend, 129
orlistat, 173
outputs, 155
    commercial, 179
    of lean thinking, 171
    policy making, 145
    poor labour, 135
overeating, 9, 11, 28, 38, 81, 90,
    107, 162, 180
overweight, 60, 81, 129
    adolescent, 81
    and obese women, 18
    and obesity, 2, 6, 61, 67, 76, 91,
        133, 138
    and obesity in children, 91
    childhood, 58
    childhood obesity and, 10
    childhood rates of, 77

Pacific Islands nations, 101
palatability, 44, 95, 103, 106
parenting, 79, 91, 105
    authoritarian, 91
    authoritative, 105
parents, 4, 8, 77, 91–2, 104, 140,
    172, 179
pathways, 45, 170
    neural, 169

    to obesity, 128
people, 2, 11, 18, 27, 29, 48, 85, 102,
    137, 178, 182
    and institutions, 108
    and objects, 79
    appropriate, 70
    decisions, 147
    everyday, 181
    everyday lives, 52
    free-living, 38, 40
    healthy eating, 176
    in society, 179
    making healthier choices, 168
    obese, 67, 128
    of low socioeconomic status, 84,
        88, 93, 152
    of Nauru, 62
    old, 71
    Pacific Islander, 82
    poorer, 96, 139
    slimmer, 74
    taller, 59
    wealthy, 21
    young, 105
phylogenies, viii
physical activity, 41, 157
    across the world, 71
    differences, 78
    environment, 156
    habits, 3
    in everyday life, 49
    levels, 120
    norms, 81
    patterns, 3
    programmes, 4
    regular, 3
    vigorous, 128
pleasure, 36, 95, 104, 107–8
    and pain, 36
    in food, 28
    seeking, 107
policy, 28, 32, 52, 72, 100, 131, 133,
    146, 177
    and practice, 33
    and regulation, 35
    approaches, 52, 143
    cacophony, 168
    concern, 6
    discourse, 142
    documents, 145
    evaluation, 144

policy (cont.)
  evidence-based, 69, 142
  food, 100
  formation, 147, 182
  goals, 93
  government, 108–9
  governmental, 141, 148
  intervention, 164
  level playing field, 92
  levers, 174
  makers, 131, 137, 143, 148, 151
  making, 178
  -making models, 148
  national planning, 158
  neoliberal, 92
  nutrition, 181
  obesity, 6, 20, 33, 54, 67, 92, 133,
    135, 142–3, 145–7, 149, 151,
    165, 170–1, 174, 176, 179
  obesity science and, 1, 133, 149,
    168
  objectives, 93
  objects, 150
  operationalization, 35
  process, 147
  public, 145, 180
  regulation, 170
  reports, 92
  responses, 5, 95
  scenarios, 158
  science and, 167
  soft, 175
  spatial, 21
  state, 8
  UK government, 166
  US, 136
  use, 34
  workplace, 104
policy makers, 142
political
  advice, 156
  arguments, 53
  ecology of childhood obesity, 135
  forces, 95
  framing of obesity, 165
  ideology, 158, 160
  liberalization, 120
  norms, 88
  party, 160
  philosophy, 103
  position, 147–8, 180

pressure, 177
process, 145
processes, 52
regulation, 56
science, 134
system, 20, 160
theory, 107
will, 133, 149
political applications, 148
political systems
  neoliberal, 166
politics, 7, 24, 33, 99, 104, 107, 131,
    148, 163, 170
  complete ecology of, 135
  domestic, 151
  pressures of, 145
  UK, 162
polyrationality, 21, 169, 181
population, 5, 7, 23, 136, 141, 144
  adult, 9
  African, 47
  Asian, 64
  body fatness in, 181
  body size, 179
  health, 181
  obesity, 8, 164, 172
  past, 129
  regional, 10
  representativeness, 31
  samples, 134
  size, 54, 122
  world, 2, 19
population obesity
  emergence of, 11
potential
  flooding, 21
  for longevity, 126
  futures, 153
  individual and community, 93
  regulators of obesity, 146
  reproductive, 42
  rewards, 107
power, 140, 154, 166
  corporate, 92
  economic, 52, 109
  global, 85, 95
  imbalances, 122
  nuclear, 28
  of brands, 103
  purchasing, 158
  regulatory, 180

practice, 24, 154, 164
  anthropometric, 56
  clinical, 135
  consumer, 172
  cultural and social, 18
  epidemiological, 56
  everyday, 23, 32, 143
  general, 143
  institutional, 26
  medical, 36
  of epidemiology, 15
  public health, 65, 69
  regulatory, 24
  scientific, 26
  statistical, 31
predation pressure, 47
predictive adaptive response, 20,
    125
predisposition
  biological, 172
  epigenetic, 94, 169
  evolutionary, 106
  nutritional, 113
preference
  in food, 85
pregnancy, 11, 36, 44, 77, 91, 124,
    126, 130
prestige
  employment, 74, 79
  occupational, 72
price, 72, 96, 103
  market, 57
  of food, 53
  stability, 101
  subsidy, 139
primates, 44
private industry, 164, 175
processing, 29, 94, 96, 101, 109,
    155, 174
  food, 19
  of food, 3
  of food, primary, 14
  secondary, 14
products
  commercial, 69
  extremely palatable, 102
  food, 14, 71, 85, 101, 103, 165
  high-energy-density food, 140
  high-sugar, 139
  meal replacement, 4
  meat, 181

milk and dairy, 118
  unhealthy, 139
  weight-loss, 56
  weight management, 55
profit, 55, 109, 170, 174, 178
programming
  developmental, 35, 66, 73, 124,
    126, 130
  early-life, 155, 173
protein
  agouti-related, 45
  intake, 39
  leverage, 38
  uncoupling, 46
Prozac (fluoxetine), 91
public health, 2, 8–9, 14, 19, 34, 92,
    104, 111, 137
  approaches, 135
  research, 50
  response, 51
  rhetoric, 93
Public Health Responsibility Deal,
    165

randomized controlled trials, 42,
    144, 174
rates of obesity
  future, 124, 154, 161
  rapid increases in, 118
rational choice theory, 26
rational consumption
  model, 11
rationality, viii, 11, 23–4, 72, 168,
    176, 180
  bounded, 11, 26, 180
  bureaucratic, 182
  collaborative, 177
  economic, 109
  evolutionary, 79, 130, 180
  formal, 19, 93, 124, 179
  governmental, 146, 180
  instrumental, 24
  Kantian, 26
  practical, 24, 33, 170, 179
  principle of, 24
  substantive, 33, 92, 124
  theoretical, 43, 166, 173, 182
  value, 24
  Weber's forms of, 25
reality, 160
  empirical, 29

of policy making, 172
  physical, 65
recession
  economic, 86
recommended daily allowance, 41
regulation, 144, 174
  epigenetic, 49, 73, 130
  governmental, 52, 160
  obesity, 149, 166, 181
  of energy balance, 41
  of food intake, 169
  of food systems, 109
  of gene expression, 126
  of macronutrient intake, 44
  of new drugs, 171
  of obesity, 137, 177
  of urbanism, 176
  of weight status, 72
  physiological, 173
  self-, 140
relations
  international, 151
  interpersonal, 81
  land-use, 21
  logical or normative, 30
  power, 166
  social, 82, 170
relationship
  causal, 49
  complex, 174
  discursive, 170
  ecological, 36, 67
  energetic, 171
  interpersonal, 18, 82
  J-shaped, 67
  parent–child, 91
Report of the Commission on Ending
    Childhood Obesity, 135
representation, 89
  abstract, 30
  media, 80
  union, 88
reproduction
  controlled, 131
  of social class, 102
research, 31, 133, 142, 145, 147–8,
    178
  adult health and disease, 125
  agendas, 149
  and policy, 171
  councils, 156, 163

discipline, 149, 169
  genetic, 45
  joined-up, 154
  obesity, 33, 150, 153
  operational, 155
  scientific, 126
  siloed, 162
  world-leading, 154
resilience, 94
  against obesogenic
    environments, 51
resistance, 176
  indigenous agricultural, 176
  insulin, 9, 116, 125
resources, 79, 146
  capital, 105
  economic, 11
  energy, 36
  homogeneous, 97
  mental, 131
responsibility, 93, 109, 137
  backward-looking, 136
  corporate, 109
  ethical, 92
  for obesity, 95
  for the future, 152
  forward-looking, 136
  individual, 2, 20, 24, 135, 176
  individualized, 174
  personal, 93, 108, 149
  social, 167
  state, 110
retail, 15
retailers
  food, 94–5
  supermarket, 92
risk, 152
  cardiovascular, 65
  chronic disease, 66
  disease, 131
  ecological and environmental,
    149
  factor, 162, 170
  factor approach, 150
  factors, 54, 153, 158
  future, 153
  groups, 136
  measurement, 67
  mitigation, 153
  obesity, 74
  of cardiovascular disease, 3

risk (cont.)
  of metabolic disease, 126
  of morbidity and mortality, 61
  of mortality, 61
  of obesity, 28, 49, 122, 135, 164
  of premature mortality, 65
  perception of, 28
  Type 2 diabetes, 67

sanitation, 35, 175
satiation, 38, 95, 169
satiety, 38, 95, 158, 169
Saving Lives: Our Healthier Nation, 6
school
  children, 138
  primary, 33
  programmes, 138
  relations at, 82
schools, 4, 82, 104, 138, 140, 144,
    172
  state-funded primary, 162
science, 25–6, 141, 149, 163, 170,
    178
  and policy, 7, 23, 151, 163
  and technology, 24
  biological and medical, 156
  brain, 152
  critique of, 34
  developmental life course, 112
  epidemiological, 67, 124
  food, 174
  into policy, 179
  obesity, 3, 18, 26, 32, 35, 44, 133,
    135, 142, 148, 150, 154, 168–9,
    171, 177, 181
  obesity policy and, 141
  social, 33, 153, 164
  strategic, 142
  theoretically rational, 179
  translation of, 20
seasonality, 44, 130
secular trend, 73, 128
sedentism, 141
selection, 7
  climatic, 46
  differential, 35
  fertility, 47
  intensity of, 47
  mortality, 47
  natural, 36, 45, 47
  of genes, 47
  positive, 46
  pressure, 107

selective serotonin reuptake
    inhibitors, 91
self-monitoring
  of food intake, 108
self-organization, 14, 152
sensitivity
  ecological, 128
  taste, 35
  to stress, 104
set-point, 38, 41
  hypothesis, 38
  model, 38, 40
settling point
  model, 41
shock
  economic, 86
Silk Road, 97
Simon, Herbert, 11
'Six Characters in Search of an
    Author', viii
skills
  coping, 91
  lack of, 105
slimness, 11, 79
smoking, 10, 90, 136
  bans, 181
  cessation, 137
snacking, 106, 181
  among children, 106
social brain hypothesis, 28
social change
  consumer-driven, 164
social conventions, 108
social evolutionism, 24
societies
  traditional, 47
society, 8, 20, 72, 80, 134, 137, 160,
    170
  civil, 104
  fluid notions of, 104
  Kuwaiti, 82
  late modern, 50, 167, 175
  medieval, 147
  modern, 49, 147
  neoliberal, 92, 109, 168
  secular, 102
sociology, 23, 33, 134, 156, 168
Socratic philosophy, 36
solidarity
  social, 160
Spanish conquests, 99
special interests, 148
stability, 175

personal, 88
  weight, 38
state
  city, 97
  communist, 120
  disease, 8
  functions of, 109
  healthcare, 89
  intervention, 140
  nation, 38, 86, 170
  nutritional, 73
  of energy stores, 41
  regulation, 8
  steady, 38
  support, 105
  the, 55, 69, 79, 104
state
  nation, 54
State, Washington, 179
States
  of the US, 137
stature, 59
  and socioeconomic status, 56
  increased, 129
  measures of, 56
status, 16, 77, 79, 84, 102–3, 134
  ambivalent, 136
  economic, 72
  educational, 73
stigma, 10, 18, 65, 80, 146, 154
  social, 6, 93
  weight, 33, 81, 135
stimulus
  hunger, 108
stratification, 18
stress, 81, 90, 107, 123, 128, 171
  alleviation, 86, 104
  management, 90
  measures, 134
  of everyday life, 109
  psychological, 88, 176
  psychosocial, 81, 86
structural
  and upstream issues, 166
  change, 52
  complexity, 162
  factors, 69
  forces, 49
  policies, 148
  processes, 146
  realism, 32
structure
  and function of towns and cities, 21

complex, 40
demographic, 54
family, 123
legal, 88
meal, 106
occupational, 102
of domination, 25
of high European cuisine, 99
of power, 177
physical, 51
social, 154, 160–1
sociodemographic, 35
sublime
    rational mapping of, viii
subordinate status, 90
subsistence
    traditional, 42
suburbanization, 51
success
    reproductive, 106
sugar, 3, 19, 32, 78, 95–6, 102, 181
    blood, 36
    lobby, 167
    sweetened beverages, 5, 100, 175
Sugar Reduction: The Evidence for
    Action, 166
supermarkets
    and restaurants, 85, 181
    large, 50
    petrol stations and, 51
supplies
    food, 97
    food energy, 111
    national food, 114
surgery
    bariatric, 4, 9
    obesity, 34, 171
    weight-loss, 128
surplus, 37, 97
    food, 74
    of grain, 97
surveillance, 3, 137, 144, 146, 179
    and monitoring, 137
    obesity, 57, 133, 161, 179
Survey of Economic Risk
    Perceptions and Insecurity, 86
survivorship, 18, 44, 47, 106, 108,
    130
susceptibility
    epigenetic, 50
    genes, 45, 48
    obesity, 71, 172
    to branding and advertising, 105

to metabolic dysfunction, 125
Sweden, 67, 86, 97
systems, 26, 134, 150, 162, 166,
    168, 171, 175–6
    approach, 21, 163
    baroque-complex, 173
    biological, 14, 150
    business, 171
    cognitive, 152–3
    complex, 32, 141, 151, 153, 155,
    173
    distribution, 176
    economic, 18, 92, 120
    endocrine, 125
    expert, viii, 7, 14, 21, 35, 52, 109,
    164, 166, 170, 172, 175
    expert interactive, 180
    food, 94, 96, 102, 109, 174, 179
    formal, 29
    global, 151
    intelligent infrastructure, 152,
    163
    interactive expert, 14
    neoliberal, 18, 106, 176
    non-equilibrium, 40
    of evidence production, 69
    political, 99
    social, 20
    soft, 155
    supply, 171
    thinking, 163
    urban planning, 171
systems, 151
systems and processes
    global, 151
systems modelling, 167

Tackling Obesities: Future Choices,
    7, 20, 149–50
Tackling Obesity in England, 6
taste, 85, 108
    acquired, 158
    and distinction, 102
    neurophysiology of, 174
    preferences, 102
    stimulus, 96
taxation, 5, 33, 53, 90, 92, 96, 136,
    139, 175–6, 178
    regimes, 30
taxonomy
    group–grid, 160
Ten Facts About Obesity, 146
The Health of the Nation, 6

thermodynamics, 40
    laws of, 36
The Surgeon General's Call to
    Action to Prevent and Decrease
    Overweight and Obesity, 6, 141
The Surgeon General's Vision for a
    Healthy and Fit Nation, 6
thyroid extract, 173
trade, 88, 96
    agreements, 92
    deregulation of, 116
    global, 99, 116
    global food, 101
    integration of, 122
    international, 133
    liberalization, 117
    mercantile, 100
    policy, 100
    routes, 97
    slave, 58
tradition, 34, 94, 96, 131, 180
transformation
    economic, 111, 123
    energy, 36
    evolutionary, 96
    global, 23
    technological, 101
transport, 163, 166, 171, 180
    active, 139, 145
    motorized, 7, 158
    physically active, 7
    public, 14–15, 137
    system, 172
transportation, 14–15, 109
    physical, 20
    physically active, 50
treatment, 4, 9, 31–2, 69, 81, 151, 162
    life-long, 7
    medical, 1, 150
    obesity, 43, 95, 173
Type 2 diabetes, 9, 36, 45, 58, 103,
    113, 116, 120

ultraprocessed foods, 118
uncertainty, 31, 85–6, 90, 148, 152
    food, 106
undernutrition, 36
under-reporting
    of obesity, 61
Unit for Biocultural Variation and
    Obesity, viii
United Kingdom (UK), 95, 133, 145,
    156

United States (US), 1, 53, 90, 94–5,
126, 133
  facts about obesity, 4
  food system, 100
  obesity inequality in, 90
United States Anxiety Disorder
    Industry, 90
university
  educated, 154
  students, 120
University
  Deakin, 50
  of Bristol, 157
  of Oxford, viii, 157
urban
  deprivation, 84
  diets, 101
  geographical space, 84
  landscape, 50
  places, 69
  planning, 3, 7, 15, 21, 175
  planning and regulation, 49
  rural inequalities, 120
  US, 101
urbanism, 35
urbanization, 19, 71, 99, 103, 111, 122
  rapid, 111

values, 5, 116, 141, 146–8, 154, 160,
177

clusters of, 25
health, 172
individualist, 104
non-ordered, 30
sets of, 24
social, 165
surrounding health, 70

waist circumference, 31, 48
waist:height ratio, 57, 67
waist:hip ratio, 57, 66–7
water, 14, 35, 175
  carbonation of, 103
  regulation, 21
  systems, 176
wealth, 56, 129, 131
  financial, 72
  imbalance, 122
  of nations, 15
  shock, 86
weaning, 44, 130
Weber, 24–5
  Max, viii
weight bias, 72, 80–1
weight for height
  standard tables, 60
weight gain, 2, 39, 81, 86, 91, 154,
164, 169
  childhood, 72
  individual, 96

weight loss, 4, 9, 37, 42, 49, 81,
173
  intervention, 128
  products, 55
welfare, 14, 99
  human, 56
  provision, 15, 86
  regimes, 86, 134
  social, 86
Westernization, 19, 111
wicked problems, 153, 177
work
  loss, 69
  obesity, 15
  of government, 177
  productivity, 6
  productivity analysis, 15
  representational, 29
  time off, 55
workplace, 10
World Bank, 15–16, 57
  categories of income, 77
world views, 33, 148, 160
World War II, 101, 174, 179
  obesity rates after, 19
  servicemen, 51
WS systems design team,
157

zoology, 47